Pericardial Diseases

Editors

JAE K. OH
WILLIAM R. MIRANDA
TERRENCE D. WELCH

CARDIOLOGY CLINICS

www.cardiology.theclinics.com

Consulting Editors

JORDAN M. PRUTKIN
DAVID M. SHAVELLE
TERRENCE D. WELCH
AUDREY H. WU

November 2017 • Volume 35 • Number 4

ELSEVIER

1600 John F. Kennedy Boulevard • Suite 1800 • Philadelphia, Pennsylvania, 19103-2899

http://www.theclinics.com

CARDIOLOGY CLINICS Volume 35, Number 4
November 2017 ISSN 0733-8651, ISBN-13: 978-0-323-54873-1

Editor: Stacy Eastman
Developmental Editor: Sara Watkins

Cardiology Clinics (ISSN 0733-8651) is published quarterly by Elsevier Inc., 360 Park Avenue South, New York, NY 10010-1710. Months of issue are February, May, August, and November. Business and Editorial Offices: 1600 John F. Kennedy Blvd., Ste. 1800, Philadelphia, PA 19103-2899. Customer Service Office: 3251 Riverport Lane, Maryland Heights, MO 63043. Periodicals post-age paid at New York, NY and additional mailing offices. Subscription prices are $326.00 per year for US individuals, $604.00 per year for US institutions, $100.00 per year for US students and residents, $398.00 per year for Canadian individuals, $758.00 per year for Canadian institutions, $464.00 per year for international individuals, $758.00 per year for international institutions and $220.00 per year for Canadian and international students/residents. To receive student/resident rate, orders must be accompanied by name of affiliated institution, data of term, and the *signature* of program/residency coordinator on institution letterhead. Orders will be billed at individual rate until proof of status is received. Foreign air speed delivery is included in all *Clinics* subscription prices. All prices are subject to change without notice. **POSTMASTER:** Send address changes to *Cardiology Clinics*, Elsevier Health Sciences Division, Subscription Customer Service, 3251 Riverport Lane, Maryland Heights, MO 63043. **Customer Service: 1-800-654-2452 (U.S. and Canada); 314-447-8871 (outside U.S. and Canada). Fax: 314-447-8029. E-mail: journalscustomerservice-usa@ elsevier.com (for print support); journalsonlinesupport-usa@elsevier.com (for online support).**

Reprints. For copies of 100 or more, of articles in this publication, please contact the Commercial Reprints Department, Elsevier Inc., 360 Park Avenue South, New York, NY 10010-1710. Tel.: 212-633-3874; Fax: 212-633-3820; E-mail: reprints@elsevier.com.

Cardiology Clinics is also published in Spanish by McGraw-Hill Interamericana Editores S. A., P.O. Box 5-237, 06500, Mexico D. F., Mexico; in Portuguese by Reichmann and Alfonso Editores Rio de Janeiro, Brazil; and in Greek by Dimitrios P. Lagos, 8 Pondon Street, GR115-28 Ilissia, Greece.

Cardiology Clinics is covered in *MEDLINE/PubMed (Index Medicus)*, *Excerpta Medica*, *The Cumulative Index to Nursing and Allied Health Literature* (CINAHL).

Contributors

EDITORIAL BOARD

JORDAN M. PRUTKIN, MD, MHS, FHRS
Assistant Professor of Medicine, Division of
Cardiology/Electrophysiology, University of
Washington Medical Center, Seattle,
Washington, USA

DAVID M. SHAVELLE, MD, FACC, FSCAI
Associate Professor, Keck School of Medicine,
Director, General Cardiovascular Fellowship
Program, Director, Cardiac Catheterization
Laboratory, Los Angeles County + USC
Medical Center, Division of Cardiovascular
Medicine, University of Southern California,
Los Angeles, California, USA

TERRENCE D. WELCH, MD
Assistant Professor, Department of Medicine,
Section of Cardiology, Dartmouth-Hitchcock
Medical Center, Lebanon, New Hampshire,
USA; Department of Internal Medicine, Geisel
School of Medicine at Dartmouth, Hanover,
New Hampshire, USA

AUDREY H. WU, MD
Assistant Professor, Internal Medicine,
University of Michigan, Ann Arbor, Michigan,
USA

EDITORS

JAE K. OH, MD, FACC, FASE, FAHA
Samsung Professor of Cardiovascular
Diseases, Director of Pericardial Diseases
Clinic, Co-Director, Integrated CV Imaging,
Department of Cardiology, Mayo Clinic,
Rochester, Minnesota, USA; General Director,
Heart Vascular Stroke Institute (HVSI),
Samsung Medical Center, Seoul, Republic of
Korea

WILLIAM R. MIRANDA, MD
Instructor in Medicine, Department of
Cardiology, Mayo Clinic, Rochester,
Minnesota, USA

TERRENCE D. WELCH, MD
Assistant Professor, Department of Medicine,
Section of Cardiology, Dartmouth-Hitchcock
Medical Center, Lebanon, New Hampshire,
USA; Department of Internal Medicine, Geisel
School of Medicine at Dartmouth, Hanover,
New Hampshire, USA

AUTHORS

NANDAN S. ANAVEKAR, MB, BCh
Associate Professor of Medicine, Department
of Cardiovascular Diseases, Division of
Cardiac Radiology, Department of Radiology,
Mayo Clinic, Rochester, Minnesota, USA

CHRISTOPHER APPLETON, MD
Professor, Department of Medicine, Mayo
Clinic School of Medicine, Division of
Cardiovascular Diseases, Mayo Clinic,
Scottsdale, Arizona, USA

AMIR AZARBAL, MD
Fellow, Cardiology Unit, University of Vermont
Medical Center, University of Vermont,
Burlington, Vermont, USA

SUNG-A CHANG, MD, PhD
Division of Cardiology, Department of
Medicine, Samsung Medical Center, School of
Medicine, Sungkyunkwan University, Heart
Vascular Stroke Institute, Gangnam-gu, Seoul,
Republic of Korea

FIORENZO GAITA, MD
Department of Medical Sciences, University Cardiology, AOU Città della Salute e della Scienza di Torino, Torino, Italy

LINDA GILLAM, MD, MPH
Chair, Department of Cardiovascular Medicine, Morristown Medical Center/Atlantic Health System, Professor of Medicine, Sidney Kimmel Medical College, Thomas Jefferson University, Morristown, New Jersey, USA

KEVIN L. GREASON, MD
Associate Professor of Surgery, Department of Cardiovascular Surgery, Mayo Clinic, Rochester, Minnesota, USA

POUYA HEMMATI, MD
Joint General and Thoracic Surgery Resident, Department of Cardiovascular Surgery, Mayo Clinic, Rochester, Minnesota, USA

BRIAN D. HOIT, MD
Professor, Department of Medicine (Cardiology), Case Western Reserve University, UH Harrington Heart & Vascular Institute, Director of Echocardiography, University Hospitals Cleveland Medical Center, Cleveland, Ohio, USA

MASSIMO IMAZIO, MD, FESC
Department of Medical Sciences, University Cardiology, AOU Città della Salute e della Scienza di Torino, Torino, Italy

ALLAN L. KLEIN, MD
Section of Cardiovascular Imaging, Center for the Diagnosis and Treatment of Pericardial Diseases, Heart & Vascular Institute, Cleveland Clinic, Cleveland, Ohio, USA

KONSTANTINOS KOULOGIANNIS, MD
Department of Cardiovascular Medicine, Morristown Medical Center/Atlantic Health System, Morristown, New Jersey, USA

ITZHAK KRONZON, MD, FASE, FACC, FACP, FESC, FAHA
Department of Cardiovascular Medicine, Lenox Hill Hospital, Northwell Health, New York, New York, USA

DEBORAH H. KWON, MD
Section of Cardiovascular Imaging, Center for the Diagnosis and Treatment of Pericardial Diseases, Heart & Vascular Institute, Cleveland Clinic, Cleveland, Ohio, USA

MARTIN M. LeWINTER, MD
Professor of Medicine and Molecular Physiology and Biophysics, Cardiology Unit, The University of Vermont Medical Center, The University of Vermont, Burlington, Vermont, USA

BERNHARD MAISCH, MD, FESC, FACC
Faculty of Medicine, Heart and Vessel Center, Philipps-Universität Marburg, Marburg, Germany

JOSEPH J. MALESZEWSKI, MD
Professor, Department of Medicine, Professor, Departments of Laboratory Medicine and Pathology, Cardiovascular Diseases, and Clinical Genomics, Mayo Clinic, Rochester, Minnesota, USA

WILLIAM R. MIRANDA, MD
Instructor in Medicine, Department of Cardiology, Mayo Clinic, Rochester, Minnesota, USA

JAE K. OH, MD, FACC, FASE, FAHA
Samsung Professor of Cardiovascular Diseases, Director of Pericardial Diseases Clinic, Co-Director, Integrated CV Imaging, Department of Cardiology, Mayo Clinic, Rochester, Minnesota, USA; General Director, Heart Vascular Stroke Institute (HVSI), Samsung Medical Center, Seoul, Republic of Korea

SABINE PANKUWEIT, PhD
Faculty of Medicine and Cardiology Clinic, UKGM, Marburg, Germany

YUVRAJSINH J. PARMAR, MD
Department of Cardiovascular Medicine, Lenox Hill Hospital, Northwell Health, New York, New York, USA

MICHAEL POON, MD, FACC
Department of Cardiovascular Medicine, Lenox Hill Hospital, Northwell Health, New York, New York, USA

ARSEN D. RISTIĆ, MD, PhD, FESC
Department of Cardiology, Clinical Centre of Serbia, University of Belgrade School of Medicine, Belgrade, Serbia

HARTZELL V. SCHAFF, MD
Stuart W. Harrington Professor of Surgery, Department of Cardiovascular Surgery, Mayo Clinic, Rochester, Minnesota, USA

PETAR SEFEROVIC, MD, FESC
Department of Cardiology, Clinical Centre of
Serbia, University of Belgrade School of
Medicine, Belgrade, Serbia

†**RALPH SHABETAI, MD**
Emeritus Professor, Department of Medicine,
University of California San Diego, La Jolla,
California, USA

ANKIT B. SHAH, MD, MPH
Division of Cardiology, Massachusetts General
Hospital, Boston, Massachusetts, USA

TERRENCE D. WELCH, MD
Assistant Professor, Department of Medicine,
Section of Cardiology, Dartmouth-Hitchcock
Medical Center, Lebanon, New Hampshire,
USA; Department of Internal Medicine, Geisel
School of Medicine at Dartmouth, Hanover,
New Hampshire, USA

BO XU, MB BS (Hons), FRACP
Section of Cardiovascular Imaging, Center for
the Diagnosis and Treatment of Pericardial
Diseases, Heart and Vascular Institute,
Cleveland Clinic, Cleveland, Ohio, USA

†Deceased.

PETAR SEFEROVIC, MD, FESC
Department of Cardiology, Clinical Centre of Serbia, University of Belgrade School of Medicine, Belgrade, Serbia

RALPH SHABETAI, MD
Emeritus Professor, Department of Medicine, University of California San Diego, La Jolla, California, USA

ANKIT B. SHAH, MD, MPH
Division of Cardiology, Massachusetts General Hospital, Boston, Massachusetts, USA

TERRENCE D. WELCH, MD
Assistant Professor, Department of Medicine, Section of Cardiology, Dartmouth-Hitchcock Medical Center, Lebanon, New Hampshire, USA; Department of Internal Medicine, Geisel School of Medicine at Dartmouth, Hanover, New Hampshire, USA

BO XU, MB BS (Hons), FRACP
Section of Cardiovascular Imaging, Center for the Diagnosis and Treatment of Pericardial Diseases, Heart and Vascular Institute, Cleveland Clinic, Cleveland, Ohio, USA

Contents

Constrictive pericarditis and cardiac tamponade cause severe diastolic dysfunction, but do not depress systolic function until the agonal state has been reached. Multi-modality cardiovascular imaging has brought the nuances of pericardial disease to the domain of the practicing cardiologist. This introduction is a revised article originally written by the late Dr Shabetai for a pericardial diseases textbook that was not published. As he was the editor of a previous *Pericardial Diseases* issue for *Cardiology Clinics* in the 1980s, it is most appropriate to begin our issue with his insights. The remaining articles describe advances in diagnosis and management, focusing on clinically important aspects of pericardial diseases.

The pericardium consists of a visceral mesothelial monolayer (epicardium) that reflects over the great vessels and joins an outer, relatively inelastic fibrous parietal layer of organized collagen and elastin fibers, between which is a potential space that normally contains up to 50 mL of plasma filtrate. Although not essential for life, the pericardium serves important, albeit subtle, functions in the euvolemic healthy individual that become increasingly important in hypervolemic states and conditions in which the heart enlarges acutely. The pericardial functions can be divided into the mechanical, reflex, membranous, metabolic, and ligamentous.

 Video content accompanies this article at http://www.cardiology.theclinics.com.

Pericardial diseases represent diverse conditions, ranging from painful inflammatory states, such as acute pericarditis, to life-threatening tamponade and chronic heart failure due to constrictive pericarditis. Multimodality cardiovascular imaging plays important roles in diagnosis and management of pericardial conditions. This review provides a clinical update on multimodality cardiovascular imaging of the pericardium, incorporating echocardiography, multidetector computed tomography, and cardiac MRI, focusing on guiding clinicians about when each cardiac imaging modality should be used in each relevant pericardial condition.

Acute and recurrent pericarditis are the most common pericardial syndromes encountered in clinical practice either as an isolated process or as part of a systemic disease. The diagnosis is based on clinical evaluation, electrocardiogram, and echocardiography. The empiric therapy is based on nonsteroidal anti-inflammatory drugs plus colchicine as first choice, resorting to corticosteroids for specific indications (eg, systemic inflammatory disease on corticosteroids, pregnancy, renal failure, or concomitant oral anticoagulants), for contraindications, or failure of the first-line therapy. The most common complication is recurrence, occurring in up to 30% of cases after a first episode of pericarditis.

The normal pericardial sac contains up to 50 mL of fluid, which consists of a plasma ultrafiltrate. Anything greater constitutes a pathologic effusion. The curvilinear pressure-volume relationship of the pericardial sac dictates hemodynamic consequences of a pericardial effusion and is responsible for rapidly accumulating fluid that causes cardiac tamponade. A variety of diseases and complications cause pericardial effusion. The most common are idiopathic pericarditis, cancer, connective tissue disorders, and hemorrhage. Management of pericardial effusion is dictated by whether tamponade is present or threatened. If it is, urgent/emergent pericardiocentesis is indicated. If not, a systematic approach to diagnosis and management should be undertaken.

 Video content accompanies this article at http://www.cardiology.theclinics.com.

Cardiac tamponade is caused by an abnormal increase in fluid accumulation in the pericardial sac, which, by raising intracardiac pressures, impedes normal cardiac filling and reduces cardiac output, sometimes dramatically so. This article outlines the pathophysiology, clinical features, and treatment of this important clinical condition, highlighting the important role played by echocardiography in diagnosis and management.

Constrictive pericarditis is a potentially treatable cause of diastolic heart failure that arises because a diseased, inelastic pericardium restricts ventricular diastolic expansion. Affected patients present with heart failure with predominant right-sided symptoms and signs. The key to diagnosis is identification of the unique hemodynamic properties associated with constriction: dissociation of intrathoracic and intracardiac pressures and enhanced ventricular interaction. Comprehensive echocardiography with Doppler imaging is useful, but invasive hemodynamic assessment and cross-sectional imaging may be required for confirmation. Cardiac MRI provides an opportunity to evaluate for pericardial inflammation. Most cases of chronic constriction are progressive and life limiting, and require surgical pericardiectomy.

Effusive-constrictive pericarditis (ECP) corresponds to the coexistence of a hemodynamically significant pericardial effusion and decreased pericardial compliance. The hallmark of ECP is the persistence of elevated right atrial pressure postpericardiocentesis. The prevalence of ECP seems higher in tuberculous pericarditis and lower in idiopathic cases. The diagnosis of ECP is traditionally based on invasive hemodynamics but the presence of echocardiographic features of constrictive pericarditis post-pericardiocentesisis can also identify ECP. Data on the prognosis and optimal treatment of ECP are still limited. Anti-inflammatory agents should be the first line of treatment. Pericardiectomy should be reserved for refractory cases.

Pouya Hemmati, Kevin L. Greason, and Hartzell V. Schaff

Pericardiectomy is a potentially curative treatment for constrictive pericarditis. We use a median sternotomy and believe that adequate resection involves removal of the diaphragmatic pericardium and the anterior pericardium. Late outcomes depend on severity of right-sided heart failure preoperatively, the etiology of constrictive pericarditis, and adequate pericardial resection. Late results are excellent in patients with idiopathic disease or those with pericarditis secondary to prior cardiac operations. However, survival is reduced in those with radiation-induced constrictive pericarditis, primarily owing to additional secondary effects of radiation on cardiac valves, epicardial coronary arteries, and ventricular myocardium where fibrosis may cause associated restrictive cardiomyopathy.

Bernhard Maisch, Arsen D. Ristić, Sabine Pankuweit, and Petar Seferovic

Interventional procedures for pericardial diseases include pericardiocentesis, drainage of pericardial effusion, intrapericardial therapy, and percutaneous balloon pericardiotomy or percutaneous pericardiostomy. Echocardiographic and fluoroscopic guidance have greatly increased safety and feasibility. Several devices for pericardiocentesis have been tested (PerDucer, PeriAttacher, visual puncture systems, Grasper, Scissors, and Reverse slitter), mainly to facilitate access to the pericardium in the absence of effusion for epicardial ablations or left atrial appendage ligation. In selected patients with pericardial effusions that cannot be managed medically or with prolonged drainage, various medications can be applied intrapericardially to prevent further recurrences or induce sclerosis of the pericardial space.

Joseph J. Maleszewski and Nandan S. Anavekar

Pericardial tumors are rare lesions that include a range of neoplastic conditions that may arise within the pericardium or metastasize to involve it secondarily. Understanding the spectrum of lesions that are included in the differential diagnosis of a pericardial mass-lesion is critical to making timely, accurate diagnoses and getting the appropriate therapy should one be necessary. This article summarizes the radiologic and pathologic findings of the most commonly encountered of these entities.

Yuvrajsinh J. Parmar, Ankit B. Shah, Michael Poon, and Itzhak Kronzon

Congenital abnormalities of the pericardium are a rare group of disorders that include congenital absence of the pericardium, pericardial cysts, and diverticula. These congenital defects result from alterations in the embryologic formation and structure of the pericardium. Although many cases are incidentally found, they can present as symptomatic, life-threatening disease. Owing to their rarity, many cases are inappropriately diagnosed. Alterations in the embryologic formation and structure may result in the formation of these congenital abnormalities. We review the presentation, diagnosis, and management of congenital absence of the pericardium, pericardial cysts, and diverticula. A summary of multimodality imaging features is provided.

Sung-A Chang

Viral pericarditis is the most common cause of acute pericarditis and it is typically responsive to aspirin or nonsteroidal anti-inflammatory drugs. Tuberculous pericarditis is common in immunocompromised patients or in immunocompetent patients in endemic areas. The diagnosis of tuberculous pericarditis usually requires a multidisciplinary approach, and presumptive treatment should be started for people with suspected infections living in endemic areas. Antituberculous treatment along with corticosteroid therapy can reduce complications from constrictive pericarditis. Purulent pericarditis is fatal if untreated. Bacterial and fungal cultures from pericardial fluid and blood are essential to determine the best treatment.

CARDIOLOGY CLINICS

THE CLINICS ARE AVAILABLE ONLINE!
Access your subscription at:
www.theclinics.com

Preface
The Pericardium: Simple and Innocent, but Complex and Fascinating

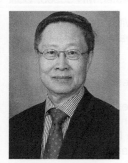 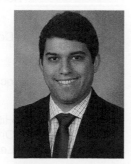 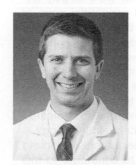

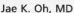

Jae K. Oh, MD   William R. Miranda, MD   Terrence D. Welch, MD

Editors

The pericardium is a simple, two-layered, thin membranous structure covering the heart and the proximal portion of the great vessels without an essential function. However, when this innocent organ is attacked by inflammation, infection, or scarring, it may lead to fascinating, although clinically undesirable, hemodynamic derangements.

Pericardial disorders have intrigued physicians and physiologists since the sixteenth century when cardiac tamponade was recognized as a cause of death after a chest wound or stabbing. However, clinical presentations of cardiac tamponade were not fully described until the nineteenth century. Since the introduction of cardiac catheterization in the 1940s and the progress in cardiovascular imaging over the last 40 years, we have witnessed a revolution in the understanding, diagnosis, and treatment of pericardial diseases. Invasive and noninvasive hemodynamic characteristics of cardiac tamponade and constriction have been well established with respiratory variation in ventricular filling. Pericardial anatomy, effusion, thickness, calcification, and inflammation can be reliably assessed by echocardiography, computed tomography, MRI, and PET. The detection of pericardial diseases as well as their management has advanced with nonsteroidal anti-inflammatory drugs/colchicine combination for acute pericarditis to reduce its recurrence, safe pericardiocentesis under echocardiographic guidance, and pericardiectomy to potentially cure disabling heart failure from constrictive pericarditis.

Despite many advances in the diagnosis and the management of various pericardial disorders, we still do not know the exact natural history of acute pericarditis, how to prevent pericardial inflammation after a cardiac procedure injuring the pericardium, who develops constrictive pericarditis or pericardial calcification, and the optimal treatment of recurrent pericarditis. Although there are guidelines for pericardial diseases by the European Society of Cardiology, currently there is no guideline published in the United States. It is hoped that this special issue in pericardial diseases can serve as a guideline to detect, diagnose, and manage various pericardial diseases.

In this issue, we cover the whole spectrum of pericardial disorders, ranging from pericardial

Cardiol Clin 35 (2017) xiii–xiv
http://dx.doi.org/10.1016/j.ccl.2017.09.001
0733-8651/17/© 2017 Published by Elsevier Inc.

anatomy and physiology to the rare congenital anomalies and tumors. The following articles review the developments in the diagnosis and management of "old pericardial disorders," such as constriction, cardiac tamponade, and acute pericarditis. We also discuss transient constriction and effusive-constrictive pericarditis, increasingly recognized clinical entities that were largely unknown at the time of the last pericardial issue of *Cardiology Clinics*, edited by the late Dr Shabetai almost 30 years ago. These articles provide state-of-art overviews on medical, surgical, and percutaneous therapy of pericardial diseases as well as cardiac imaging. In the introduction article, we, as co-editors, also pay a tribute to the late Dr Shabetai, a world-renowned expert who dedicated his career to the study of pericardial physiology.

We would like to thank all the authors who found time in their busy schedules to contribute to this issue with their expertise. Like us, they share a passion for care of patients with pericardial disorders, a challenging but uniquely rewarding part of cardiology. Last, we would like to thank *Cardiology Clinics*. We were deeply honored by their invitation to be the guest editors for this issue.

Jae K. Oh, MD
Department of Cardiology
Mayo Clinic
200 1st Street, SW
Rochester, MN 55905, USA

William R. Miranda, MD
Department of Cardiology
Mayo Clinic
200 1st Street, SW
Rochester, MN 55905, USA

Terrence D. Welch, MD
Dartmouth-Hitchcock Medical Center
One Medical Center Drive
Lebanon, NH 03756, USA

E-mail addresses:
oh.jae@mayo.edu (J.K. Oh)
miranda.william@mayo.edu (W.R. Miranda)
Terrence.D.Welch@hitchcock.org (T.D. Welch)

Pericardial Effusion and Compressive Disorders of the Heart
Influence of New Technology on Unraveling its Pathophysiology and Hemodynamics

Ralph Shabetai, MD[a,†], Jae K. Oh, MD[b,*]

KEYWORDS

- Pericardium • Pericardial effusion • Cardiac tamponade • Constrictive pericarditis

KEY POINTS

- Constrictive pericarditis and cardiac tamponade cause severe diastolic dysfunction, but do not depress systolic function until an extreme, end-stage state has been reached.
- Although physiologic and hemodynamics features of pericardial disorders have been studied for more than two centuries, recent advances in cardiovascular imaging (in particular echo-Doppler) have revolutionized the diagnosis and understanding of pericardial diseases.
- The concept of ventricular interdependence is the hallmark of both cardiac tamponade and constrictive pericarditis. However, their underlying pathophysiology is significantly different.
- Techniques used for pericardiocentesis have signicantly evolved the past decades and echocardiographic-guidance has markedly improved its safety.

"This introduction is a revised article originally written by the late Dr Shabetai for a pericardial diseases textbook which was not published. He was the editor of previous Pericardial Diseases issue for Cardiology Clinics in the 1980s, it is most appropriate to begin our issue with his insights. The remaining articles describe advances in diagnosis and management, focusing on clinically important aspects of pericardial diseases."

Clinicians now take it for granted that when the question of a pericardial effusion arises, it is quickly settled by echocardiography. Before the advent of echocardiography, one relied on the notoriously inaccurate physical examination, an unexplained increase in heart size on a chest radiogram, or evidence of pericarditis. The chest radiogram alone, despite signs such as a double density along the cardiac edge, or a posterior bulge on the lateral view, is seldom sufficient for a firm diagnosis of pericardial effusion. Other techniques used in the preechocardiographic era included cardiac fluoroscopy, which disclosed absence of cardiac pulsations, and cardiac catheterization, during which the catheter failed to reach the edge of what

[a] Department of Medicine, University of California, San Diego, La Jolla, CA 92093, USA; [b] Department of Cardiovascular Diseases, Mayo Clinic, 200 First Avenue Southwest, Rochester, MN 55905, USA
[†] Deceased
[*] Corresponding author.
E-mail address: oh.jae@mayo.edu

Cardiol Clin 35 (2017) 467–479
http://dx.doi.org/10.1016/j.ccl.2017.07.001
0733-8651/17/© 2017 Elsevier Inc. All rights reserved.

seemed to be the right atrial border. Angiography disclosed a stationary water density surrounding an actively beating heart. Another method for diagnosing pericardial effusion that has been replaced by echocardiography was to inject carbon dioxide intravenously. The patient was placed in the left decubitus position and the radiolucent bubble was observed fluoroscopically and documented by a cross-table radiograph. The size of the effusion was estimated from the width of the water density over the gas bubble. Compare the effort and discomfort of the procedure with that of performing a limited echocardiogram to rule out pericardial effusion. In fact, reliable detection of pericardial effusion was the first clinical application of A-mode echocardiography by Dr Feigenbaum and colleagues[1] (Fig. 1).

The etiology of pericardial effusion has changed over the recent decades, in part because of the development of effective antibiotics. Tuberculosis and other pyogenic infections have become much less common as the cause of pericardial effusion, with or without tamponade; purulent pericarditis is now rare, although only a little less sinister than it used to be. Pericardial effusions complicating invasive cardiac procedures and therapy, or in acquired immune deficiency syndrome (AIDS) have become more common. Moreover, nowadays pericardial effusion occurs more often against a background of myocardial or systemic disease, a factor that may make evaluation and treatment more difficult. Young cardiologists will not know this, but cardiac tamponade used to be the scourge of dialysis units, until about a decade ago when the changed dialyzing membrane blocked transmission of whatever agent was responsible. On a medical service and in the clinic, cardiac tamponade is now more often subacute than either acute or chronic.

Serial echocardiography has demonstrated that silent pericardial effusion is common in pregnancy and after myocardial infarction or cardiac surgery. Although Dressler's syndrome is becoming less frequent, cardiac tamponade continues to be an important complication after heart surgery. Tamponade, often occurring after the patient has been discharged from hospital, may be a manifestation of pericardial injury, or owing to hemorrhage, often localized and sometimes organized, most commonly behind the right atrium. Echocardiography and computer-assisted tomography have been useful in characterizing localized effusions. Even after pericardial effusion resolves, the pericardium remains inflamed, resulting in constrictive hemodynamics. The extent of pericardial inflammation can be determined from delayed

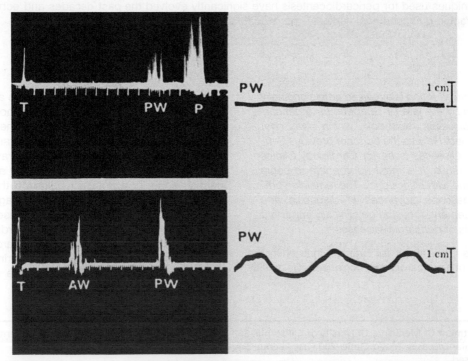

Fig. 1. (*Top*) A-mode echocardiography detecting pericardial effusion between posterior wall (PW) and the pericardium (P). The systolic and diastolic motion of PW is lost. (*Bottom*) After draining of pericardial effusion, the space is no longer present and the motion of PW is restored. (*From* Feigenbaum H, Waldhausen JA, Hyde LP. Ultrasound diagnosis of pericardial effusion. JAMA 1965;191:713; with permission.)

gadolinium enhancement on magnetic resonance imaging (MRI) (**Fig. 2**). Pericardial inflammation may resolve spontaneously or progress to form a scar with or without calcification.

The changes in constrictive pericarditis that have occurred in the same time period and their diagnostic and therapeutic consequences are particularly dramatic. Gone are the days of chronic constrictive pericarditis in the developed countries, often of tuberculous etiology, with a heavily calcified pericardium, anasarca, cachexia, and atrial fibrillation. It is now more common to find subacute pericarditis, often idiopathic, without calcification and with much less wasting and fluid retention. Imaging techniques are so advanced that constrictive pericarditis can be diagnosed without invasive hemodynamics, often only after an echocardiogram. One can expect to find radiographically evident calcification in about one-quarter of the cases (see **Fig. 2**). Calcific constrictive pericarditis, compared with noncalcific, is more apt to be associated with an audible knock, and more atrial enlargement. These changes have increased the difficulties of diagnosis, but also have contributed significantly to the safety of pericardiectomy. Radiation-induced constrictive pericarditis was more common before optimal shielding and radiation ports had been developed. When radiation-induced constriction advances to the point where pericardiectomy is required, the operative risk is higher than in pericardiectomy for constrictive pericarditis of other etiology, and in the survivors, the outcome is less satisfactory.[2] This worse prognosis is largely owing to concomitant radiation damage to the myocardium.

EVOLUTION OF THE KNOWLEDGE OF THE PATHOPHYSIOLOGY

It has been known for centuries that cardiac tamponade and constrictive pericarditis are disorders of diastolic function, caused by vastly increased pericardial restraint. Richard Lower (1631–1691)[3] described an "intermittent pulse" in a case of constrictive pericarditis. He noted that the pulse disappeared with inspiration and attributed this phenomenon to descent of the diaphragm, which would tighten the application of the pericardium to the heart. Norman Chevers was a contemporary of the illustrious William Harvey. After the battle of Edgehill ended with the victory of the Roundheads, Harvey formed a group of physiologists to work with him in an environment congenial to Royalists at Oxford University. Lower was prominent among them. Chevers described several cases of constrictive pericarditis seen at Guys hospital early in the 19th century. His writings include descriptions of the pathophysiology that display a remarkable comprehension of diastolic dysfunction, perhaps acquired during his long sojourn in India.[4] Neither of these brilliant clinical investigators, of course, had access to the stethoscope, still less to measurements of cardiac volumes and pressures, nor any kind of imaging. Their deductions were made from astute clinical observations and correlation with autopsy findings.

In earlier writings, the features common to cardiac tamponade and constrictive pericarditis, such as substantial elevation and equalization of ventricular diastolic pressures on the 2 sides of the heart, were stressed, but subsequently, the importance of features such as the different patterns of ventricular filling and the waveform of atrial and ventricular diastolic pressure was increasingly recognized.

Ventricular Interaction

Perhaps the most important key to understanding the pathophysiology of cardiac tamponade and constrictive pericarditis is the concept of ventricular interaction, the concept of which also is not

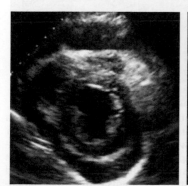 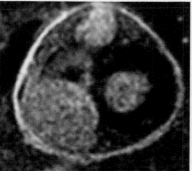 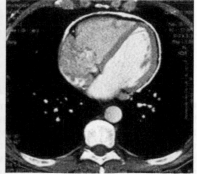

Fig. 2. A composite of transthoracic echocardiography (*left*), cardiac MRI (*center*) with delayed enhancement of the pericardium, and computed tomography (*right*) showing moderate amount of pericardial effusion, pericardial inflammation, and calcification, respectively.

as modern as many would imagine.[5] That overdistension of 1 ventricle compresses, thereby making the diastolic pressure–volume of the opposite ventricle steeper, was shown by Taylor and colleagues[6] in 1967, using postmortem canine hearts without an intact pericardium. Even the normal pericardium strengthens ventricular interaction to some degree,[7] but cardiac tamponade and constrictive pericarditis increase ventricular interaction by orders of magnitude.[8] Later investigators have shown that this greatly enhanced ventricular interaction is an important mechanism underlying many of the clinical, echo Doppler, and magnetic resonance findings of constrictive pericarditis and cardiac tamponade[9–12] (**Fig. 3**)

Greatly enhanced ventricular interaction is common to cardiac tamponade and constrictive pericarditis because, in both, pericardial compliance is greatly reduced, so that total cardiac volume is virtually constant throughout the cardiac cycle. Any significant change in the volume of 1 side of the heart therefore induces an equal and opposite change in the volume of the contralateral side. But once more, there is an important difference between the 2 conditions. In cardiac tamponade, inspiration increases right heart volume at the expense of the left heart volume, whereas in constrictive pericarditis, inspiration decreases left heart volume, allowing the right heart volume to expand. The reason for this difference is that, in

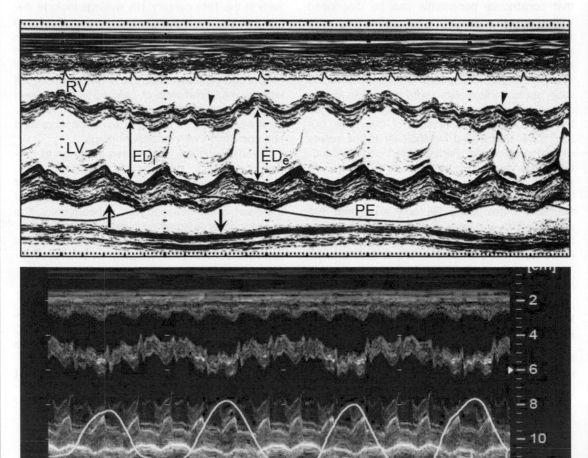

Fig. 3. (*Top*) M-mode echocardiogram from the parasternal window in a patient with cardiac tamponade and a large circumferential pericardial effusion (*PE*). The M-mode was recorded simultaneously with the respirometer tracing at the bottom (*upward arrow*, onset of inspiration; *downward arrow*, onset of expiration). The left ventricular (*LV*) dimension during inspiration (ED_i) becomes smaller than with expiration (ED_e). The opposite changes occur in the right ventricle (*RV*). The ventricular septum (*arrowheads*) moves toward the LV with inspiration and toward the RV with expiration, accounting for the abnormal ventricular septum in patients with cardiac tamponade. (*Bottom*) M-mode echocardiogram from a patient with constrictive pericarditis. There is an abrupt change in ventricular septal motion with the onset of inspiration and expiration. ([*Top*] *From* Oh JK, Seward JB, Tajik AJ. The echo manual. 3rd edition. Philadelphia: Lippincott, Williams and Wilkins; 2006; with permission.)

cardiac tamponade, much (although not all) of the respiratory variation in intrathoracic pressure is transmitted to the cardiac chambers, despite pericardial effusion under increased pressure, thereby allowing the physiologic increase in systemic venous return during inspiration to occur (**Fig. 4**). This interventricular septum is the only wall of the right ventricle that can move to accommodate its increased volume, because the remaining walls are restrained by the high pericardial pressure. The interventricular septum bulges toward the left side because of the increase right heart volume.

In constrictive pericarditis, in contradistinction to cardiac tamponade, the pericardial cavity is obliterated; therefore, respiratory variations of intrathoracic pressure are completely blocked from the heart with the result that the physiologic increase in systemic venous return with inspiration cannot occur. Inspiration, however, decreases left ventricular volume because pulmonary venous pressure, but not left ventricular diastolic pressure, decreases. The consequence of this inspiratory diminution of the pressure gradient responsible for left ventricular filling is that left ventricular volume declines. Ventricular interaction dictates that the right ventricular volume can increase. But how does this come about if systemic venous return does not increase? The answer is that the interventricular septum is deviated to the left, but in this case not by increased right ventricular volume, but because of the decreased left ventricular volume. These 2 different mechanisms are well-demonstrated by echo Doppler studies showing in cardiac tamponade, inspiration increases systemic venous return and right heart volume. The latter is manifested by a gradual leftward displacement of the interventricular septum, best appreciated in M-mode (see **Fig. 3**). In constrictive pericarditis, in contrast, inspiration fails to increase systemic venous return and lower

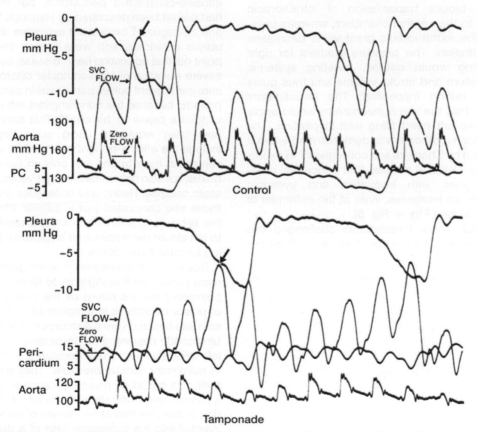

Fig. 4. The effect of inspiration on superior vena caval flow in a dog. (*Top*) Control. (*Bottom*) Acute cardiac tamponade. During tamponade, note severe pulsus paradoxus. Superior caval flow, measured with a snugly fitted flow probe, increases shortly after inspiration begins in both control and tamponade (*downward arrows*). In the control state, inspiration lowers both pleural and pericardial pressures by 9 mm Hg. During tamponade, inspiration lowers pleural pressure 8 mm Hg, but pericardial pressure only 5 mm Hg; thus, transpericardial pressure increases during inspiration. Pc, pericardium; SVC, superior vena cava. (*From* Shabetai R, Fowler NO, Fenton JC, et al. Pulsus paradoxus. J Clin Invest 1965;44:1883; with permission.)

systemic venous pressure, but makes the interventricular septum bounce sharply to the left (see **Fig. 3**). This motion was not apparent until the advent of real-time echocardiography.

Pulsus Paradoxus

How pulsus paradoxus got its name is now well-known. It will be recalled that the original description of the phenomenon attributed to Kussmaul,[13] who named it paradoxic, because the pulse was irregular (disappeared at the height of inspiration) whereas the heart beat was regular. Kussmaul's description long preceded experimental demonstration of ventricular interaction, but interaction is implicit to some of the mechanisms proposed in the middle of the subsequent century to explain pulsus paradoxus. In 1924, Katz and colleagues[14] proposed a hypothesis unrelated to ventricular interdependence, but based on pressure measurements obtained with the insensitive instruments of the day, that elevated intrapericardial pressure blocks transmission of intrathoracic pressure to the cardiac chambers, whereas pressure in the extrathoracic great veins decreases with inspiration. The pressure gradient for right heart filling would decline, lowering systemic venous return and stroke volume and thus pulse pressure during inspiration. The investigators assumed that the same mechanism would apply to impaired left heart filling with inspiration. The flaw in this hypothesis was demonstrated when it was shown by Shabetai and colleagues[15] in experimental and clinical studies, that pericardial pressure declines with inspiration and systemic venous return increases, even at the extremes of tamponade (see **Fig. 4**; **Fig. 5**).

By 1952, some investigators challenged this idea, believing that inspiration does increase systemic venous return even in the presence of tamponade and is necessary for pulses paradoxus to develop in cardiac tamponade. Accepting the truth of these ideas, Dornhorst and colleagues[16] built a mechanical model to demonstrate that inspiration increases the volume of the right heart, which further increases pericardial pressure. Increased pericardial pressure together with increased right heart volume compressed the left ventricle during inspiration (ventricular interaction). Sharp and colleagues[17] measured pulmonary wedge and pericardial pressures during surgery in a patient with malignant pericardial effusion. They varied pericardial pressure by aspiration and infusion and found that cardiac increasing of the pericardial pressure prevented transmission of respiratory variations of intrathoracic pressure to the left. They concluded that the cause of pulsus paradoxus is a decrease in the pressure gradient from pulmonary veins to the left heart during inspiration. Unfortunately, their patient most likely had effusive–constrictive pericarditis, but this entity had not yet been described by Hancock.[18] Reddy and colleagues[19] carried out extensive studies on pulsus paradoxus and were among the first to point out that coexisting heart disease, by causing severe elevation of left ventricular diastolic pressure can prevent pulses paradoxus in cardiac tamponade, because the noncompliant left and right ventricles cease to be equal. This concept has now been expanded using echo Doppler to include the effects of right heart failure and right ventricular hypertrophy, not only on pulses paradoxus, but also right atrial and right ventricular diastolic collapse. Reddy and colleagues are among those who concluded that in cardiac tamponade the pressure gradient from the pulmonary veins to left atrium decreases with inspiration, accounting for pulsus paradoxus.

Golinko and colleagues[20] were perhaps the most persuasive investigators to favor decreased pulmonary venous return as the principal cause of pulsus paradoxus in tamponade. Their conclusion was based on animal studies in which cardiac tamponade prevented the inspiratory decrease in left atrial and pericardial pressures, but not that in pulmonary venous pressure. They backed up their data based on pressure measurements with a fluoroscopic study showing the effect of respiration on the direction of movement of an oil bubble injected into the pulmonary vein of a dog. In the control state, the bubble moved from the pulmonary vein to the left atrium throughout the respiratory cycle. After they had produced tamponade, inspiration caused the bubble either to remain stationary, or else to move in the reverse direction, that is, from the left atrium to the pulmonary vein.

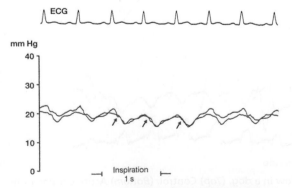

Fig. 5. Pressures recorded from the superior vena cava and pericardium on a patient with cardiac tamponade. Note absence of the *y* descent in early diastole from the venous pressure tracing but preserved *x* descent at midsystole (*arrows*). Both pressures are lower during inspiration.

The key findings in our own studies of tamponade are that, during inspiration, superior and inferior vena caval blood flow increases, both left and right heart pressures decrease, and that although pericardial pressure also decreases, transmural pericardial pressure increases, indicating substantial but incomplete transmission of the inspiratory decrease in thoracic pressure through the pericardium to the heart. In an experiment using an occlusive extracorporeal pump in closed chest dogs, we showed that a constant return of blood to the left atrium prevented pulsus paradoxus in tamponade. In addition, increased systemic venous return not only is maintained despite tamponade, but must be present for pulsus paradoxus to occur. We conclude that increased right heart volume is the major mechanism responsible for cardiac tamponade, acting through left heart-to-right heart interaction, and that decreased pressure gradient for left ventricular filling plays a lesser role. Unlike Golinko and colleagues,[20] we found that the gradient for left ventricular filling plays a lesser role and that inspiration does lower left atrial and left ventricular diastolic pressure despite the presence of tamponade (**Fig. 6**). The requisite technology has improved substantially since any

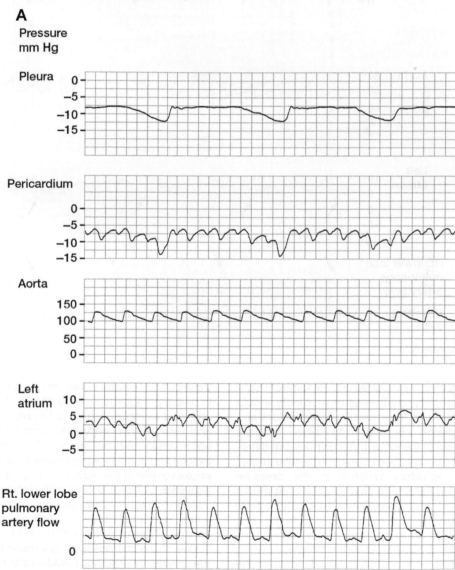

Fig. 6. Hemodynamic effects of respiration in acute cardiac tamponade in a dog. (*A*) Control, for comparison. (*B*) Tamponade. Inspiration lowers left atrial and pericardial pressures, although pericardial pressure was raised 14 mm Hg greater than the control level. Left atrial and pericardial pressures decline at the onset of inspiration (*upward arrows*). Note also hypotension, pulsus paradoxus and augmentation in the percent increase in pulmonary arterial flow (*downward arrows*).

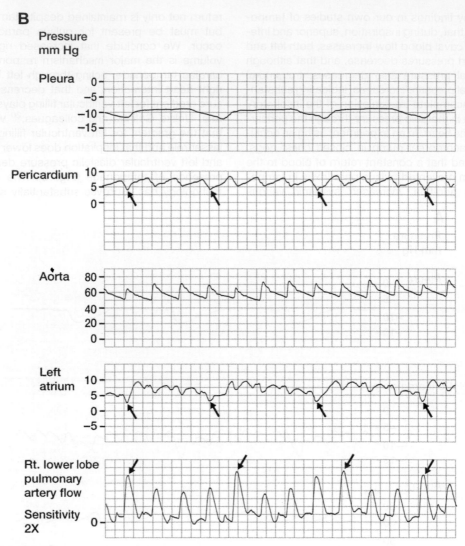

Fig. 6. (*continued*)

of these reports were published. Respiratory variation in these very small pressure gradients should be measured with intravascular manometers and analog-to-digital conversion to allow accurate determination of the instantaneous pressure differences. After this has been done, the relative importance of respiratory variation is the pressure gradient from the venae cavae to the right atrium and from the pulmonary veins to the let atrium can be settled.

Dock[21] reverted to the older and simpler theory proposed by Chevers centuries before, namely, that when the pericardium is lax, descent of the diaphragm has minimal hemodynamic effect, but when it is tense, traction by the pericardio–diaphragmatic ligaments increases when the diaphragm descends, compressing the heart and reducing cardiac filling and stroke volume.

Ventricular interaction plays the predominant role in pulsus paradoxus, but the effects of respiration are most complex, which is the reason why left and right ventricular peak systolic pressures are not precisely 180° out of phase.[14,22] Other effects include phase delay, which causes the increase in stroke volume of the right heart to be delayed until expiration before it occurs in the left heart, transmission of changing thoracic and abdominal pressures to the circulation, and the mechanical consequences of descent of the diaphragm.

One of the still unsolved questions pertains to the prevalence of pulsus paradoxus in constrictive pericarditis. The original description of pulsus paradoxus was based on clinical observation of a case of constrictive pericarditis, but, although this phenomenon is present in almost all cases of severe tamponade, it is reported in only one-quarter of the papers on constrictive pericarditis published in this and the previously century. The enigma is why pulsus paradoxus is frequently absent in constrictive pericarditis despite pronounced respiratory variation in atrioventricular inflow. Pulsus paradoxus, however, is present in almost all cases of significant cardiac tamponade, and the exceptions are readily explained. Why the prevalence of pulsus paradoxus in the 2 compressive diseases of the heart differs remains to be solved.

The studies summarized were undertaken before the advent of imaging other than chest radiography and fluoroscopy; therefore, changes in cardiac chamber volume had to be inferred. To measure intracardiac and vascular pressures and blood flow velocities required invasive techniques. Modern imaging modalities, especially echocardiography, have revolutionized the evaluation of pericardial function and diseases. The volumes or dimensions of the cardiac chambers, ventricular inflow and outflow velocities, and the approximate volume of a pericardial effusion have been measured routinely by echocardiography for many years now. Pulmonary arterial pressure stroke volume and systemic and pulmonary venous pressures are readily estimated with acceptable accuracy. Respiratory variation in transmitral early diastolic blood flow velocity and pulmonary venous blood flow velocity has become an established means to differentiate constrictive pericarditis from restrictive cardiomyopathy. Pericardial structure is easily imaged by computed tomography, MRI, or transesophageal echocardiography. In some cases transthoracic echocardiograms suffice for the recognition of an abnormally thick pericardium, especially when the pericardium seems to be tethered to the heart.

The consequences of these advances, mainly brought about in echocardiographic laboratories, are profound. Cardiac catheterization and angiography are no longer needed, or indeed desired, for the diagnosis of cardiac tamponade. Knowledge of the pathophysiology has passed from a few interested clinicians and investigators to all competent cardiologists and is the basis of their diagnosis and treatment.

PERICARDIAL PRESSURE AND TRANSMURAL CARDIAC PRESSURE

For a long time, pericardial pressure was measured in the standard way using a fluid filled catheter and an external transducer. Pressure (so-called liquid pressure) obtained in this manner is virtually identical to pleural pressure and therefore several millimeters of mercury lower than the right atrial and right ventricular diastolic pressure. Transmural diastolic cardiac pressures are, therefore, significantly greater than pressure measured with respect to atmospheric pressure. Transmural diastolic pressure is a true measure of preload. In the mid 1980s, it was proposed that only a potential pericardial space exists over the flat surfaces of the heart so that the true external restraint imposed by the pericardium is the contact pressure of the pericardium on the heart, not the liquid pressure within the pericardial space. Contact pressure cannot be measured by a catheter inserted into the pericardial space, but is determined via an unstressed flat balloon placed in the pericardial sac, through which the force of the pericardium against the heart is measured.

Smiseth and Tyberg and colleagues[23] validated contact pressure in canine experiments in which the pericardium was removed and the decrease in left ventricular diastolic pressure observed with the chamber volume unchanged from its preipericardiectomy value was considered as the true pericardial restraining force; they called this pressure decrease the theoretic pericardial pressure. Pericardial contact pressure, measured via a balloon, was almost identical to the theoretic pericardial pressure and was considered higher than the liquid pressure, being almost equal to right atrial and right ventricular diastolic pressures over a wide range of ventricular volumes. The result would be that the heart operates over a large range of volumes at a transmural pressure close to zero, a construct that is not in accord with the concept of the critical role of preload in regulating cardiac function. A small amount of fluid in the pericardium separates the pericardium from the heart, so that a contact force no longer exists. Pericardial pressure can then be measured in the conventional manner.

Contact pressure is not an issue when the pericardium is tapped for the relief of a large effusion or cardiac tamponade. After the fluid has been evacuated, pericardial pressure is restored to a value close to that of pleural pressure, because the previously distended pericardium cannot immediately shrink to its normal size.

Clinicians do not normally puncture the pericardium unless it contains excess fluid; therefore, although contact pressure is relevant for physiologists, it is much less so for clinicians. Currently however, techniques are being developed to catheterize the normal pericardium. An instrument, the "PerDUCER"[24] is advanced via the triangle of safety (the trigone) as far as the pericardium, which is viewed through the instrument. Suction is applied to create a bubble and draw it to the needle tip. The bubble is pierced, allowing passage of a guide wire and catheter into the pericardium (**Fig. 7**). Alternative techniques that have not yet been applied clinically include puncture of the right atrial appendage.[25] Interest in accessing the normal pericardium is stimulated by the concept of delivering cardiovascular therapeutic agents, such as viral agents, to deliver vascular growth factors to the myocardium. None of the agents would be lost into the circulation as occurs with intracoronary administration, but it remains to be seen how efficient transfer to the endomyocardium will be.

Why, then, does it matter whether a small fluid-containing pericardial cavity, in which liquid pressure can be measured, is present in health, or whether there is no true cavity and only contact pressure is relevant? This issue is important for determining left ventricular diastolic compliance, which requires knowledge of the true pressure surrounding the left ventricle. Transmural pressure is also important for hemodynamic interpretation. For example, conventionally measured pulmonary arterial pressure normally decreases during inspiration, but when measured transmurally, it increases. In cardiac tamponade, where right heart diastolic transmural pressure, by definition, is zero, pulmonary arterial pressure increases during inspiration. An equivalent phenomenon occurs in constrictive pericarditis, in which pulmonary arterial pressure also increases with inspiration.

A thin layer of pericardial fluid would provide uniform restraint even with the heart is subject to gravitational stress,[26] whereas regional differences in contact pressure are present at rest and are magnified in response to acute dilation of one or the other sides of the heart.[27] Acute volume overload greatly increases right atrial pressure, but a conventional pressure measuring system shows that a substantial proportion of this increase is born by the pericardium and the increase in right atrial transmural pressure is far less (**Fig. 8**).[28] These observations were reported for dogs without pericardial effusion and have been confirmed for all cardiac chambers in numerous subsequent studies.[29] To circumvent the dilemma, other investigators have sought to assess pericardial restraint in human subjects without invading the pericardium. For example, balloon occlusion of the inferior vena cava lowered the left ventricular pressure by one-third in patients with normal systolic function, dilated cardiomyopathy, coronary heart disease, or left ventricular hypertrophy.[30] Similarly, left ventricular dilatation and hypertrophy has been reported as a consequence of pericardiectomy performed to enable coronary artery bypass grafting.[31]

Upright exercise in patients with heart failure may induce pericardial constraint if the heart enlarges sufficiently. When patients with severe heart failure exercise, the initial response is a progressive increase in the pulmonary wedge pressure that is steeper than that of the right atrial pressure. Also, stroke volume increases progressively. As exercise progresses, the 2 pressures increase at the same rate and stroke volume ceases to increase, suggesting that dilation of the heart has caused it to engage the pericardium, creating pericardial constraint.[32]

It has been suggested that patients with intractable heart failure with a severely dilated heart may benefit from pericardiectomy by reducing filling pressure after withdrawing pericardial constraint. Although case reports were published, this idea has long since been abandoned. Indeed the opposite approach—fitting a prosthetic device around the dilated heart to limit further dilation—is now being investigated.[33]

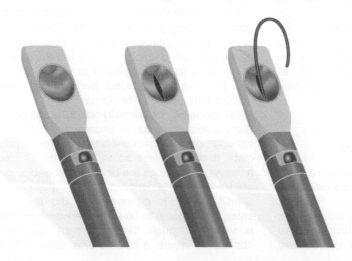

Fig. 7. The PerDUCER. (*Left*) Needle retracted during capture of a pericardial bubble. (*Center*) Needle advanced, bevel up, to puncture the bubble. (*Right*) Bevel down to allow guidewire to be advanced into the pericardium. (*Reproduced from* Reiger PJ, Beaurline CM, Grabek JR. Intrapericardial therapeutics and diagnostics. In: Seferovic PM, Spodick DH and Maisch B, editors. Pericardiology. Belgrade (Serbia): Science; 2000. p. 393–405; with permission.)

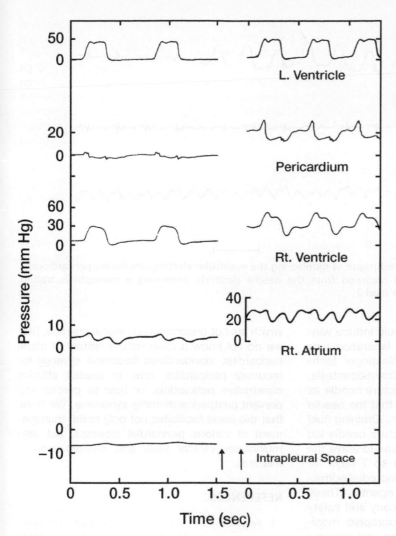

Fig. 8. The effect of rapid infusion of 1000 mL of dextran on pericardial and cardiac pressures. (*Left*) At baseline state. (*Right*) After rapid dextran infusion. Pericardial pressure is increased, but pleural pressure is unaffected. (*Reproduced from* the American Heart Association, with permission; and *From* Holt JP, Rhode EA, Kines H. Pericardial and ventricular pressure. Circ Res 1960;8:1174, with permission.)

Pericardiocentesis

Pericardiocentesis provides another example of dramatic advance both in technique and as to when it is indicated. For too long, the procedure was not carried out for tamponade until patients were severely hypotensive, and had pronounced pulsus paradoxus and severely depressed cardiac output. These are the signs of decompensated cardiac tamponade. It is now recognized that even pulsus paradoxus is a relatively late sign of tamponade and that tamponade becomes hemodynamically important when right heart collapse is present echocardiographically and before marked pulsus paradoxus has developed.[34]

From the blind tap, often performed by unsupervised junior staff at the bedside in a large open ward with minimal aseptic technique, we have progressed through pericardiocentesis performed by the cardiac catheterization team who used fluoroscopy to guide them through the procedure, almost invariably via the subxiphoid route, because the operators lacked the means to determine the distribution of the effusion. These developments improved the safety of pericardiocentesis because right heart pericardial and systemic arterial pressures were monitored, aseptic techniques were used, the intrapericardial location of the needle or trochar could be verified by injecting radiopaque contrast and emergencies could be treated much more rapidly and effectively. Aspirating fluid via the puncture needle exposed the patient to the risk of laceration of a coronary vessel or the myocardium, a danger that led to the introduction of electrocardiographic monitoring by means of an electrode attached to the needle (**Fig. 9**). Monitoring the electrogram in this way has fallen into disuse after the introduction of improved guidance, also because it carried

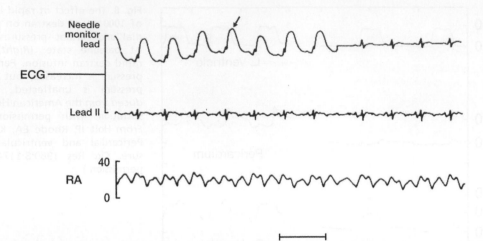

Fig. 9. The now largely abandoned technique of monitoring the ventricular electrogram during pericardiocentesis. Note the ST elevation (*arrow*) recorded from the needle electrode producing a monophasic tracing, compared with the minor increase in lead 2.

the risk of a current leak, which could induce ventricular fibrillation. The danger of laceration was reduced significantly when the Seldinger technique was introduced for pericardiocentesis, which allowed removal of the puncture needle as soon as the operator was certain that the needle tip was securely in the pericardium. Draining fluid via a catheter instead of the puncture needle led logically to the next step, which was to leave the catheter in the pericardium for 1 to 7 days for prolonged drainage, or the intrapericardial administration of chemotherapeutic agents. These changes further improved the efficacy and safety of pericardiocentesis. Echocardiographic monitoring was the next major advance and became increasingly popular as the resolution of the ultrasound devices continued to improve. Among the many advantages of echoguidance are (1) avoiding ionizing radiation, (2) the ability to determine the thickness of the effusion and where it is most abundant and closest to the skin, and (3) the ease with which the proper location of the intrapericardial needle can be verified by injecting microbubbles.[35]

SUMMARY

It is clear that tremendous progress has been made in the understanding, diagnosis, and management of various pericardial diseases thanks to many giant clinicians, physiologists, and multimodality cardiovascular imaging specialists. The current state and knowledge in all forms of pericardial diseases are well articulated in this issue of the pericardial diseases. However, we still have a lot of work to do for pericardial diseases,

which are not uncommon in clinical practice. Still, we do not know a clear natural history of acute pericarditis, standardized treatment strategy for recurrent pericarditis, how to predict effusive constrictive pericarditis, or how to predict and prevent postpericardiotomy syndrome. We hope that this issue facilitates not only better management of various pericardial diseases, but also multicenter clinical trials and investigations in this area.

REFERENCES

1. Feigenbaum H, Waldhausen JA, Hyde LP. Ultrasound diagnosis of pericardial effusion. JAMA 1965;191:711–4.
2. Ling LH, Oh JK, Tei C, et al. Pericardial thickness measured with transesophageal echocardiography: feasibility and potential clinical usefulness. J Am Coll Cardiol 1997;29:1317–23.
3. Lower R. Tractatus de Corde, Item de Motu, et Colare Sanguinius et Chyli in Sum Transiti, London J. Allestry, 1969, quoted by Boyd LJ and Elias H, in Contributions to diseases of the heart and pericardium. 1. Historical introduction. Bull NY Med Coll 1955;18:1–37.
4. Chevers N. Observations on the disease of the orifice and valves of the aorta. Guys Hosp Rep 1842;7:387–439.
5. Henderson Y, Prince AL. Relative systolic discharges from the right and left ventricles and their bearing upon pulmonary congestion and depletion. Heart 1914;5:217–26.
6. Taylor RR, Covell JW, Sonnenblick EH, et al. Dependence of ventricular distensibility on filling of the opposite ventricle. Am J Physiol 1967;213(3):711–8.

7. Glantz SA, Misbach GA, Moores WY, et al. The pericardium substantially affects the left ventricular diastolic pressure-volume relationship in the dog. Circ Res 1978;42:433–41.

8. Santamore WP, Bartlett R, VanBuren SJ, et al. Ventricular coupling in constrictive pericarditis. Circulation 1986;74:597–602.

9. Hatle LK, Appleton CP, Popp RL. Differentiation of constrictive pericarditis and restrictive cardiomyopathy by Doppler echocardiography. Circulation 1989;79:357–70.

10. Oh JK, Hatle LK, Seward JB, et al. Diagnostic role of Doppler echocardiography in constrictive pericarditis. J Am Coll Cardiol 1994;23:154–62.

11. Welch TD, Ling LH, Espinosa RE, et al. Echocardiographic diagnosis of constrictive pericarditis: Mayo clinic criteria. Circ Cardiovasc Imaging 2014;7(3):526–34.

12. Anavekar NS, Wong BF, Foley TA, et al. Index of biventricular interdependence calculated using cardiac MRI: a proof of concept study in patients with and without constrictive pericarditis. Int J Cardiovasc Imaging 2013;29(2):363–9.

13. Kussmaul A. Ueber schwielige mediastinopericarditis und den paradoxen puls. Berliner. Klin Wochenschr 1878;10:461–4.

14. Katz LN, Gauchat HW. Observations on pulsus paradoxus (with special reference to pericardial effusions). Arch Intern Med 1924;33:371–93.

15. Shabetai R, Fowler NO, Fenton JC, et al. Pulsus paradoxus. J Clin Invest 1965;44(11):1882–98.

16. Dornhorst AC, Howard P, Leathart GI. Pulsus paradoxus. Lancet 1952;1:746–8.

17. Sharp JT, Bunnell IL, Holland JF, et al. Hemodynamics during induced cardiac tamponade in man. Am J Med 1960;29:640–6, 1960.

18. Hancock EW. Subacute effusive-constrictive pericarditis. Circulation 1971;43:183–92.

19. Reddy PS, Curtis EI, O'Toole JD, et al. Cardiac tamponade: hemodynamic observations in man. Circulation 1978;58:265–72.

20. Golinko RJ, Kaplan N, Rudolph AM. The mechanism of pulsus paradoxus during acute pericardial tamponade. J Clin Invest 1963;42:249–57.

21. Dock W. Inspiratory traction on the pericardium: the cause of pulsus paradoxus in pericardial disease. Arch Intern Med 1961;108:837–40.

22. Shabetai R, Fowler NO, Gueron M. The effects of respiration on aortic pressure and flow. Am Heart J 1963;65:525–33.

23. Smiseth OA, Frais MA, Kingma I, et al. Assessment of pericardial constraints in dogs. Circulation 1985;116:322–32.

24. Seforovic PM, Ristic AD, Maskimovic R, et al. Initial experience with Per Ducer device in the diagnosis and treatment of pericardial disease. Clin Cardiol 1999;22(Suppl 1):30–5.

25. Verrier RL, Waxman S, Lovette EG, et al. Transatrial access to the normal pericardial space: a novel approach for diagnostic sampling, pericardiocentesis, and therapeutic interventions. Circulation 1998;98:2331–3.

26. Banchero N, Rutishauser WJ, Tsakiris AG, et al. Pericardial pressure during transverse acceleration in dogs without thoracotomy. Circ Res 1967;20:65–77.

27. Hoit BD, Lew WY, LeWinter M. Regional variation in pericardial contact pressure in the canine ventricle. Am J Physiol 1988;255:H1370–7.

28. Holt JP, Rhode EA, Kines H. Pericardial and ventricular pressure. Circ Res 1960;8:1171–81.

29. Shirato K, Shabetai R, Bhargava V, et al. Alterations of the left ventricular diastolic pressure-segment length relation produced by the pericardium. Circulation 1978;57:1191–8.

30. Dauterman K, Pak PH, Maughan WL, et al. Contribution of external forces to left ventricular diastolic pressure. Implications for the clinical use of the Starling Law. Ann Intern Med 1995;122:737–42.

31. Tichler MD, Rowan AM, LeWinter MM. Increased left ventricular mass after thoracotomy and pericardiectomy. A role for relief of pericardial constraint. Circulation 1993;87:1921–7.

32. Janicki J. Influence of the pericardium and ventricular interdependence on left ventricular diastolic and systolic function. Circulation 1980;81(2 Suppl). III-15–20.

33. Kung RT, Rosenberg M. Heart booster: a pericardial support device. Ann Thorac Surg 1999;6:764–7.

34. Klopfenstein HS, Schuchard GH, Wann LS, et al. The relative merits of pulsus paradoxus and right ventricular diastolic collapse in the early detection of cardiac tamponade: an experimental echocardiographic study. Circulation 1985;71:829–33.

35. Tsang TSM, Barnes ME, Hayes SN, et al. Clinical and echocardiographic characteristics of significant pericardial effusions following cardiothoracic surgery and outcomes of echo-guided pericardiocentesis for management: Mayo Clinic experience, 1979-1998. Chest 1999;116:322–31.

Anatomy and Physiology of the Pericardium

Brian D. Hoit, MD

KEYWORDS

• Pericardium • Ventricular interaction • Mesothelium • Hemodynamics

KEY POINTS

- The pericardium is composed of visceral (epicardial) and parietal (fibrous pericardial) components: the former reflects over the great vessels, creating sinuses and recesses (a major component of the pericardial reserve volume), and becomes the serosal layer of the latter, which has ligamentous attachments to the sternum, spine, and diaphragm.
- Histologically, the relatively inelastic fibrous pericardium is composed of functionally arranged compact collagen layers interspersed with short elastin fibers; the visceral pericardium is a mesothelial monolayer with numerous microvilli, which provide friction-bearing surfaces and increase surface area.
- The pericardium is not essential for life, but serves important mechanical functions (eg, constraint of ventricular filling, ventricular interaction) that are subtle in healthy individuals, but are critical in disease states characterized by a rapid increase in heart size.
- Other functions of the pericardium include membranous (equalizing gravitational, hydrostatic, and inertial forces and reducing friction over the surface of the heart, and serving as a barrier to infection); metabolic; ligamentous (limiting excessive displacement of the heart); and reflexive (hemodynamic neuromodulation).
- The mesothelium of the pericardium is metabolically active and produces prostacyclins and other substances that modulate epicardial coronary arterial tone, fibrinolysis, and sympathetic neurotransmission.

ANATOMY OF THE PERICARDIUM

The pericardium is composed of visceral and parietal components. The visceral pericardium is a mesothelial cell monolayer that adheres firmly to the epicardium, reflects over the origin of the great vessels, and becomes the serosal layer of the parietal pericardium, a tough, fibrous tissue that envelops the heart. The pericardial space is enclosed between these 2 layers and normally contains up to 50 mL of pericardial fluid. Pericardial fluid is largely a plasma ultrafiltrate, but may include myocardial interstitial fluid and lymph drainage.[1] Pericardial fluid volume is greatest over the atrioventricular and interventricular grooves; over the flatter surfaces of the heart, there is only a thin film of fluid. Thus, only a potential space is present over most of the cardiac surface, a fact that has implications for how pericardial pressure is measured and for how the restraining effect of the pericardium on cardiac volumes is estimated. The thickness of the pericardium varies by region ($\sim$0.8–1.0 mm thick on anatomic specimens) and is slightly greater on imaging studies (0.7–1.2 mm by cardiac computed tomography [CT] and 1.5 to 2.0 mm by cardiac magnetic resonance [CMR]).[2,3]

There are no disclosures to report.
Department of Medicine (Cardiology), Case Western Reserve University, Harrington Heart and Vascular Center, University Hospitals Cleveland Medical Center, 11100 Euclid Avenue, Cleveland, OH 44106-5038, USA
E-mail address: bdh6@cwru.edu

Cardiol Clin 35 (2017) 481–490
http://dx.doi.org/10.1016/j.ccl.2017.07.002
0733-8651/17/© 2017 Elsevier Inc. All rights reserved.

cardiology.theclinics.com

Pericardial Sinuses and Recesses

Pericardial reflections around the great vessels and pulmonary veins result in the formation of the oblique sinus, a U-shaped midline cul-de-sac behind the left atrium between the pulmonary veins and inferior vena cava; the transverse sinus, a tunnellike passageway between the anterior and posterior pericardial cavity, which is bounded anteriorly by the aorta and main pulmonary artery, and posterolaterally by the atria and their append-ages, and the superior venal cava; and extensions of the transverse sinus, the pericardial recesses (**Fig. 1**, **Table 1**). Recesses can be seen on advanced imaging studies (CT, CMR, and transe-sophageal echocardiography) and surgical or postmortem examination. These potential spaces (particularly the oblique sinus) are major contribu-tors to the pericardial reserve volume (ie, the differ-ence between unstressed pericardial volume and cardiac volume) that accommodates physiologic changes in ventricular filling. The phrenic nerves and pericardiophrenic vessels are contained in a bundle between the fibrous pericardium and the mediastinal pleura that courses anterior to the pul-monary hilum.

Attachments of the Pericardium

The fibrous pericardium is attached to the adven-titia of the great arteries, cervical fascia, and the central tendon of the diaphragm; it is more loosely attached to the esophagus and the descending aorta posteriorly and to the left leaf of the dia-phragm inferiorly. Several pericardial ligaments firmly affix the pericardium in the thorax: antero-superiorly to the manubrium by the superior peri-cardiosternal ligament, antero-inferiorly to the xiphoid process by the inferior pericardiosternal ligament, posteriorly to the vertebral column, and inferiorly to the central tendon of the diaphragm (**Fig. 2**). The fibrous pericardium contacts the chest wall behind the fifth to seventh costal carti-lages, an area known because of pericardiocente-sis as the "triangle of safety."

The Epicardium

Between the visceral pericardium (epicardium) and the subjacent myocardium is an inconstant amount of epicardial fat (most prominent in the atrioventricular and interventricular grooves and right ventricular [RV] free wall) that contains

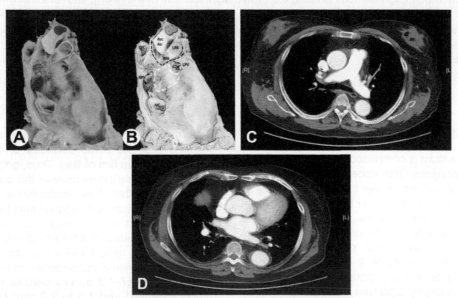

Fig. 1. (*A*) Lateral dorsal and diaphragmatic aspects of the pericardial sac after removal of the anterior portion of the pericardial sac and heart. The aorta and pulmonary trunks are enclosed in one sheath and the pulmonary veins and venae cavae are covered in another. (*B*) The transverse sinus (*dashed black arrow*) forms a tunnel be-tween the arterial and venous pericardial reflections, creating access between the right and left sides of the peri-cardial cavity. The inverted U-shaped cul-de-sac behind the left atrium between the pulmonary veins is the oblique sinus (*dashed white line*). (*C*) Contrast-enhanced CT axial image demonstrating the superior aortic recess of the transverse sinus (*arrow*). (*D*) Contrast-enhanced CT axial image demonstrating the oblique sinus (*arrow*). Asc Ao, ascending aorta; IVC, inferior vena cava; LPA, left pulmonary artery; LPV, left pulmonary vein; RPA, right pulmonary artery; RPV, right pulmonary vein; SVC, superior vena cava. (*Reproduced from* Klein AL, Abbara S, Agler DA, et al. American Society of Echocardiography clinical recommendations for multimodality cardiovascular imaging of patients with pericardial disease. J Am Soc Echocardiogr 2013;26:965–1012; with permission.)

Table 1
Pericardial recesses

Recess	Location
Superior aortic	Between the Ao and SVC
Inferior aortic	Between the ascending Ao and the right atrium
Postcaval recess	Behind and to the right of the SVC
Left and right pulmonic recesses	Inferior to the proximal left and right PA

Abbreviations: Ao, aorta; PA, pulmonary artery.

the coronary arteries and veins, nerves, and lymphatics.

The arterial supply of the pericardium originates from the pericardiophrenic and musculophrenic arteries, branches of the internal thoracic (mammary) arteries, and the descending thoracic aorta. Venous drainage is from the pericardiophrenic veins, branches of the superior intercostal and internal thoracic veins, which arise from the innominate veins. Lymphatics drain from multiple pathways: the parietal pericardium drains into anterior and posterior mediastinal nodes, and the visceral pericardium drains into tracheal and brachial mediastinal nodes.

Parasympathetic innervation is supplied by the vagus and the left recurrent laryngeal nerves and branches from the esophageal plexus. Sympathetic nerve supply is derived from the first dorsal ganglion, stellate ganglion, and aortic, cardiac, and diaphragmatic plexi.[4] Sensory nerves from the phrenic nerve supply sensation to the pericardium, only approximately one-sixth of which is directly responsive to painful stimuli.[5]

Histology of the Pericardium

Histologically, the pericardium is composed predominantly of compact collagen layers (primarily type 1 and 3 collagen) interspersed with short elastin fibers (**Fig. 3**). The abundance and orientation of the collagen fibers are responsible for the characteristic viscoelastic mechanical properties of the pericardium, namely, stress relaxation and creep and hysteresis. Pericardial mechanics can be modeled as 2 sets of springs arranged in parallel that represent the thick collagen and thin elastin fibers, respectively.[6] Although small, low-pressure effusions compress only the thin elastic springs, in cardiac tamponade, the heavier collagen springs are compressed, resulting in the typical steep portion of the J-shaped pericardial pressure-volume relation.

The fibrous parietal pericardium contains superficial, middle, and deep layers of collagen fibers that are interlaced with elastin fibers. Mesothelial cells are attached to the fibrous pericardium by delicate connective tissue rich in elastin. In humans, the collagen fibers are straight at birth, become progressively wavy until young adulthood, and progressively straighten with increasing age. Elastin fibers, initially numerous early in life, are less densely distributed later in life. Although these data suggest that the pericardium is less compliant in the elderly, the contribution of increased pericardial stiffness to altered diastolic function in the elderly is unclear.[7]

Despite its simple histology, electron microscopy of the pericardium reveals surprisingly detailed cytoarchitecture. Mesothelial cells interdigitate and overlap, which facilitates stretching of the mesothelium in diastole and permits changes in surface configuration; mechanical stability is assured by a cytoskeleton of fine filamentous bundles.[8] Mesothelial cells completely cover the serosal layers from which numerous microvilli, and in smaller numbers, single cilia protrude, providing friction-bearing surfaces and an increase in the surface area for bulk fluid transport. With sweeping motions, the microvilli and cilia distribute pericardial fluid and allow the pericardium to accommodate to changes in the cardiac-cycle–dependent size and shape of the heart.

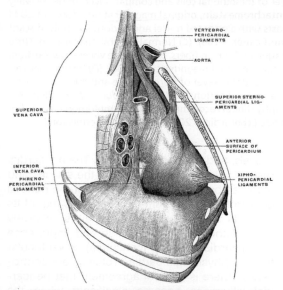

Fig. 2. Ligamentous attachments of the pericardium to the sternum, diaphragm, and vertebral column. (*Reproduced from* ClipArt ETC. Available at: www.etc.usf.edu/. Accessed January 5, 2017.)

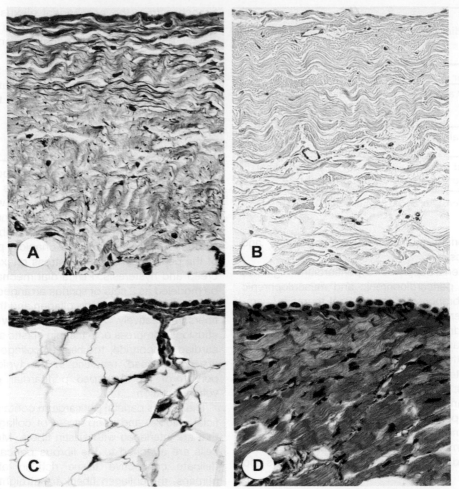

Fig. 3. (*A*) Normal parietal pericardium. Note the single layer of mesothelial cells and compact layers of dense wavy collagen (*yellow*) and short elastic fibers (*black*) (Movat pentachrome stain, original magnification ×100). (*B*) CD34 immunostaining of the parietal pericardium shows fibroblasts with elongated nuclei and endothelial cells of scant thin blood vessels (CD 34 immunoperoxidase, original magnification ×100). (*C*) Normal visceral pericardium. Note the mesothelial cell layer and thin subepithelial layer of collagen and elastin fibers. Beneath the visceral pericardium is abundant epicardial adipose tissue (Movat pentachrome stain, original magnification ×100). (*D*) Visceral pericardium without adipose tissue. Note the mesothelial monolayer and thin layer of fibrous tissue and the immediately subjacent myocardium (Movat pentachrome stain, original magnification ×100). (*Reproduced from* Klein AL, Abbara S, Agler DA, et al. American Society of Echocardiography clinical recommendations for multimodality cardiovascular imaging of patients with pericardial disease. J Am Soc Echocardiogr 2013;26:970; with permission.)

PHYSIOLOGY OF THE PERICARDIUM

The pericardium is not essential for life, and no adverse consequences follow congenital absence or surgical removal of the pericardium. However, the pericardium serves important albeit subtle functions (**Box 1**) that can be divided into the mechanical, reflexive, membranous, metabolic, and ligamentous.

Mechanical Effects

The total pericardial volume includes the cardiac volume, the intrapericardial portions of the great vessels, and the pericardial fluid. The pericardial reserve volume (owing largely to the sinuses and recesses but also to the elasticity of the parietal pericardium), the volume that exceeds that of its contents in the euvolemic state, is relatively small. Although the magnitude and importance of pericardial restraint (constraint) of ventricular filling at physiologic cardiac volumes are controversial, there is general agreement that pericardial influences become significant when the reserve volume is exhausted. The limits of the pericardial reserve volume may be reached with rapid increases in blood volume (hypervolemia)

Box 1
Functions of the pericardium

Mechanical

Limits short-term cardiac distention

Facilitates cardiac chamber coupling and interaction

Maintains pressure-volume relations of the cardiac chambers and their output

Reflex

Hemodynamic modulation via neuroreceptors, mechanoreceptors, and chemoreceptors

Membranous/serosal

Lubricates, reduces friction

Equalizes gravitational, hydrostatic, and inertial forces

Mechanical barrier to infection

Metabolic

Vasomotor

Modulates sympathetic neurotransmission and contractility

Fibrinolytic

Immunologic

Ligamentous

Limits displacement of the heart

Neutralizes the effects of respiration and change of body position

Contributes to apparent compliance of the pericardium

and in disease states characterized by rapid increases in heart size (eg, acute mitral and tricuspid regurgitation, pulmonary embolism, RV infarction). When this happens, the pericardium limits distension of the cardiac chambers and facilitates interaction and coupling of the ventricles and atria.[6] Conversely, hypovolemia abrogates or abolishes these pericardial effects. Limitation of cardiac filling volumes by the pericardium may also limit cardiac output and oxygen delivery during exercise; for example, it was shown that removing the pericardium of greyhound dogs caused a 25% increase in Vo_{2max} and cardiac output.[9]

Ventricular interaction and restraint are closely related phenomena. The normal pericardium constrains cardiac filling, particularly the thin-walled atria and right ventricle and is an important contributor to resting ventricular diastolic pressure and atrial function. Ventricular interaction describes the change in volume, pressure, or filling of a cardiac chamber that results from changes in an adjacent chamber (**Fig. 4**). For example, an increase in RV volume results in an increase in left ventricular (LV) diastolic stiffness. Although the right and left ventricles interact because of their common septum, the pericardium further "couples" the chambers, heightening their interaction. Cardiac chamber interactions occur primarily during diastole, although systolic interactions can be detected. Ventricular interaction maintains the pressure-volume relations of the cardiac chambers and assures a balanced output from the right and left ventricles, allows both ventricles to generate greater isovolumic pressure at a given diastolic volume, and helps maintain the normal geometry of the heart.

The pressure-volume relation of the pericardium is nonlinear; that is, the relation is initially flat, producing little to no change in pressure for changes in volume, and when the pericardial reserve volume is outstripped, develops a "bend" or "knee" and terminates in a steep slope, producing large changes in pressure for small changes in volume (**Fig. 5**). Thus, acutely, relatively small pericardial

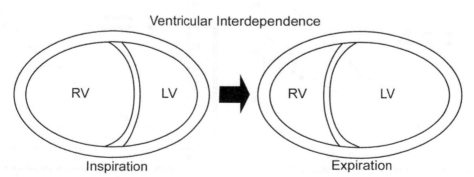

Fig. 4. Schematic diagram of ventricular interdependence. With inspiration, there is a shift of the ventricular septum toward the left ventricle that is reversed with expiration. (*Reproduced from* Klein AL, Abbara S, Agler DA, et al. American Society of Echocardiography clinical recommendations for multimodality cardiovascular imaging of patients with pericardial disease. J Am Soc Echocardiogr 2013;26:978; with permission.)

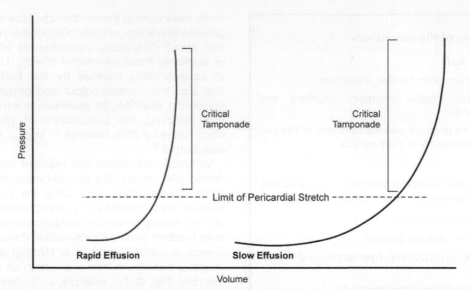

Fig. 5. Pericardial pressure-volume curves from a rapidly developing (*left*) and more slowly developing (*right*) effusion. The flat, initial segment of the curves is the pericardial reserve volume that, once exceeded, causes a steep increase in pressure. (*Reproduced from* Klein AL, Abbara S, Agler DA, et al. American Society of Echocardiography clinical recommendations for multimodality cardiovascular imaging of patients with pericardial disease. J Am Soc Echocardiogr 2013;26:978; with permission.)

effusions may cause cardiac tamponade. In contrast, adaptation to chronic stretching of the pericardium involves stress-relaxation, pericardial hypertrophy, and an increase in pericardial surface area, which results in a rightward shift of the pressure-volume relation; this explains why large but slowly developing effusions may not produce tamponade (see **Fig. 5**).

The pericardium also influences quantitative and qualitative aspects of ventricular filling, that is, the thin-walled right ventricle and atrium are more subject to the influence of the pericardium than is the more resistant, thick-walled left ventricle.[10] In open-chest dogs, removal of the pericardium

influenced differently the filling of the right and left ventricles (early to late diastolic velocity filling ratios increased across the mitral valve and decreased across the tricuspid valve, a response explained by the differences between right and left atrial compliances) and decreased the slope of the RV but not LV pressure-volume relation, suggesting regional pericardial effects (**Fig. 6**).[11] In another canine model, pericardiectomy increased atrial compliance and was associated with greater relative increases in conduit than reservoir function, suggesting fundamentally different pericardial effects on left atrium vis-à-vis the left ventricle.[12]

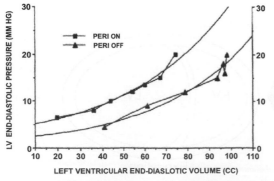
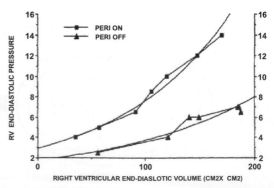

Fig. 6. LV (*left*) and RV (*right*) end-diastolic pressure-volume curves before and after pericardiectomy from a single animal. Note the parallel rightward shift of the left and the nonparallel rightward shift of the RV end-diastolic pressure-volume relations. (*Reproduced from* Hoit BD, Dalton N, Bhargava V, et al. Pericardial influences on right and left ventricular filling dynamics. Circ Res 1991;68:197–208; with permission.)

Measuring pericardial pressure

Surprisingly, the manner in which pericardial pressure should be measured remains unresolved. In the absence of a pericardial effusion, determining pericardial pressure with a fluid-filled catheter may be inappropriate because the pericardial "cavity" is largely a potential space.

When incised, the normal parietal pericardium retracts, indicating that the pericardium exerts a constitutive stress on the underlying myocardium (ie, an epicardial radial stress), and it has been argued that contact force using a flat gas- or liquid-filled unstressed balloon be used to measure pericardial constraint.[13] Indeed, pressures measured with flat balloons are essentially the same as the theoretic pericardial pressure (ie, the fall of LV diastolic pressure upon widely opening the pericardium when measured at the same ventricular volume) in the absence of a pericardial effusion.[13]

Although it is generally assumed that except for hydrostatic difference, conventional pericardial pressure over the cardiac surface is uniform, it cannot be assumed a priori that pericardial contact pressure (the normal force exerted by the pericardium per unit area of balloon) is uniform over the heart. In fact, using flat, air-filled balloons, the author showed that pericardial contact pressure is greater over the left than right heart, increasing over the left ventricle with aortic compression and volume loading and increasing over the right ventricle with pulmonary artery compression and volume loading.[14,15]

These concepts have important implications for normal pericardial physiology insofar as fluid pericardial pressure, like pleural pressure, is negative; as a result, transmural pressure (cavity minus pericardial pressure, which is the distending or true filling pressure of a chamber) is higher than pressure measured in the chamber itself. For example, during ventricular ejection, the resultant decrease in pericardial pressure increases atrial transmural pressure and filling. However, when there is a pericardial effusion, conventional fluid-filled pressures are appropriate (in cardiac tamponade transmural chamber pressures are near zero), and in constrictive pericarditis, obliteration of the pericardial space makes evaluating pericardial pressure moot.

Pathophysiologic role of pericardium in heart failure

Acute heart failure and volume overload increase pericardial restraint once the pericardial reserve volume is surpassed; when this occurs, a significant proportion of the increase in ventricular diastolic pressure is shouldered by the pericardium.

In hemodynamic terms, transmural distending pressure in a cardiac chamber is less than intracavitary pressures recorded with a catheter in that chamber.

Hemodynamic studies of vasodilators in acute decompensated heart failure using high-fidelity pressure manometry and ventriculography serendipitously demonstrated that the pericardium contributed significantly to the observed elevations of LV diastolic pressure.[16] Thus, the venodilator nitroglycerine, which decreased ventricular volume, shifted the entire diastolic LV pressure-volume relation downward, whereas the arteriolar dilator amyl nitrate, which had little effect on LV volume, lowered pressure along the trajectory of the initial pressure-volume curve.

The effect of chronic pericardial restraint was demonstrated in chronically instrumented canine experiments, in which infrarenal aortocaval anastomoses were constructed and the effect of pericardiectomy on the diastolic pressure-segment length was examined both acutely (3 days) and after several weeks of shunting.[17] Acutely, the pressure-segment length curve shifted to the right after pericardiectomy, but chronically, the rightward shift upon opening the pericardium was abrogated, indicating the loss of pericardial restraint and reduced ventricular interaction; this could be accounted for by chronic volume overload causing an increase in pericardial chamber compliance. This change in compliance was later shown in vitro with biaxial stretching of the pericardium and measurement of stress-strain curves to be due to a change in the biomechanical properties of the pericardial tissue itself.[18]

Reflex Effects

Neuroreceptors, mechanoreceptors, and chemoreceptors in the pericardium alter heart rate and blood pressure in response to lung inflation, ventricular distention, and pericardial fluid constituents, respectively. These reflexes provide "pericardial servomechanisms" that modulate the mechanical functions of the pericardium.[19,20]

Membranous Effects

The thin layer of pericardial fluid equalizes gravitational, hydrostatic, and inertial forces over the surface of the heart, so that transmural cardiac pressures neither change during acceleration nor differ regionally within cardiac chambers. Pericardial fluid and surfactant phospholipids reduce friction on the epicardium. The pericardium also acts as an anatomic barrier to the spread of infection from contiguous structures.

Metabolic Effects

The mesothelium of the pericardium is metabolically active and produces endothelin, prostaglandin E_2, eicosanoids, and prostacyclin in response to pericardial stretch, increases in myocardial work, angiotensin II, and bradykinin. These substances modulate epicardial coronary arterial tone, cardiac function, and by inhibiting efferent sympathetic effects, sympathetic neurotransmission.[19,21] Prostacyclin also inhibits platelet aggregation and may influence coronary thrombosis and prevent clotting of intrapericardial blood. Both atrial natriuretic peptide and brain natriuretic peptide (BNP) are present in the pericardial fluid at levels exceeding those found in the plasma; the level of BNP is a sensitive and accurate indicator of ventricular volume and pressure and may play an autocrine-paracrine role in modifying heart failure–induced ventricular remodeling.[22] Complement and other immune-related substances are normally found in the pericardium, and levels increase in pericarditis with an immune-mediated etiopathogenesis.

Epicardial fat

Epicardial fat (**Figs. 7** and **8**) is a marker of cardiovascular risk and is associated with the cardiovascular risk factors, obesity, diabetes, age, and hypertension.[23] It differs from pericardial fat (external to the parietal pericardium and also known as paracardial, intrathoracic, or mediastinal fat) in biochemical and molecular properties. Pericardial fat receives its vascular supply from the pericardiophrenic artery, and epicardial fat is nourished from the coronary arteries. Epicardial fat is involved in the local distribution and regulation of vascular flow, and inflammatory and mechanical protection of the myocardium and coronary arteries; serves as an immune barrier and local source of fatty acids for myocardium at times of high demand; and has thermogenic effects. It is involved in triglyceride and glucose-insulin metabolism, low-grade chronic inflammation, and the production of proinflammatory and anti-inflammatory cytokines. Epicardial fat may have paracrine effects and accelerate atherosclerosis by enhancing endothelial dysfunction, smooth muscle cell proliferation, increased oxidative stress, and plaque instability.

Ligamentous Effects

Superior and inferior pericardiosternal and diaphragmatic ligaments prevent excessive torsion and limit displacement of the pericardium and its contents within the chest and neutralize the effects of respiration and change of body position.[24] In

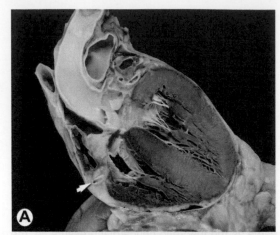
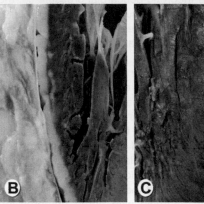

Fig. 7. Epicardial fat. (A) Abundant epicardial fat in the right atrioventricular groove (note the right coronary artery; *arrow*), and a variable amount in the RV free wall, which outlines the pericardium. (B) Epicardial and pericardial fat over the right ventricle delineates the parietal pericardium. (C) A paucity of epicardial fat over the left ventricle results in poor visualization of the pericardium in this area on imaging studies. (*Reproduced from* Klein AL, Abbara S, Agler DA, et al. American Society of Echocardiography clinical recommendations for multimodality cardiovascular imaging of patients with pericardial disease. J Am Soc Echocardiogr 2013;26:971; with permission.)

addition, these attachments contribute to the apparent compliance of the pericardial pressure-volume relation.[25]

IMPLICATIONS FOR PATHOPHYSIOLOGY

In view of the pericardium's simple structure, clinicopathologic processes involving it are understandably few, and the response to injury is limited to exudation of fluid, fibrin, and inflammatory cells. Healing may result in obliteration of the pericardial space by adhesions between the visceral and parietal layers, and later, calcification, either focal or extensive, may occur.

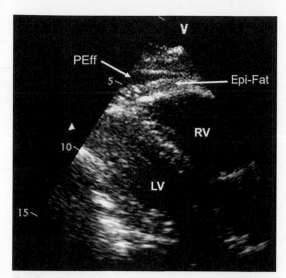

Fig. 8. Epicardial fat (Epi-Fat) and pericardial effusion (PEff) on 2-dimensional echocardiography. Epicardial fat is brighter than myocardium, tends to have uniform thickness, and moves with the heart, distinguishing it from effusion. (*Reproduced from* Klein AL, Abbara S, Agler DA, et al. American Society of Echocardiography clinical recommendations for multimodality cardiovascular imaging of patients with pericardial disease. J Am Soc Echocardiogr 2013;26:982; with permission.)

Pericardial heart disease includes pericarditis, which may be an acute, subacute, or chronic fibrinous, "noneffusive," or exudative process; tamponade and its variants; and constriction, which may be an acute, subacute, or chronic adhesive or fibrocalcific response. However, despite a limited number of clinical syndromes, the pericardium is affected by virtually every category of disease, including infectious, neoplastic, immune-inflammatory, metabolic, iatrogenic, traumatic, and congenital causes. A brief consideration of the anatomic and physiologic implications in pericardial disease follows. These conditions will be discussed in detail later in this issue.

Pathophysiology of Pericardial Effusion and Cardiac Tamponade

The clinical presentations of patients with pericardial effusion are diverse and depend on the volume of the effusion and its rate of accumulation, the nature and cause of the effusion, the thickness and compliance of the pericardium, and the presence of coexisting heart disease.

The primary abnormality is compression of the cardiac chambers due to increased pericardial pressure that is exerted throughout the cardiac cycle.[26] The pericardium has some degree of elasticity, but once the elastic limit is reached, the heart must compete with the intrapericardial fluid for a fixed intrapericardial volume, and heightened ventricular interaction (interdependence) rapidly ensues. As the total pericardial volume reaches the stiff portion of its pressure-volume relation, tamponade rapidly follows, and as cardiac tamponade progresses, the cardiac chambers become smaller, and diastolic chamber compliance is reduced. Very little fluid needs to accumulate to produce cardiac tamponade once the pericardium can no longer stretch.[26] At this point, the initial removal of fluid during pericardiocentesis produces the greatest reduction in intrapericardial pressure.

Although tamponade has been shown to compress the epicardial coronary arteries, ischemia does not occur because it is balanced by a reduction in preload (and hence, myocardial oxygen demand) and does not contribute to the pathophysiology of cardiac tamponade.[7]

Pathophysiology of Constrictive Pericarditis

Constrictive pericarditis is a condition in which a thickened, inelastic, scarred, and often calcified pericardium limits diastolic filling and constrains the upper limit of cardiac volume.[27] The thickened, rigid pericardium prevents the normal inspiratory decrease in intrathoracic pressure from being transmitted to the heart chambers, causing a dissociation of intracardiac and intrathoracic pressures; as a result, venous pressure does not decrease, and systemic venous return fails to increase with inspiration.

Because the left atrium and the terminal portions of the pulmonary veins are intrapericardial, pulmonary venous, but not left atrial pressure declines during inspiration, the pulmonary venous-to-left atrial gradient and flow decreases, leading to a reduction in LV volume. Because of ventricular interaction, the right heart volume expands via a shift of the interventricular septum. As in cardiac tamponade, with expiration, the opposite changes occur.

With constrictive pericarditis, early diastolic filling is even more rapid than normal. Compression does not occur until the cardiac volume approximates that of the constraining pericardium, which occurs in middiastole, at which point filling abruptly stops. Consequently, as constrictive pericarditis becomes more severe, ventricular volumes and stroke volumes are reduced.

Pathophysiology of Effusive-Constrictive Pericarditis

Although the pericardial cavity is typically obliterated in patients with constrictive pericarditis, pericardial effusion may be present in some cases. In this setting, the scarred pericardium not only constricts the cardiac volume but can also increase the pericardial fluid pressure, leading to signs suggestive of cardiac tamponade. Pericardial abnormality consistent with constrictive pericarditis with a concomitant effusion is called effusive-constrictive pericarditis.[28] Such patients may be mistakenly thought to have only cardiac tamponade; however, elevation of the right atrial and pulmonary wedge pressures after drainage of the pericardial fluid points to the underlying constrictive process.

REFERENCES

1. Miller AJ, Pick R, Katz LN. The production of acute pericardial effusion. The effects of varying degrees of interference with venous blood and lymph drainage from the heart muscle in the dog. Am J Cardiol 1971;28:463–6.

2. White CS. MR evaluation of the pericardium. Top Magn Reson Imaging 1995;7:258–66.

3. Bull RK, Edwards PD, Dixon AK. CT dimensions of the normal pericardium. Br J Radiol 1998;71:923–5.

4. Holt JP. The normal pericardium. Am J Cardiol 1970; 26:455–65.

5. Spodick DH. Acute pericarditis. New York: Grune & Stratton; 1959.

6. Rabkin SW, Ping HH. Mathematical and mechanical modeling of stress strain relationship of pericardium. Am J Physiol 1975;229:896–900.

7. Shabetai R. The pericardium. Norwell (MA): Kluwer Academic; 2003.

8. Spodick DH. Macrophysiology microphysiology, and anatomy of the pericardium: a synopsis. Am Heart J 1992;124:1046–51.

9. Stray-Gunderen J, Musch TL, Haidet GC, et al. The effect of pericardiectomy on maximal oxygen consumption and maximal cardiac output in untrained dogs. Circ Res 1986;58:523–30.

10. Assanelli D, Lew WYW, Shabetai R, et al. Influence of the pericardium on right and left filling in the dog. J Appl Physiol (1985) 1987;63:1025–32.

11. Hoit BD, Dalton N, Bhargava V, et al. Pericardial influences on right and left ventricular filling dynamics. Circ Res 1991;68:197–208.

12. Hoit BD, Shao Y, Gabel M, et al. Influence of pericardium on left atrial compliance and pulmonary venous flow. Am J Physiol 1993;264:H1781–7.

13. Tyberg V, Misbach GA, Glanz SA, et al. A mechanism for shifts in the diastolic left ventricular pressure-volume curve: the role of the pericardium. Eur J Cardiol 1978;7(Suppl):163–75.

14. Hoit BD, Lew WYW, LeWinter M. Regional variation in pericardial contact pressure in the canine ventricle. Am J Physiol 1988;255:H1370–7.

15. Smiseth OA, Scott-Douglas NW, Thompson CR, et al. Non-uniformity of pericardial surface pressure in dogs. Circulation 1987;75:1229–36.

16. Ludbrook PA, Byrne JD, McKnight RC. Influence of right ventricular hemodynamics on left ventricular diastolic pressure-volume relations in man. Circulation 1979;59:21–31.

17. LeWinter MM, Pavelec R. Influence of the pericardium on left ventricular end-diastolic pressure-segment relations during early and late stages of experimental chronic volume overload in dogs. Circ Res 1982;50:501–9.

18. Lee MC, LeWinter MM, Freeman G, et al. Biaxial mechanical properties of the pericardium in normal and volume overload dogs. Am J Physiol 1985;249: H222–30.

19. Spodick DH. Physiology of the normal pericardium: functions of the pericardium. In: The pericardium. A comprehensive textbook. New York: Marcel Dekker, Inc.; 1997. p. 15–26.

20. Cinca J, Rodriguez-Sinovas A. Cardiovascular reflex responses induced by epicardial chemoreceptor stimulation. Cardiovasc Res 2000;45: 63–71.

21. Miyazaki T, Pride HP, Zipes DP. Prostaglandins in the pericardial fluid modulate neural regulation of cardiac electrophysiological properties. Circ Res 1990;66:163–75.

22. Tanaka T, Hasegawa K, Fujita M, et al. Marked elevation of brain natriuretic peptide levels in pericardial fluid is closely associated with left ventricular dysfunction. J Am Coll Cardiol 1998;31: 399–403.

23. Bertaso AG, Bertol D, Duncan BB, et al. Epicardial fat: definition, measurements and systematic review of main outcomes. Arq Bras Cardiol 2013;101: 18–28.

24. Klein AL, Abbara S, Agler DA, et al. American Society of Echocardiography clinical recommendations for multimodality cardiovascular imaging of patients with pericardial disease. J Am Soc Echocardiogr 2013;26:965–1012.

25. Freeman GL, LeWinter MM. Pericardial adaptations during chronic cardiac dilation in dogs. Circ Res 1984;54:294–300.

26. Spodick DH. Acute cardiac tamponade. N Engl J Med 2003;349:684–90.

27. Adler Y, Charron P, Imazio M, et al. 2015 ESC Guidelines for the diagnosis and management of pericardial diseases: the Task Force for the Diagnosis and Management of Pericardial Diseases of the European Society of Cardiology (ESC) endorsed by: the European Association for Cardio-Thoracic Surgery (EACTS). Eur Heart J 2015;36:2921–64.

28. Hancock EW. A clearer view of effusive-constrictive pericarditis. N Engl J Med 2004;350:435–7.

Imaging of the Pericardium
A Multimodality Cardiovascular Imaging Update

Bo Xu, MB BS (Hons), FRACP, Deborah H. Kwon, MD, Allan L. Klein, MD*

KEYWORDS

- Pericardium • Acute pericarditis • Recurrent pericarditis • Constrictive pericarditis
- Pericardial tamponade • Echocardiography • Multidetector computed tomography • CMR imaging

KEY POINTS

- Pericardial diseases represent diverse conditions, ranging from painful inflammatory states, such as acute pericarditis, to life-threatening tamponade and chronic heart failure due to constrictive pericarditis.
- Echocardiography is generally the first-line imaging investigation for the assessment of pericardial disorders.
- Multidetector cardiac computed tomography can be useful for the assessment of the location and extent of pericardial calcification in end-stage chronic constrictive pericarditis, as well as delineating congenital anomalies of the pericardium.
- Cardiac magnetic resonance (CMR) imaging can be used to demonstrate pericardial edema and pericardial late gadolinium enhancement, an imaging correlate of active inflammation with neovascularization and fibroblast proliferation.
- CMR imaging may help guide and modulate therapy decision, and monitor response to treatment in patients with pericarditis.

 Video content accompanies this article at http://www.cardiology.theclinics.com.

INTRODUCTION

Pericardial conditions ranging from acute pericarditis and constrictive pericarditis to cardiac tamponade represent an important group of cardiovascular disorders; increased morbidity and mortality are associated with many of these conditions.[1,2] Multimodality cardiovascular imaging is critical in the diagnosis and management of pericardial conditions, providing structural, functional, and hemodynamic information characteristic of pericardial diseases.[3,4]

This review presents a clinically focused update on multimodality cardiovascular imaging of pericardial conditions. A focus is on forming a framework on when and how each cardiovascular imaging modality is helpful in each pericardial condition. An emphasis is given on how multimodality cardiovascular imaging may affect the diagnosis and management of patients with pericardial conditions.

ANATOMY OF THE PERICARDIUM

The pericardium is composed of the visceral and parietal layers, 2 avascular layers that surround the

Section of Cardiovascular Imaging, Center for the Diagnosis and Treatment of Pericardial Diseases, Heart and Vascular Institute, Cleveland Clinic, Desk J1-5, 9500 Euclid Avenue, Cleveland, OH 44195, USA
* Corresponding author.
E-mail address: kleina@ccf.org

Cardiol Clin 35 (2017) 491–503
http://dx.doi.org/10.1016/j.ccl.2017.07.003
0733-8651/17/© 2017 Elsevier Inc. All rights reserved.

heart and proximal great vessels (**Fig. 1**). The outer, parietal layer is fibrous, containing predominantly collagen, with interspersed elastin fibrils.[3] The parietal layer is normally ≤2 mm thick. The inner, visceral layer is composed of a single layer of mesothelial cells, collagen and elastin (**Fig. 2**). Normally, there is a physiologic potential space between the visceral and parietal pericardial layers, which may contain up to 50 mL of fluid. Alterations in the thickness, elasticity of the pericardium, and accumulation of excessive pericardial fluid in disease states, can significantly alter normal cardiac filling.

ACUTE PERICARDITIS

Acute pericarditis is a frequently encountered clinical condition. Although the exact incidence of acute pericarditis is not known, it has been reported to account for a notable proportion (approximately 5%) of nonacute myocardial infarction–related chest pain cases presenting to the emergency department.[5,6] However, the reported

incidence of acute pericarditis is likely underestimated, because there is no established gold standard for its diagnosis. The diagnosis of acute pericarditis is made clinically, based on the presence of 2 or more established diagnostic criteria (classical pleuritic-type chest pain on clinical history, supportive features on physical examination, such as a pericardial friction rub, typical electrocardiographic changes including diffuse, concave upward ST-segment elevation and PR depression, and the finding of a new pericardial effusion).[3–5,7]

Transthoracic echocardiography (TTE) should be the initial cardiac imaging investigation for patients with suspected acute pericarditis (**Table 1**). The presence of a pericardial effusion on TTE, supported by the appropriate clinical context, is suggestive of acute pericarditis.[1,2,5] However, it should be noted that most frequently, in acute pericarditis, TTE is unremarkable.[1,6] Despite this, TTE should be performed in all patients with suspected acute pericarditis.[8] Suspected acute pericarditis represents part of the clinical syndrome

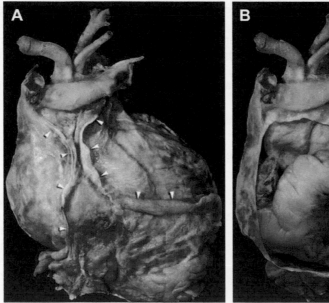
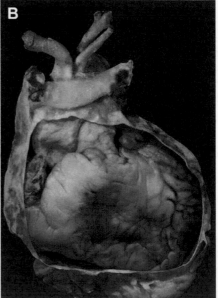

Fig. 1. Anatomy of the pericardium. Anterior view of the intact parietal pericardial sac (*A*). The attachment of the fibrous sac to the diaphragm is seen at the base. Abundant epipericardial fat is conspicuously present at the pericardial-diaphragm junction. The mediastinal pleura invest the lateral portion of fibrous pericardium. The anterior reflections of the mediastinal pleura are indicated by the white arrowheads. The space between the arrowheads corresponds to the attachment of the pericardium to the posterior surface of the sternum. Superiorly, the left innominate vein is seen merging with the superior vena cava. The arterial branches of the aortic arch are just dorsal to the innominate vein. The anterior portion of the pericardial sac has been removed to show the heart and great vessels in anatomic position (*B*). It distinctly shows how the proximal segments of the great arteries are intrapericardial. At that point, there is fusion of the adventitia of the great vessels with the fibrous pericardium. (*Adapted from* Klein AL, Abbara S, Agler DA, et al. American Society of Echocardiography clinical recommendations for multimodality cardiovascular imaging of patients with pericardial disease: endorsed by the Society for Cardiovascular Magnetic Resonance and Society of Cardiovascular Computed Tomography. J Am Soc Echocardiogr 2013;26:969; with permission.)

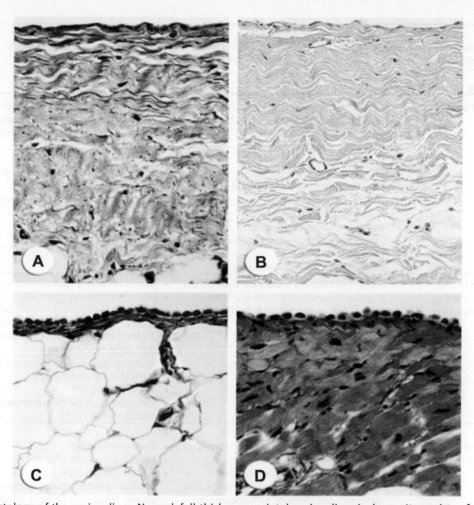

Fig. 2. Histology of the pericardium. Normal, full-thickness parietal pericardium is shown It consists of a layer of mesothelial cells and compact layers of dense wavy collagen (*yellow*) with interspersed short elastic fibers (*black*) (*A*). Fibroblasts with elongated nuclei and scant thin blood vessels are normally present in the parietal pericardium. CD34 immunostaining highlights the endothelial cells of capillaries (*B*). The visceral pericardium (also called epicardium) consists of a mesothelial cell layer and a thin subepithelial layer of collagen with elastic fibers. The mesothelial cells show distinct microvilli. Beneath the visceral pericardium is epicardial adipose tissue (*C*). In other areas of the visceral pericardium (or epicardium), only a thin layer of fibrous tissue (*yellow*) separates the mesothelial cells from the myocardium with absence of epicardial fat. Original magnifications ×400; A, C, D: Movat pentachrome stain; B: CD34 immunoperoxidase. (*Adapted from* Klein AL, Abbara S, Agler DA, et al. American Society of Echocardiography clinical recommendations for multimodality cardiovascular imaging of patients with pericardial disease: endorsed by the Society for Cardiovascular Magnetic Resonance and Society of Cardiovascular Computed Tomography. J Am Soc Echocardiogr 2013;26:970; with permission.)

of acute chest pain and not infrequently acute pericarditis is interpreted as ST-elevation myocardial infarction due to diffuse ST elevation on ECG. TTE can effectively assess for the absence of regional wall motion abnormalities to exclude ST-segment elevation myocardial infarction. This may reduce unnecessary invasive coronary angiography.[9] Additionally, TTE can be used for risk stratification. Tamponade physiology has been reported in 3% of patients with acute pericarditis.[3] Furthermore, TTE can help identify features of constrictive physiology early on, such as an abnormal diastolic septal bounce and increased pericardial brightness or thickening. Such patients may warrant closer clinical follow-up and serial echocardiographic monitoring.

Multidetector cardiac computed tomography (MDCT) should not be used as a first-line imaging investigation in suspected acute pericarditis. With increasing use of computed tomography (CT) of the chest in the emergency department, the pericardium may be imaged, albeit the scan may have been done for a different indication. CT can help evaluate pericardial thickness. A thickened,

Table 1
Multimodality cardiovascular imaging investigations used in the evaluation of patients with pericardial conditions, and their relative strengths and limitations

Imaging Modality	Strengths	Limitations
Echocardiography	• First-line imaging investigation in the diagnostic evaluation of patients with pericardial disease • Readily available • Portable • Low cost • Can be performed at bedside and during an emergency • Respirometer available for respiro-phasic assessment • Transesophageal echocardiogram available as adjunct echocardiographic modality	• Relatively narrow field of view • Technically difficult ultrasound windows (eg, obesity, emphysema, and postoperative settings) • Operator dependent • Low signal-to-noise ratio of the pericardium • Limited tissue characterization
Multidetector computed tomography	• Adjunct imaging modality that offers improved anatomic delineation • Evaluation of extracardiac disease • Preoperative planning • Assessment of pericardial calcification	• Use of ionizing radiation • Use of iodinated contrast • Functional evaluation only possible with retrospectively gated studies (higher radiation dose; suboptimal temporal resolution) • Imaging acquisition affected by arrhythmias and ectopy • Need for breath-hold • Patients must be hemodynamically stable
Cardiac magnetic resonance imaging	• Adjunct imaging modality for improved anatomic delineation • Superior tissue characterization • Ability to assess for pericardial inflammation (pericardial edema and delayed gadolinium enhancement)	• High cost • Time-consuming • Calcification not well seen • Use of gadolinium contrast contraindicated in patients with severe renal impairment (glomerular filtration rate <30 mL/min) • Patients must be hemodynamically stable

Adapted from Klein AL, Abbara S, Agler DA, et al. American Society of Echocardiography clinical recommendations for multimodality cardiovascular imaging of patients with pericardial disease: endorsed by the Society for Cardiovascular Magnetic Resonance and Society of Cardiovascular Computed Tomography. J Am Soc Echocardiogr 2013;26:967; with permission.

but noncalcified pericardium may be a feature of acute pericarditis.[10] CT also may detect the presence of a pericardial effusion. The presence of a small pericardial effusion may be a supportive feature of acute pericarditis in the appropriate clinical setting. However, the presence of a large pericardial effusion should prompt the clinician to corroborate with other imaging modalities (typically TTE), and assess its hemodynamic consequences. The attenuation value of the pericardial fluid on CT could help differentiate the type of pericardial effusion: typically, an attenuation value >60 Hounsfield units supports the presence of blood; an attenuation value between 20 and 60 Hounsfield units supports the presence of an exudate;

an attenuation value <10 Hounsfield units supports the presence of a transudate.[11,12]

Cardiac magnetic resonance (CMR) imaging is probably the most sensitive imaging technique for diagnosing acute pericarditis by demonstrating pericardial inflammation using delayed gadolinium enhancement. Pericardial thickness and the extent of a pericardial effusion can be measured using T1-weighted black blood sequences.[13,14] The findings of a thickened, but noncalcified pericardium supports the diagnosis of acute pericarditis.[13] The acuity of inflammation can be assessed using CMR. An increased signal on T2-weighted short tau inversion recovery (STIR) sequences supports an acute inflammatory process associated with edema.[15] Additional valuable information can be obtained from pericardial late gadolinium enhancement (LGE) imaging. The histologic correlates of pericardial LGE have been studied; the presence of LGE suggests increased vascular permeability, neovascularization, and fibroblast proliferation in the pericardium.[16] The sensitivity of pericardial LGE for detection of pericardial inflammation is high (reported to range from 94% to 100%).[15,17] This could provide valuable information in management of patients with difficult to treat acute pericarditis, resistant to conventional treatment with nonsteroidal anti-inflammatory drugs and colchicine. The presence of pericardial LGE in patients with ongoing symptoms should prompt the clinician to consider up-titration of medical therapy, as well as prolongation of standard medical therapy duration. However, data on how long LGE persists after a treated episode of acute pericarditis are still lacking.

RECURRENT PERICARDITIS

Recurrent pericarditis occurs in up to one-third of patients following an initial episode of acute pericarditis.[6,7,18,19] The rate of further recurrences after a first recurrent episode of pericarditis is higher, up to 50%.[6,7,18,19] Recurrent pericarditis is diagnosed when a documented first episode of acute pericarditis is followed by a symptom-free period of 4 to 6 weeks or longer, and evidence of subsequent recurrence of pericarditis is present.[4] By definition, when the duration of symptoms exceeds 3 months, it is defined as chronic pericarditis. In clinical practice, there may be some overlap in the classification of patients according to these definitions.

Although TTE is usually performed in patients with suspected recurrent pericarditis, the most useful diagnostic imaging test is CMR, unless there is clinical evidence of associated constrictive pericarditis, which is not common in this situation. The presence and extent pericardial LGE could help guide the institution of anti-inflammatory therapy.[20] CMR is also helpful in excluding recurrent pericarditis by observing the absence of pericardial inflammation.

CONSTRICTIVE PERICARDITIS

Constrictive pericarditis has been considered a challenging condition to diagnose, but comprehensive multimodality imaging currently available makes its diagnosis much easier (see Terrence D. Welch and Jae K. Oh's article, "Constrictive Pericarditis," in this issue). Accurate diagnosis is important, as this is a curable cause of diastolic heart failure, and a subset of the patients with an early stage of constriction with pericardial inflammation can be treated medically. The most common etiologies for constrictive pericarditis include idiopathic, postviral, and postcardiac surgery.[21,22] In the developing world, infectious etiologies, such as tuberculosis, remain important.[23]

In constrictive pericarditis, the cardiac chambers are encased in a "rigid cage," with significant respiratory variation in cardiac filling.[1,2,14,24] One of the hallmarks of constrictive pericarditis by echocardiography is a restrictive pattern of transmitral filling profile, characterized by very rapid filling of the left ventricle during early diastole, before the constraint imposed by the rigid pericardial cage limits further left ventricular filling from mid-diastole onward (**Fig. 3**, Video 1).[3,13]

Echocardiography is the first-line imaging investigation for patients with suspected constrictive pericarditis, with a class I recommendation in the European Society of Cardiology guidelines for the diagnosis and management of pericardial diseases.[4] Ventricular interdependence is a key feature of constrictive pericarditis, which should be carefully assessed with echocardiography and the use of a respirometer. The M-mode signs of ventricular interdependence include (1) movement of the ventricular septum toward the left ventricle on inspiration; and (2) movement of the ventricular septum toward the right ventricle on expiration.[21] Diastolic septal bounce is an additional feature of ventricular interdependence that could be examined by both 2-dimensional and M-mode echocardiography. On M-mode echocardiography, this is manifested by a septal notch. Significant respiratory variation in the transmitral inflow profile can be seen in constrictive pericarditis: (1) the mitral E wave velocity usually decreases by ≥25% on inspiration; and (2) the tricuspid E wave velocity usually decreases by ≥40%.[25,26] Hepatic vein Doppler flow profile provides helpful clues to the presence of constrictive physiology. On expiration, there is prominent diastolic flow reversal within hepatic vein Doppler profile. This contrasts with increased hepatic vein flow reversal on inspiration, seen in patients with restrictive cardiomyopathy.[3] Tissue Doppler imaging provides additional clues to the presence of constrictive physiology. Mitral annulus early diastolic velocity (e′), especially from the medial annulus, is relatively normal or even augmented, and is usually, but not always, higher than lateral annulus e′ (annulus reversus) (**Fig. 4**).[27,28]

A relatively simple approach to the echocardiographic diagnosis criteria (Mayo Clinic diagnostic criteria) of constrictive pericarditis was established

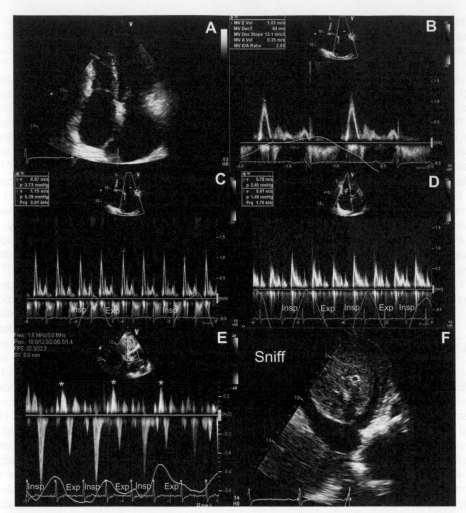

Fig. 3. Echocardiographic findings in constrictive pericarditis. Moderate biatrial enlargement with evidence of septal bounce (*A*: apical 4-chamber view; septal bounce is better appreciated on cine loop: Video 1). Restrictive pattern of diastolic filling characterized by rapid early diastolic filling, with atrial contraction contributing minimally to left ventricular filling (*B*). Respirophasic variation in mitral inflow Doppler profile, with a typical decrease in peak E wave velocity on the first beat following inspiration (*C*). Respirophasic variation in tricuspid inflow Doppler profile, with a typical increase in peak E wave velocity on the first beat after inspiration (*D*). Prominent diastolic flow reversal within hepatic vein on expiration (*E: white asterisks*). Dilated inferior vena cava that fails to collapse on inspiration, suggestive of elevated right atrial pressure (*F*).

by an important, single-center study.[29] Patients with surgically confirmed constrictive pericarditis were compared with patients with restrictive cardiomyopathy or severe tricuspid regurgitation.[29] The echocardiographic features that were found to be independently associated with constrictive pericarditis were as follows: (1) the presence of ventricular septal shift during respiration, (2) increased medial early diastolic mitral annular velocity, and (3) increased hepatic expiratory diastolic reversal ratio on pulsed-wave Doppler.[29] The combination of ventricular septal shift and a medial early diastolic mitral annular velocity ≥9 cm/s, or a hepatic vein expiratory

diastolic reversal to forward velocity ratio of ≥0.79 yielded the highest diagnostic sensitivity (87%) and specificity (91%).[29]

Advanced echocardiographic imaging, including the assessment of ventricular mechanics with strain imaging provides valuable pathophysiologic and diagnostic insights. Using 2-dimensional speckle-tracking echocardiography, global longitudinal strain is generally preserved, whereas circumferential strain, torsion, and early diastolic twisting are reduced.[30,31] Tethering of the pericardium in patients with constrictive pericarditis can lead to reduced left ventricular anterolateral wall and right ventricular free wall strain, with

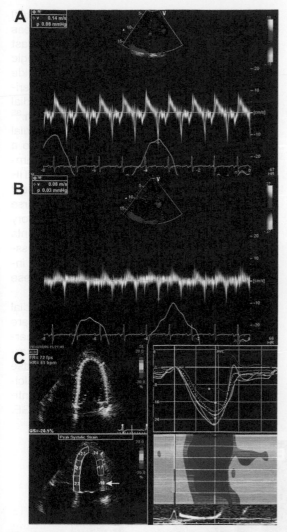

Fig. 4. Annulus reversus. Medial early diastolic mitral annular velocity (e′) is increased (*A*: 14 cm/s), while lateral early diastolic mitral annular velocity (e′) is reduced (*B*: 8 cm/s). The phenomenon of annulus reversus also can be demonstrated on strain imaging using 2-dimensional speckle tracking, with the peak systolic strain in the basal anterolateral segment being significantly lower (*C: white arrow*) than the septum in this example.

preservation of septal strain.[31] Interestingly, pericardiectomy results in improvement of longitudinal strain in the previously tethered ventricular segments.[31]

For many patients, a comprehensive clinical and echocardiographic assessment incorporating M-mode, Doppler, 2-dimensional, and strain imaging can help clench the diagnosis of constrictive pericarditis. For certain groups of patients, MDCT and CMR may provide additional information. MDCT is very useful in the assessment of the

location and extent of pericardial calcification (**Fig. 5**).[32] The presence of pericardial calcification indicates persistent, chronic pericardial inflammation, resulting in irreversible fibrosis and calcific change.[16] Information derived from MDCT is particularly helpful for the subset of patients with previous cardiac surgery or radiation heart disease, for the purpose of preoperative planning. MDCT can also

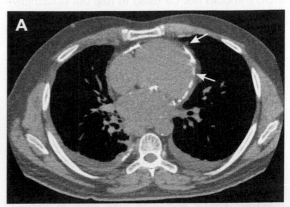

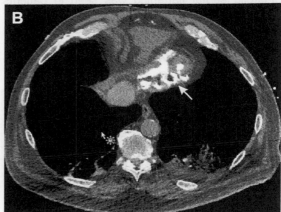

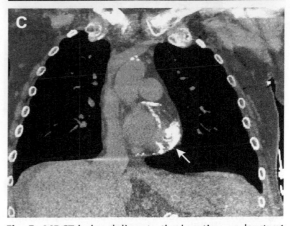

Fig. 5. MDCT helps delineate the location and extent of pericardial calcification (*arrows* in *A–C*). The presence of pericardial calcification suggests end-stage chronic fibrotic changes.

demonstrate pericardial thickening. It should be noted that although MDCT provides useful anatomic assessment of the pericardium, it does not provide hemodynamic assessment, which is key in diagnosing constrictive pericarditis. MDCT can effectively assess pericardial thickness. In constrictive pericarditis, the parietal pericardial layer may become as thick as 20 mm.[3] However, it should be noted that the absence of pericardial thickening on MDCT should not be used to rule out constrictive pericarditis. In a study of 143 patients with surgically confirmed constrictive pericarditis, 18% of patients had normal pericardial thickness on histologic examination, and 28% of patients had normal pericardial thickness on MDCT.[23]

CMR, like echocardiography, can demonstrate the important changes in transvalvular flow and ventricular septal motion with respiration. In a CMR study using real-time phase-contrast CMR, a ≥25% variation in transmitral flow was valuable in diagnosing constrictive pericarditis.[33] Cine CMR is useful for demonstrating ventricular septal shift. A single-center CMR study found that early diastolic septal flattening was seen in patients with constrictive pericarditis.[34] The ability of CMR to assess for fibroblast proliferation and neovascularization makes it a uniquely important imaging modality in the assessment of constrictive pericariditis.[16] An increased T2 STIR pericardial signal suggests pericardial edema,[15] whereas pericardial LGE correlates with ongoing fibroblast proliferation and neovascularization on histologic assessment.[16] Such information can help provide insights into the clinical stage of constrictive pericarditis (Fig. 6). Prominent T2 STIR and pericardial LGE support active pericardial inflammation.[35] Normal T2 STIR with the presence of pericardial LGE supports the patient has transitioned into a subacute stage.[36] Lack of ongoing active inflammation would be reflected by normal T2 STIR and lack of pericardial LGE. In this context, it could be hypothesized that the patient's disease course may no longer be modified by anti-inflammatory therapy. In a retrospective cohort of 159 patients with recurrent pericarditis, quantitative assessment of pericardial LGE provided incremental information regarding the clinical course of these patients.[37]

In a study of patients with significant pericardial LGE, it has been shown that these patients are more likely to respond to anti-inflammatory therapy, and achieve resolution of constrictive pericarditis.[38] For patients in the end-stage of disease progression with significant pericardial calcification, and nonresponders to intense anti-inflammatory therapy without pericardial LGE,

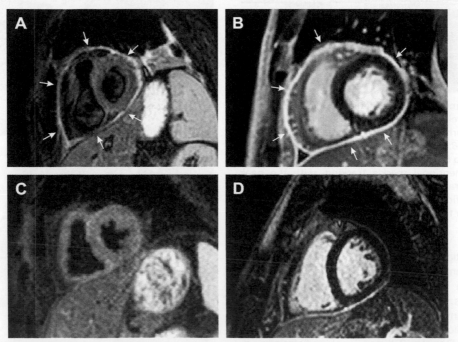

Fig. 6. Effects of intense anti-inflammatory therapy in a patient with recurrent pericarditis demonstrated on CMR. Before anti-inflammatory therapy (A, B), intense pericardial signal on T2 STIR imaging suggests pericardial edema (arrows in A), and circumferential pericardial LGE suggests ongoing inflammation with neovascularization and fibroblast proliferation (arrows in B). Following intense anti-inflammatory therapy, resolution of pericardial edema (C) and significant pericardial LGE are evident (D).

pericardiectomy may be required for definitive treatment.

TRANSIENT CONSTRICTIVE PERICARDITIS

Transient constrictive pericarditis occurs in an important subset of patients affected by constrictive pericarditis. Diagnosis of transient constrictive pericarditis has important therapeutic and management implications. Rather than fibrosis and end-stage significant pericardial calcification, the predominant pathophysiologic process involved in transient constrictive pericarditis is ongoing inflammation. Transient constrictive pericarditis is a temporary form of constriction, usually developing after pericarditis, which resolves with anti-inflammatory therapy.[4,39] The pathophysiologic process begins with pericarditis, with the most common etiologic agents in the developed world being viral idiopathic causes and post cardiac surgery.[4,39] It has been reported that 1.8% of patients with acute pericarditis progress to constrictive pericarditis.[40] The risk for progression to constrictive pericarditis varies with the etiology for acute pericarditis, with those patients suffering from purulent, bacterial pericarditis having the highest risk for progression to constrictive pericarditis.[40] The exact incidence of transient constrictive pericarditis is unknown. Transient constrictive pericarditis typically resolves within 3 months, and represents up to 17% of the constrictive pericarditis cases.[40,41] Timely and accurate diagnosis of transient constrictive pericarditis may halt progression to chronic constrictive pericarditis, by allowing the clinician to initiate and maintain appropriate anti-inflammatory therapy.

TTE is the first-line imaging investigation in the workup of patients with suspected transient constrictive pericarditis. A pericardial effusion or pericardial thickening may be seen. Additionally, dynamic features to support constrictive physiology can be assessed by echocardiography, including (1) respirophasic septal shift, (2) respirophasic septal bounce or shudder, (3) inferior vena cava plethora, (4) increased respiratory variation in the mitral and tricuspid Doppler inflow profiles, and (5) diastolic hepatic vein flow reversal during expiration.[3] Tissue Doppler imaging features of constrictive physiology include (1) annulus reversus, as described previously: a reduction in lateral early diastolic mitral annular velocity, relative to the medial early diastolic mitral annular velocity; and (2) annulus paradoxus, the usual relationship between increasing E/e′ ratio and elevated left atrial pressure is reversed, due to increased medial e′ velocity seen in constrictive pericarditis.[28,42] CMR imaging provides additional diagnostic information. Transverse black blood spin-echo images can be used to assess pericardial thickness (≥ 3 mm).[14] Cine imaging with steady-state free precession sequences can effectively assess for the presence of pericardial effusion, diastolic septal bounce, and dilated inferior vena cava. Pericardial edema as demonstrated by T2 STIR spin-echo sequences suggests acute pericardial inflammation. Pericardial LGE imaging has been reported to have high sensitivity (86%) and specificity (80%) for transient constrictive pericarditis.[38]

MDCT is less relevant for the assessment of patients with suspected transient constrictive pericarditis. MDCT is effective in the identification of pericardial calcification, which may be seen in patients with chronic, end-stage constrictive pericarditis. The goal in the assessment of patients with transient constrictive pericarditis is appropriate identification of patients at an early stage of inflammatory process, before the development of significant pericardial calcification and scarring.

Transient constriction can also be assessed by PET with fluorodeoxyglucose F 18 (^{18}F FDG-PET)/CT. Chang and colleagues[43] demonstrated in patients with tuberculosis constrictive pericarditis that ^{18}F FDG-PET/CT could predict the response to steroid therapy with a high accuracy.

PERICARDIAL EFFUSION AND TAMPONADE

There are many causes of pericardial effusion. Common causes of pericardial effusion include inflammatory states affecting the pericardium, such as acute pericarditis, malignancy, post cardiac surgery, and end-stage renal disease.[3,4] TTE is the first-line imaging investigation for the assessment of pericardial effusion (**Fig. 7**, Videos 2 and 3). Semiquantitative assessment of pericardial effusion can be performed with echocardiography.

Separation of parietal pericardium and epicardium during both systole and diastole on M-mode echocardiography has been found to be associated with effusions that are greater than 50 mL.[44] On 2-dimensional echocardiography, at end diastole, the size of pericardial effusion can be classified as small (<1 cm), moderate (1–2 cm), large (>2 cm), or very large (>2.5 cm).[45] Fibrinous stranding or the presence of clots may be detectable on echocardiography. In addition, the presence of loculated pericardial effusion may be found, which has implications when pericardiocentesis is being considered. A left-sided pleural effusion can be differentiated from a pericardial effusion by demonstrating that the pleural effusion is found between the descending aorta and the left ventricle on parasternal long-axis imaging.[3]

Additional imaging modalities, such as CT and CMR, can provide further assessment of a

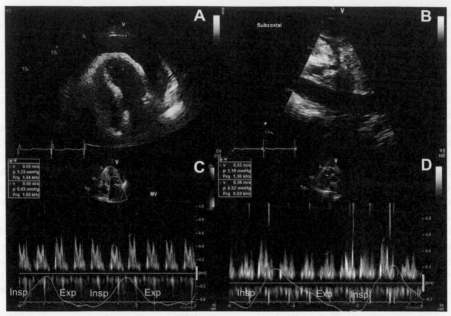

Fig. 7. Pericardial tamponade. A large circumferential pericardial effusion (*A*: apical 4-chamber view; during cine loop recording, the heart is seen to swing in the large pericardial effusion: Video 2; right ventricular diastolic chamber compression can be better appreciated on cine loop: Video 3). A dilated, fixed inferior vena cava (*B*) is an important echocardiographic sign of tamponade physiology; Significant respirophasic variation in mitral (*C*) and tricuspid (*D*) inflow Doppler profiles.

pericardial effusion. However, these imaging modalities are rarely used as the primary investigation for the diagnosis and assessment of pericardial effusion. When pericardial effusion is detected on CT and CMR, it often is an incidental finding.[46] CT imaging can provide helpful additional information in the situation of a complex, loculated pericardial effusion. Such information may help decision-making regarding the need for surgical rather than percutaneous drainage of pericardial effusion.

Cardiac tamponade occurs when a hemodynamically significant pericardial effusion causes impaired cardiac chamber filling, elevated and equal intracardiac diastolic pressures, with resultant compromise in cardiac output.[47] TTE should be performed urgently, when cardiac tamponade is suspected. Echocardiography has a very high diagnostic accuracy for the presence of pericardial effusion (approaching 100%).[3] The diagnosis of cardiac tamponade is based on clinical assessment (presence of tachycardia, elevated central venous pressure, and pulsus paradoxus), complemented by echocardiographic assessment. Important echocardiographic findings in cardiac tamponade include (1) the presence of a pericardial effusion (although clots, masses, or air in the pericardial space can also lead to tamponade), (2) dilated inferior vena cava with

minimal or no inspiratory collapse; and (3) evidence of reduced stroke volume on Doppler assessment.[3] Diastolic compression, or even collapse of the right ventricle, supports the presence of a hemodynamically significant pericardial effusion. However, it should be noted that in certain conditions, such as right ventricular hypertrophy, and severe pulmonary hypertension, despite elevated intrapericardial pressure, signs of right ventricular chamber compression may be absent.[48,49] Right atrial collapse during systole is an additional useful feature, supporting tamponade physiology. Right atrial collapse for more than one-third of the cardiac cycle has been shown to be highly sensitive and specific for tamponade.[50] Additionally, significant respiratory variation in mitral and tricuspid inflows can be seen. In cardiac tamponade, the peak mitral E velocity decreases greater than 30% during the first heart beat on inspiration, and the peak tricuspid E velocity decreases greater than 60% during the first heart beat on expiration.[51]

CONGENITAL ABSENCE OF THE PERICARDIUM

Congenital absence of the pericardium (CAP) is rare. The commonest variant is complete absence of left side of the pericardium, whereas total absence of the pericardium, or partial absence of either left or right side of the pericardium, are even more rare.[3,52,53] Most frequently, CAP is detected as an incidental finding during cardiac imaging. Patients may present with a range of symptoms. These symptoms are often atypical, including atypical chest pain, dyspnea, and palpitations.

TTE is the first-line imaging investigation in the assessment of patients with suspected CAP. Together with typical electrocardiographic changes, including the presence of right bundle branch block, and chest radiography findings, echocardiography is useful in reaching the diagnosis of CAP for many patients. Features on echocardiography that may point to CAP include (1) presence of unusual imaging windows, suggesting displacement of the heart; (2) right ventricular dilatation or the appearance of right ventricular dilatation; (3) excessive cardiac motion; and (4) paradoxic septal motion during systole.[3,53–55]

Asymptomatic patients with CAP generally do not warrant further imaging investigations. Additional cardiovascular imaging with CMR and MDCT should be considered for symptomatic patients with suspected CAP, for the purpose of potential surgical planning, exclusion of high-risk anatomy features that may predispose to strangulation, and risk stratification. On CMR and MDCT, a key finding suggestive of CAP is displacement of the heart into the left-hemithorax (levorotation), with posterolateral displacement of the left ventricular apex.

SUMMARY

Pericardial diseases represent an important group of cardiac disorders, including common conditions, such as acute pericarditis, and less common conditions, such as constrictive pericarditis, and potentially life-threatening conditions, such as pericardial tamponade. Echocardiography remains the first-line imaging investigation for the diagnosis of most of these pericardial conditions. With advances in multimodality cardiovascular imaging, CMR and MDCT provide incremental value in the diagnosis and assessment of patients with pericardial conditions. Importantly, detection of active pericardial inflammation by CMR imaging, reflected by the presence of pericardial edema and pericardial LGE in patients with constrictive pericarditis, may have important management and treatment implications. Appropriate initiation and maintenance of anti-inflammatory therapy in select patients, may halt disease progression into the irreversible stage with the development of chronic pericardial calcification, thereby avoiding the need for pericardiectomy.

SUPPLEMENTARY DATA

Supplementary data related to this article can be found online at http://dx.doi.org/10.1016/j.ccl.2017.07.003.

REFERENCES

1. Khandaker MH, Espinosa RE, Nishimura RA, et al. Pericardial disease: diagnosis and management. Mayo Clin Proc 2010;85:572–93.
2. Imazio M, Spodick DH, Brucato A, et al. Controversial issues in the management of pericardial diseases. Circulation 2010;121:916–28.
3. Klein AL, Abbara S, Agler DA, et al. American Society of Echocardiography clinical recommendations for multimodality cardiovascular imaging of patients with pericardial disease: endorsed by the Society for Cardiovascular Magnetic Resonance and Society of Cardiovascular Computed Tomography. J Am Soc Echocardiogr 2013;26: 965–1012.e15.
4. Adler Y, Charron P, Imazio M, et al. 2015 ESC guidelines for the diagnosis and management of pericardial diseases. Eur Heart J 2015;36:2921–64.
5. Motte G. Acute pericarditis. N Engl J Med 2014;371: 2410–6.
6. Troughton RW, Asher CR, Klein AL. Pericarditis. Lancet 2004;363:717–27.
7. Imazio M, Adler Y, Charron P. Recurrent pericarditis: modern approach in 2016. Curr Cardiol Rep 2016; 18:1–8.
8. Douglas PS, Garcia MJ, Haines DE, et al. ACCF/ASE/AHA/ASNC/HFSA/HRS/SCAI/SCCM/SCCT/SCMR 2011 appropriate use criteria for echocardiography. J Am Coll Cardiol 2011;57:1126–66.
9. Salisbury AC, Olalla-Gómez C, Rihal CS, et al. Frequency and predictors of urgent coronary angiography in patients with acute pericarditis. Mayo Clin Proc 2009;84:11–5.
10. Hall WB, Truitt SG, Scheunemann LP, et al. The prevalence of clinically relevant incidental findings on chest computed tomographic angiograms ordered to diagnose pulmonary embolism. Arch Intern Med 2009;169:1961–5.
11. Oyama N, Oyama N, Komuro K, et al. Computed tomography and magnetic resonance imaging of the pericardium: anatomy and pathology. Magn Reson Med Sci 2004;3:145–52.
12. Verhaert D, Gabrie RS, Johnston D, et al. The role of multimodality imaging in the management of pericardial disease. Circ Cardiovasc Imaging 2010;3: 333–43.

13. Yared K, Baggish AL, Picard MH, et al. Multimodality imaging of pericardial diseases. JACC Cardiovasc Imaging 2010;3:650–60.

14. Gentry J, Klein AL, Jellis C. Transient constrictive pericarditis: current diagnostic and therapeutic strategies. Curr Cardiol Rep 2016;18(5):41.

15. Young PM, Glockner JF, Williamson EE, et al. MR imaging findings in 76 consecutive surgically proven cases of pericardial disease with CT and pathologic correlation. Int J Cardiovasc Imaging 2012;28:1099–109.

16. Zurick AO, Bolen MA, Kwon DH, et al. Pericardial delayed hyperenhancement with CMR imaging in patients with constrictive pericarditis undergoing surgical pericardiectomy: a case series with histopathological correlation. JACC Cardiovasc Imaging 2011;4:1180–91.

17. Taylor AM, Dymarkowski S, Verbeken EK, et al. Detection of pericardial inflammation with late-enhancement cardiac magnetic resonance imaging: initial results. Eur Radiol 2006;16:569–74.

18. Imazio M, Brucato A, Cemin R, et al. Colchicine for recurrent pericarditis (CORP) a randomized trial. Ann Intern Med 2011;155:409–14.

19. Shabetai R. Recurrent pericarditis: recent advances and remaining questions. Circulation 2005;112: 1921–3.

20. Cremer PC, Tariq MU, Karwa A, et al. Quantitative assessment of pericardial delayed hyperenhancement predicts clinical improvement in patients with constrictive pericarditis treated with anti-inflammatory therapy. Circ Cardiovasc Imaging 2015;8:1–8.

21. Bertog SC, Thambidorai SK, Parakh K, et al. Constrictive pericarditis: etiology and cause-specific survival after pericardiectomy. J Am Coll Cardiol 2004;43:1445–52.

22. Ling LH, Oh JK, Schaff HV, et al. Constrictive pericarditis in the modern era. Circulation 1999;100: 1380–6.

23. Talreja DR, Edwards WD, Danielson GK, et al. Constrictive pericarditis in 26 patients with histologically normal pericardial thickness. Circulation 2003; 108:1852–7.

24. Adler Y, Charron P. The 2015 ESC guidelines on the diagnosis and management of pericardial diseases. Eur Heart J 2015;36:2873–4.

25. Hatle LK, Appleton CP, Popp RL. Differentiation of constrictive pericarditis and restrictive cardiomyopathy by Doppler echocardiography. Circulation 1989;79:357–70.

26. Oh JK, Hatle LK, Seward JB, et al. Diagnostic role of Doppler echocardiography in constrictive pericarditis. J Am Coll Cardiol 1994;23:154–62.

27. Choi JH, Choi JO, Ryu DR, et al. Mitral and tricuspid annular velocities in constrictive pericarditis and restrictive cardiomyopathy: correlation with pericardial thickness on computed tomography. JACC Cardiovasc Imaging 2011;4:567–75.

28. Reuss CS, Wilansky SM, Lester SJ, et al. Using mitral "annulus reversus" to diagnose constrictive pericarditis. Eur J Echocardiogr 2009;10:372–5.

29. Welch TD, Ling LH, Espinosa RE, et al. Echocardiographic diagnosis of constrictive pericarditis: Mayo Clinic criteria. Circ Cardiovasc Imaging 2014;7: 526–34.

30. Sengupta PP, Krishnamoorthy VK, Abhayaratna WP, et al. Disparate patterns of left ventricular mechanics differentiate constrictive pericarditis from restrictive cardiomyopathy. JACC Cardiovasc Imaging 2008;1:29–38.

31. Kusunose K, Dahiya A, Popović ZB, et al. Biventricular mechanics in constrictive pericarditis comparison with restrictive cardiomyopathy and impact of pericardiectomy. Circ Cardiovasc Imaging 2013;6: 399–406.

32. Kamdar AR, Meadows TA, Roselli EE, et al. Multidetector computed tomographic angiography in planning of reoperative cardiothoracic surgery. Ann Thorac Surg 2008;85:1239–45.

33. Thavendiranathan P, Verhaert D, Walls MC, et al. Simultaneous right and left heart real-time, free-breathing CMR flow quantification identifies constrictive physiology. JACC Cardiovasc Imaging 2012;5:15–24.

34. Francone M, Dymarkowski S, Kalantzi M, et al. Assessment of ventricular coupling with real-time cine MRI and its value to differentiate constrictive pericarditis from restrictive cardiomyopathy. Eur Radiol 2006;16:944–51.

35. Cremer PC, Kumar A, Kontzias A, et al. Complicated pericarditis: understanding risk factors and pathophysiology to inform imaging and treatment. J Am Coll Cardiol 2016;68(21):2311–28.

36. Cremer PC, Kwon DH. Multimodality imaging of pericardial disease. Curr Cardiol Rep 2015;17:24.

37. Kumar A, Sato K, Yzeiraj E, et al. Quantitative pericardial delayed hyperenhancement informs clinical course in recurrent pericarditis. JACC Cardiovasc Imaging 2017. [Epub ahead of print].

38. Feng D, Glockner J, Kim K, et al. Cardiac magnetic resonance imaging pericardial late gadolinium enhancement and elevated inflammatory markers can predict the reversibility of constrictive pericarditis after antiinflammatory medical therapy: a pilot study. Circulation 2011;124:1830–7.

39. Haley JH, Tajik AJ, Danielson GK, et al. Transient constrictive pericarditis: causes and natural history. J Am Coll Cardiol 2004;43:271–5.

40. Imazio M, Brucato A, Maestroni S, et al. Risk of constrictive pericarditis after acute pericarditis. Circulation 2011;124:1270–5.

41. Sagristá-Sauleda J, Permanyer-Miralda G, Candell-Riera J, et al. Transient cardiac constriction: an

unrecognized pattern of evolution in effusive acute idiopathic pericarditis. Am J Cardiol 2016; 59:961–6.

42. Ha HW, Oh JK, Ling LH, et al. Annulus paradoxus transmitral flow velocity to mitral annular velocity ratio is inversely proportional to pulmonary capillary wedge pressure in patients with constrictive pericarditis. Circulation 2001;104:976–8.

43. Chang SA, Choi JY, Kim EK, et al. [18F]Fluorodeoxyglucose PET/CT predicts response to steroid therapy in constrictive pericarditis. J Am Coll Cardiol 2017;69(6):750–2.

44. Galve E, Garcia-Del-Castillo H, Evangelista A, et al. Pericardial effusion in the course of myocardial infarction: incidence, natural history, and clinical relevance. Circulation 1986;73:294–9.

45. Weitzman LB. The incidence and natural history of pericardial effusion after cardiac surgery—an echocardiographic study. Circulation 1984;69:506–11.

46. Bogaert J, Centonze M, Vanneste R. Cardiac and pericardial abnormalities on chest computed tomography: what can we see? Radiol Med 2010; 115:175–90.

47. Spodick DH. Acute cardiac tamponade. N Engl J Med 2003;349:684–90.

48. Hoit BD, Gabel M, Fowler NO. Cardiac tamponade in left ventricular dysfunction. Circulation 1990;82: 1370–6.

49. Hoit BD, Fowler NO. Influence of acute right ventricular dysfunction on cardiac tamponade. J Am Coll Cardiol 1991;18:1787–93.

50. Gillam LD, Guyer DE, Gibson TC, et al. Hydrodynamic compression of the right atrium: a new echocardiographic sign of cardiac tamponade. Circulation 1983;68:294–301.

51. Appleton CP, Hatle LK, Popp RL. Cardiac tamponade and pericardial effusion: respiratory variation in transvalvular flow velocities studied by Doppler echocardiography. J Am Coll Cardiol 1988;11: 1020–30.

52. Gatzoulis MA, Munk MD, Merchant N, et al. Isolated congenital absence of the pericardium: clinical presentation, diagnosis, and management. Ann Thorac Surg 2000;69:1209–15.

53. Xu B, Betancor J, Asher C, et al. Congenital absence of the pericardium: a systematic approach to diagnosis and management. Cardiology 2017; 136:270–8.

54. Topilsky Y, Tabatabaei N, Freeman WK, et al. Images in cardiovascular medicine. Pendulum heart in congenital absence of the pericardium. Circulation 2010;121:1272–4.

55. Connolly HM, Click RL, Schattenberg TT, et al. Congenital absence of the pericardium: echocardiography as a diagnostic tool. J Am Soc Echocardiogr 1995;8:87–92.

Acute and Recurrent Pericarditis

Massimo Imazio, MD, FESC*, Fiorenzo Gaita, MD

KEYWORDS

• Pericarditis • Diagnosis • Therapy • Prognosis

KEY POINTS

- Pericarditis may be due to infectious causes (mainly viruses and tuberculosis) and noninfectious causes (especially postcardiac injury syndromes, systemic inflammatory diseases, and cancer).
- The diagnosis of pericarditis is clinical and based on the presence of a minimal number of 2 clinical criteria (pericarditis chest pain, pericardial rubs, suggestive electrocardiographic changes, and new or worsening pericardial effusion).
- A triage of patients with pericarditis is warranted to identify high-risk cases to be admitted to hospital. High-risk features of a nonviral cause and complications especially include high fever (>38°C), subacute onset, cardiac tamponade, and large pericardial effusion.
- Empirical anti-inflammatory therapies are warranted to control chest pain and reduce the risk of recurrences especially by the use of weight-adjusted doses of colchicine.
- The prognosis is related to the underlying cause. Recurrences occur in 10% to 30% of cases after a first episode, and colchicine halves the recurrence risk. The risk of constriction is very low (<1%) in viral and idiopathic pericarditis and high for bacterial causes.

INTRODUCTION

Acute and recurrent pericarditis is the most common pericardial syndrome encountered in clinical practice. Pericarditis may occur as an isolated process or as a manifestation of a systemic disease (eg, inflammatory systemic disease).

Being at the interface of different medical and surgical specialties (eg, cardiology, internal medicine, rheumatology, cardiac surgery), pericarditis has remained the Cinderella of heart diseases for decades, and only in the last 10 to 15 years has received growing interest, first clinical trials and prospective cohort studies, and international guidelines for management.

The aim of the present review is to summarize the current knowledge on the cause, diagnosis, therapy, and prognosis of pericarditis with a focus on the last 5 to 10 years of studies that were more relevant for clinical practice.

Cause

The incidence of acute pericarditis has been reported as 27.7 cases per 100,000 person-years in an Italian urban area (North Italy), with concomitant myocarditis in about 15% of cases.[1] Pericarditis is responsible for 0.1% of all hospital admissions and 5% of emergency room admissions for chest pain.[2]

The cause of acute and recurrent pericarditis varies, and causes are essentially divided into infectious and noninfectious causes (**Box 1**).[3–7] Worldwide, the most common cause of acute pericarditis is tuberculosis, because of its high frequency in developing countries, where tuberculosis is endemic and often associated with human immunodeficiency virus infection.[8,9] In developed countries with a low prevalence of tuberculosis (eg, Western Europe and North America), viral agents are presumed to be the causative

---

Disclosure Statement: None.

Department of Medical Sciences, University Cardiology, AOU Città della Salute e della Scienza di Torino, Corso Bramante 88/90, Torino 10126, Italy

* Corresponding author.

E-mail addresses: massimo.imazio@unito.it; massimo.imazio@yahoo.it

Cardiol Clin 35 (2017) 505–513
http://dx.doi.org/10.1016/j.ccl.2017.07.004
0733-8651/17/© 2017 Elsevier Inc. All rights reserved.

cardiology.theclinics.com

Box 1
Main causes of acute and recurrent pericarditis

Infectious causes:

Viral (common): Enteroviruses (coxsackieviruses, echoviruses), herpesviruses (EBV, CMV, HHV-6), adenoviruses, parvovirus B19 (possible overlap with etiologic viral agents of myocarditis)

Bacterial: Mycobacterium tuberculosis (common, other bacterial rare), *Coxiella burnetii, Borrelia burgdorferi,* rarely: *Pneumococcus* spp, *Meningococcus* spp, *Gonococcus* spp, *Streptococcus* spp, *Staphylococcus* spp, *Haemophilus* spp, *Chlamydia* spp, *Mycoplasma* spp, *Legionella* spp, *Leptospira* spp, *Listeria* spp, *Providencia stuartii*

Fungal (very rare): *Histoplasma* spp (more likely in immunocompetent patients), *Aspergillus* spp, *Blastomyces* spp, *Candida* spp (more likely in immunocompromised host)

Parasitic (very rare): *Echinococcus* spp, *Toxoplasma* spp

Noninfectious causes:

Autoimmune and autoinflammatory (common):

> *Systemic autoimmune diseases* (especially systemic lupus erythematosus, Sjögren syndrome, rheumatoid arthritis, scleroderma);

> *Systemic vasculitides* (eg,eosinophilic granulomatosis with polyangiitis or allergic granulomatosis, previously named Churg-Strauss syndrome, Horton disease, Takayasu disease, Behçet syndrome):

> *Other systemic inflammatory diseases* (eg, sarcoidosis, inflammatory bowel diseases);

> *Autoinflammatory diseases* (Familial Mediterranean fever, tumor necrosis factor [TNF] receptor TRAPS)

Neoplastic:

> Primary tumors (rare, above all pericardial mesothelioma)

> Secondary metastatic tumors (common, above all lung and breast cancer, lymphoma)

Metabolic:

> Uremia

Traumatic and iatrogenic:

> Early onset (rare):

>> *Direct injury* (penetrating thoracic injury, esophageal perforation)

>> *Indirect injury* (nonpenetrating thoracic injury, radiation injury)

> Delayed onset:

>> *Pericardial injury syndromes (common)* postmyocardial infarction syndrome, postpericardiotomy syndrome, posttraumatic, including forms after iatrogenic trauma (eg, coronary percutaneous intervention, pacemaker lead insertion, and radiofrequency ablation)

Drug-related (rare):

- Lupuslike syndrome (procainamide, hydralazine, methyldopa, isoniazid, phenytoin);
- Antineoplastic drugs (often associated with a cardiomyopathy, may cause a pericardiopathy): doxorubicin and daunorubicin, cytosine arabinoside, 5-fluorouracil, cyclophosphamide;
- Hypersensitivity pericarditis with eosinophilia: penicillins, amiodarone, methysergide, mesalazine, clozapine, minoxidil, dantrolene, practolol, phenylbutazone, thiazides, streptomycin, thiouracils, streptokinase, p-aminosalicylic acid, sulfa-drugs, cyclosporine, bromocriptine, several vaccines, granulocyte-macrophage colony-stimulating factor, anti-TNF agents

Related to management issues (for recurrences, common):

- Inappropriate dosing and/or tapering of anti-inflammatory medical therapy
- Lack of exercise restriction during the acute phase

A simple classification is to divide into infectious and noninfectious causes.
Abbreviations: HHV, human herpes virus; spp, species; TRAPS, TNF receptor associated periodic syndrome.

agent in most cases. However, definitive evidence is lacking because currently available diagnostic methods do not allow a certainty diagnosis without an invasive assessment of pericardial fluid and/or tissue (which is not warranted in most cases that are relatively benign and self-limited).[3,7] Most cases are usually preceded by or concomitant with a flulike syndrome or gastroenteritis. The most common viral agents, which may be also responsible for myocarditis, include enteroviruses (especially coxsackie viruses), herpes viruses (especially Epstein-Barr virus [EBV] and reactivation of cytomegalovirus [CMV]), parvovirus, and only in a minority of cases, influenza viruses, hepatitis C virus, and hepatitis B virus. In children, either enteroviruses or adenoviruses or herpes viruses are implicated.[3,7]

Nevertheless, in clinical practice, most cases remain "idiopathic" with a conventional diagnostic approach and account for 55% to 85% of cases according to the setting (hospitalized vs nonhospitalized).[3,7,8,10,11] In published series, the main etiologic diagnoses were tuberculosis pericarditis (4%–70%), autoimmune or postcardiac injury syndromes (2%–21%), neoplastic pericarditis (5%–10%), and purulent pericarditis (up to 3%) (Table 1).[3,7,8,10,11]

On this basis, current guidelines on the management of pericardial diseases[7] issued in 2015 by the European Society of Cardiology (ESC) suggest an epidemiologic approach to the etiologic diagnosis based on clinical presentation and aimed at the identification of the most important and common causes of pericarditis (tuberculosis, postcardiac injury syndromes, cancer, autoimmune diseases, and purulent forms).

Clinical Presentation and Diagnosis

The most common symptom is pericarditic chest pain, present in greater than 85% of cases.[1,10] It is increased by inspiration, and it has positional features: worsening when the patient is supine and improving when sitting and leaning forward. It may radiate to the shoulders, arms, and jaw and may simulate "ischemic chest pain." Pericardial rubs due to increased attrition between the inflamed pericardial layers is reported in one-third of cases, whereas a pericardial effusion, usually mild, is reported in about 60% of cases. Electrocardiogram (ECG) changes are traditionally considered a hallmark of pericarditis when PR depression and/or widespread ST segment elevation is reported. Such changes are especially reported with concomitant myocarditis and are related to subepicardial involvement rather than "pure" pericarditis.[1,10] The classical evolution of the ECG is in 4 stages: stage I (PR depression and ST segment elevation), stage II (ST normalization), stage III (T-wave inversion after ST segment normalization), and stage IV (ST-T normalization) (Fig. 1). However, this typical evolution is reported in no more than 60% of cases and is affected by the observation time (late or chronic cases may show only T-wave abnormalities) and therapy (prompt and efficacious anti-inflammatory therapy may lead to early normalization of the ECG without all stages).[3] Although ECG changes from acute

Table 1
Causes of acute pericarditis in major published series from the late 1970s to 2012

	Permanyer-Miralda (Spain)	Zayas (Spain)	Imazio (Italy)	Reuter[a] (South Africa)	Gouriet[b] (France)
Patients (n)	231	100	453	233	933
Years	1977–1983	1991–1993	1996–2004	1995–2001	2007–2012
Geographic area	Western Europe	Western Europe	Western Europe	Africa	Western Europe
Idiopathic	199 (86.0%)	78 (78.0%)	377 (83.2%)	32 (13.7%)	516 (55.0%)
Specific cause	32 (14.0%)	22 (22.0%)	76 (16.8%)	201 (86.3%)	417 (46.0%)
Neoplastic	13 (5.6%)	7 (7.0%)	23 (5.1%)	22 (9.4%)	85 (8.9%)
Tuberculosis	9 (3.9%)	4 (4.0%)	17 (3.8%)	161 (69.5%)	4 (<1%)
Autoimmune	4 (1.7%)	3 (3.0%)	33 (7.3%)	12 (5.2%)	197 (21%)
Purulent	2 (0.9%)	1 (1.0%)	3 (0.7%)	5 (2.1%)	29 (3.0%)

[a] Based on pericardial effusions.
[b] In the French study, all hospitalized patients in a tertiary referral center for cardiology and infectious diseases from Emergency Department, Cardiology, and Cardiac Surgery were included: thus, this is a selected view of hospitalized patients with a possible overrepresentation of specific causes (infections and postcardiac injury syndromes).
From Imazio M. Myopericardial diseases. Springer; 2016.

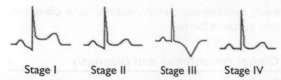

Fig. 1. Classic 4 stages of ECG evolution in acute pericarditis. (*From* Imazio M. Myopericardial diseases. Springer; 2016; with permission.)

pericarditis are characteristic and can be usually distinguished from acute myocardial infarction, a substantial portion of the patients with acute pericarditis undergo an emergent coronary angiography as ST segment elevation myocardial infarction.[12]

The clinical diagnosis of acute pericarditis is based on the following clinical criteria: (1) pericarditic chest pain, (2) pericardial rubs, (3) suggestive ECG changes (eg, widespread ST segment elevation and/or PR depression or ST-T waves abnormalities without alternative explanation, see ECG evolution in pericarditis [see **Fig. 1**]), and (4) new or worsening pericardial effusion.[7] A clinical diagnosis can be reached when 2 of 4 criteria are satisfied (**Table 2**).

Specific features at presentation have been associated with an increased risk of complications during follow-up and possible specific etiologic diagnoses (nonviral and nonidiopathic). Such features are labeled as poor prognostic predictors (**Box 2**), and these red flags should alert the clinicians to admit the patients and perform an etiologic search aimed at the identification of specific causes (eg, tuberculosis, systemic inflammatory diseases, cancer) that may warrant a targeted therapy beyond empiric anti-inflammatory therapy.[13] Their identification at presentation of a patient with pericarditis allows triage of low-risk cases (benign prognosis with good response to empiric anti-inflammatory

therapy in most cases) versus high-risk cases requiring hospital admission and cause search (**Figs. 2–4**).[7,13]

Currently, objective documentation of a viral cause is no longer recommended because the definitive demonstration of a viral cause of pericarditis would require pericardial fluid or tissue evaluation. The invasive assessment is thought not to be justified considering the relatively benign prognosis of these cases and that therapy is unaffected by the findings; there is no evidence that a specific viral therapy (if available, because often no viral therapies can be offered for some viruses) is required in an immunocompetent patient with a low-risk pericarditis.[7] The cause search should be guided by the clinical

---

Box 2
Red flags in a patient with pericarditis (features that are associated with an increased risk of complications during follow-up and a specific cause that may warrant a specific therapy beyond empiric anti-inflammatory therapy)

Major

Fever greater than 38°C

Subacute onset

Large pericardial effusion (>20 mm on echocardiography)

Cardiac tamponade

Lack of response to aspirin or NSAID after at least 1 week of therapy

Minor

Pericarditis associated with myocarditis

Immunosuppression

Trauma

Oral anticoagulant therapy

Table 2
Diagnostic criteria for acute pericarditis

Pericarditis	Definition and Diagnostic Criteria
Acute	Inflammatory pericardial syndrome to be diagnosed with at least 2 of the 4 following criteria: 1. Pericarditic chest pain 2. Pericardial rubs 3. New widespread ST elevation or PR depression on ECG 4. Pericardial effusion (new or worsening) Additional supporting findings: • Elevation of markers of inflammation (ie, CRP, ESR, and white blood cell count); • Evidence of pericardial inflammation by an imaging technique (computed tomography, cardiac magnetic resonance)

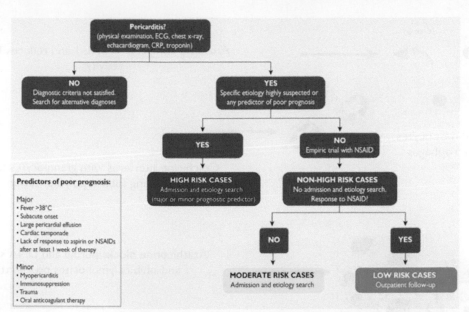

Fig. 2. Proposed triage of pericarditis according to published evidence and 2015 ESC guidelines. A large pericardial effusion is defined as an effusion with the largest telediastolic echo-free space of greater than 20 mm on echocardiography. Proposed triage of acute pericarditis according to epidemiologic background and predictors of poor prognosis at presentation (modified from Refs.[5,6,8,12]). At least one predictor of poor prognosis is sufficient to identify a high risk case. Major criteria have been validated by multivariate analysis.[9] Minor criteria are based on expert opinion and literature review. Cases with moderate risk are defined as cases without negative prognostic predictors but incomplete or lacking response to NSAID therapy. Low-risk cases include those without negative prognostic predictors and good response to anti-inflammatory therapy. Specific cause is intended as nonidiopathic cause. (*From* 2015 ESC guidelines; with permission.)

presentation and offered to high-risk cases or low-risk cases not responding to the empiric anti-inflammatory therapy within a short follow-up of 7 to 10 days.[3,7,10,13] A probabilistic approach is warranted especially excluding most common causes (eg, tuberculosis, systemic inflammatory diseases, cancer, purulent pericarditis).[3,5,7]

First level tx: Aspirin or NSAID plus colchicine

↓

Second level tx: Corticosteroids plus colchicine

↓

Third level tx: Aspirin/NSAID plus colchicine and Corticosteroids (Triple therapy)

↓

Fourth level tx: Use of alternative drugs (eg, azathioprine or IVIG or anakinra)

↓

Fifth level tx: Pericardiectomy

Fig. 3. Algorithm for medical therapy for recurrent pericarditis. tx, treatment. (*From* Imazio M. Myopericardial diseases. Springer; 2016; with permission.)

Recurrent pericarditis

In 20% to 30% of cases, pericarditis can relapse; the risk appears in patients not treated with colchicine. Recurrent pericarditis is diagnosed as acute pericarditis. Recurrent pericarditic chest pain is the most common manifestation and should be associated with at least one objective piece of evidence of disease activity (eg, pericardial rubs, new ECG changes, new or worsening pericardial effusion, and elevation of markers of inflammation). For difficult cases, the diagnosis of pericarditis can be supported by elevation of markers of inflammation (for example, C-reactive protein [CRP] or erythrocyte sedimentation rate [ESR]) or evidence of pericardial inflammation by a second-level imaging technique (eg, computerized tomography and especially cardiac magnetic resonance).

A true recurrence can occur only after a symptom-free interval of 4 to 6 weeks according to 2015 ESC guidelines[7] in order to allow the completion of anti-inflammatory therapy and its tapering for a previous episode of pericarditis (**Table 3**). According to expert opinion, "chronic pericarditis" is defined as pericarditis lasting for greater than 3 months. In clinical practice, chronic forms are represented by incessant or recurrent

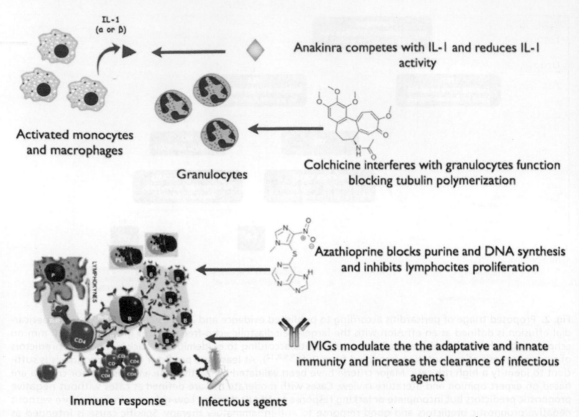

Fig. 4. Emerging options for the therapy for recurrent pericarditis with their mechanism of action. IL-1, interleukin-1. (*From* Imazio M. Myopericardial diseases. Springer; 2016; with permission.)

pericarditis cases lasting greater than 3 months, and the management of such forms follows that of incessant/recurrent pericarditis.

Therapy

Specific therapies are warranted if a specific cause is identified (eg, antibiotic therapy for tuberculous pericarditis) and are beyond the purposes of the present review. The first-line therapy for pericarditis is anti-inflammatory therapy to reduce symptoms and reduce the recurrence risk because recurrences are the most common complication of pericarditis.

A randomized controlled trial on postcardiac surgery patients with postpericardiotomy syndrome has demonstrated that anti-inflammatory therapy (ibuprofen or indomethacin) is significantly better than placebo at reducing the risk of recurrences by half during follow-up and improving the remission rate.[14] Nevertheless, exercise restriction is an important component of therapy after clinical remission for nonathletes[7] and up to 3 months for athletes according to expert consensus.[7,15,16]

The first-line therapy for patients with acute and recurrent pericarditis is nonsteroidal anti-inflammatory drugs (NSAID) at full anti-

	Definition
Incessant	Pericarditis lasting for >4–6 wk but <3 mo[a] without remission
Recurrent	Recurrence of pericarditis after a documented first episode of acute pericarditis and a symptom-free interval of 4–6 wk or longer[b]
Chronic	Pericarditis lasting for >3 mo[a]

Table 3
Definitions of recurrent, incessant, and chronic pericarditis

[a] Arbitrary term defined by experts.
[b] Usually recurrences occur within 18 to 24 mo for the index attack.
Modified from Imazio M. Myopericardial diseases. Springer; 2016.

Table 4
Empiric anti-inflammatory therapy for acute and recurrent pericarditis

Drug	Usual Dosing	Duration	Tapering[a]
Aspirin	750–1000 mg every 8 h	1–2 wk	Decrease doses every week: for example, 750 mg TID for 1 wk, then 500 mg TID for 1 wk, then stop
Ibuprofen	600 mg every 8 h	1–2 wk	Decrease doses every week: for example, 600 mg plus 400 mg plus 600 mg for 1 wk, then 600 mg plus 400 mg plus 400 mg for 1 wk, then 400 mg TID for 1 wk then stop
Colchicine	0.5 mg once (<70 kg) or 0.5 mg BID (≥70 kg)	3 mo (acute) 6 mo (recurrent)	Not mandatory, alternatively 0.5 mg every other day (<70 kg) or 0.5 mg once (≥70 kg) in the last weeks

Therapy duration is individualized when guided by symptoms and CRP normalization: the attack dose is maintained until symptoms resolution and CRP normalization.

[a] Tapering is proposed (class IIa recommendation, level of evidence B).

Modified from Imazio M. Myopericardial diseases. Springer; 2016.

inflammatory doses plus colchicine, which has been shown to halve the subsequent recurrence rate when used also in the first episode of acute pericarditis (**Table 4**).[17–21] The duration of anti-inflammatory therapy is guided by symptoms and inflammatory markers (eg, CRP) for normalization.[22]

If NSAID and colchicine are not sufficient, or for specific indications (eg, pregnancy, renal failure, specific systemic inflammatory diseases on corticosteroids, possible interference of NSAID with oral anticoagulants), corticosteroids can be used as a second-line option at low to moderate doses (eg, prednisone 0.2–0.5 mg/kg/d) with slow tapering (eg, reduce the dose by 2.5 mg every 2 weeks) only after remission and CRP normalization (**Table 5**; Ref.[23]).

For recurrent cases, symptoms control can be achieved by combining multiple drugs (an NSAID plus colchicine plus low-dose corticosteroids). If the patients have recurrences despite the outlined therapy, alternative therapies are possible (eg, azathioprine, intravenous immunoglobulins, and biological agents, especially anakinra) but are based on less solid evidence (case reports, case series, small randomized controlled trials) (**Table 6**; Refs.[24–29]).

As a last option for refractory cases, pericardiectomy should be considered in tertiary centers with specific expertise in this surgery.[30] Compared with continuing medical therapy, patients who had pericardiectomy were found to have markedly lower relapses at longer than 5-year follow-up. In addition, medical therapy, including steroid, could

Table 5
Suggested tapering of prednisone in pericardial inflammatory syndrome

Prednisone dose[a]	Starting Dose 0.25–0.50 mg/kg/d[a]	Tapering[b]
Prednisone daily dose	>50 mg	10 mg/d every 1–2 wk
	50–25 mg	5–10 mg/d every 1–2 wk
	25–15 mg	2.5 mg/d every 2–4 wk
	<15 mg	1.25–2.5 mg/d every 2–6 wk

Calcium intake (supplement plus oral intake) 1200 to 1500 mg/d and vitamin D supplementation 800 to 1000 IU/d should be offered to all patients receiving glucocorticoids. In case of recurrent symptoms during tapering, do not increase corticosteroids doses but keep the maintenance dose for a longer time, trying to control symptoms by NSAID and colchicine, and then consider slower tapering as needed.

[a] Avoid higher doses except for special cases, and only for a few days, with rapid tapering to 25 mg/d. Prednisone 25 mg is equivalent to methylprednisolone 20 mg.

[b] Every decrease in prednisone dose should be done only if the patient is asymptomatic and CRP is normal, particularly for doses less than 25 mg/d.

Modified from Imazio M. Myopericardial diseases. Springer; 2016.

Table 6
Azathioprine, intravenous immunoglobulin, and anakinra dosing

Drug	Dosing
Azathioprine	Starting with 1 mg/kg/d, then gradually increased to 2–3 mg/kg/d for several months
Intravenous immunoglobulin	400–500 mg IV daily for 5 d
Anakinra	1–2 mg/kg/d up to 100 mg/d in adults for several months

be tapered or reduced more significantly after pericardiectomy.

Prognosis

The most common complication of pericarditis is recurrence, which may occur in 20% to 30% of cases after a first episode of acute pericarditis, and up to 50% of cases in patients after a first recurrence according to historical series before colchicine therapy.[17–21]

Currently, the adjunct of colchicine to anti-inflammatory therapy may halve this recurrence rate. Despite several recurrences, the prognosis is good for "idiopathic" cases because no evolution toward constrictive pericarditis has been reported.[31]

The risk of complications is related to the cause and not to the number of recurrences.[32] The most feared complication is constrictive pericarditis. In Western Europe, the risk of constrictive pericarditis is high for bacterial causes (20%–30% for tuberculous and purulent pericarditis), intermediate for systemic inflammatory diseases and cancer (2%–5%), and low for viral and idiopathic pericarditis (<1%).[32]

An Emerging Form of Pericarditis: Postcardiac Injury Syndromes

An emerging form of pericarditis is represented by postcardiac injury syndromes that have been reported in up to 25% of more recent series of hospitalized cases.[11] Pericarditis resulting from injury to the pericardium constitutes postcardiac injury syndrome, a designation comprising postmyocardial infarction pericarditis (Dressler syndrome), the postpericardiotomy syndrome, and posttraumatic pericarditis.[33] These different clinical scenarios share an inciting cardiac injury involving the pericardium and/or pleura and a subsequent pleuro-pericardial syndrome characterized by pericarditis (with or without pericardial effusion) and pleural effusion with or without pulmonary infiltrates.

The therapy for postcardiac injury syndrome is based on empiric anti-inflammatory drugs and adjunctive use of colchicine, which may be useful

for the prevention of recurrences.[33] Corticosteroids may be helpful for those patients on oral anticoagulant therapies to avoid interference with NSAIDs.[3] The risk of constriction for such cases is intermediate (2%–5%) as for neoplastic and autoimmune diseases.[32]

SUMMARY

Current knowledge and management of acute and recurrent pericarditis have improved over the last few years thanks to randomized controlled trials, prospective cohort studies, and new updated guidelines. Nevertheless, many issues are still to be solved: (1) How is it possible to refine the etiologic classification beyond "idiopathic pericarditis," and what is it really? (2) What are the mechanisms underlying incessant and recurrent pericarditis? (3) Are there new therapeutic options for corticosteroid-dependent and colchicine-resistant cases? (4) What is the role of pericardiectomy for refractory recurrent pericarditis?

Ongoing research will probably help in the near future to provide replies to the questions, but in the meantime, pericardial diseases are no longer neglected and are on the road to evidence-based medicine.

REFERENCES

1. Imazio M, Cecchi E, Demichelis B, et al. Myopericarditis versus viral or idiopathic acute pericarditis. Heart 2008;94:498–501.
2. Kytö V, Sipilä J, Rautava P. Clinical profile and influences on outcomes in patients hospitalized for acute pericarditis. Circulation 2014;130:1601–6.
3. Imazio M. Myopericardial diseases. Springer; 2016.
4. Imazio M. Contemporary management of pericardial diseases. Curr Opin Cardiol 2012;27:308–17.
5. Imazio M, Gaita F. Diagnosis and treatment of pericardis. Heart 2015;101(14):1159–68.
6. Imazio M, Spodick DH, Brucato A, et al. Controversial issues in the management of pericardial diseases. Circulation 2010;121:916–28.
7. Authors/Task Force Members, Adler Y, Charron P, Imazio M, et al. 2015 ESC guidelines for the

diagnosis and management of pericardial diseases: the Task Force for the diagnosis and management of pericardial diseases of the European Society of Cardiology (ESC) endorsed by: the European Association for Cardio-Thoracic Surgery (EACTS). Eur Heart J 2015;36:2921–64.

8. Mayosi BM. Contemporary trends in the epidemiology and management of cardiomyopathy and pericarditis in sub-Saharan Africa. Heart 2007;93: 1176–83.

9. Sliwa K, Mocumbi AO. Forgotten cardiovascular diseases in Africa. Clin Res Cardiol 2010;99:65–74.

10. Imazio M, Demichelis B, Parrini I, et al. Day-hospital treatment of acute pericarditis: a management program for outpatient therapy. J Am Coll Cardiol 2004;43:1042–6.

11. Gouriet F, Levy PY, Casalta JP, et al. Etiology of pericarditis in a prospective cohort of 1162 cases. Am J Med 2015;128(7):784.e1-8.

12. Salisbury AC, Olalla-Gomez C, Rihal CS, et al. Frequency and predictors of urgent coronary angiography in patients with acute pericarditis. Mayo Clin Proc 2009;84(1):11–5.

13. Imazio M, Cecchi E, Demichelis B, et al. Indicators of poor prognosis of acute pericarditis. Circulation 2007;115:2739–44.

14. Horneffer PJ, Miller RH, Pearson TA, et al. The effective treatment of postpericardiotomy syndrome after cardiac operations. A randomized placebo-controlled trial. J Thorac Cardiovasc Surg 1990; 100:292–6.

15. Seidenberg PH, Haynes J. Pericarditis: diagnosis, management, and return to play. Curr Sports Med Rep 2006;5:74–9.

16. Pelliccia A, Corrado D, Bjørnstad HH, et al. Recommendations for participation in competitive sport and leisure-time physical activity in individuals with cardiomyopathies, myocarditis and pericarditis. Eur J Cardiovasc Prev Rehabil 2006;13: 876–85.

17. Imazio M, Bobbio M, Cecchi E, et al. Colchicine in addition to conventional therapy for acute pericarditis: results of the COlchicine for acute PEricarditis (COPE) trial. Circulation 2005;112:2012–6.

18. Imazio M, Brucato A, Cemin R, et al. ICAP Investigators. A randomized trial of colchicine for acute pericarditis. N Engl J Med 2013;369:1522–8.

19. Imazio M, Bobbio M, Cecchi E, et al. Colchicine as first-choice therapy for recurrent pericarditis: results of the CORE (COlchicine for REcurrent pericarditis) trial. Arch Intern Med 2005;165: 1987–91.

20. Imazio M, Brucato A, Cemin R, et al. CORP (COlchicine for Recurrent Pericarditis) Investigators. Colchicine for recurrent pericarditis (CORP): a randomized trial. Ann Intern Med 2011;155:409–14.

21. Imazio M, Belli R, Brucato A, et al. Efficacy and safety of colchicine for treatment of multiple recurrences of pericarditis (CORP-2): a multicentre, double-blind, placebo-controlled, randomised trial. Lancet 2014;383(9936):2232–7.

22. Imazio M, Brucato A, Maestroni S, et al. Prevalence of C-reactive protein elevation and time course of normalization in acute pericarditis: implications for the diagnosis, therapy, and prognosis of pericarditis. Circulation 2011;123:1092–7.

23. Imazio M, Brucato A, Cumetti D, et al. Corticosteroids for recurrent pericarditis: high versus low doses: a nonrandomized observation. Circulation 2008;118:667–71.

24. Imazio M, Lazaros G, Brucato A, et al. Recurrent pericarditis: new and emerging therapeutic options. Nat Rev Cardiol 2016;13:99–105.

25. Vianello F, Cinetto F, Cavraro M, et al. Azathioprine in isolated recurrent pericarditis: a single centre experience. Int J Cardiol 2011;147:477–8.

26. Imazio M, Lazaros G, Brucato A, et al. Intravenous human immunoglobulin for refractory recurrent pericarditis. A systematic review of all published cases. J Cardiovasc Med (Hagerstown) 2016;17:263–9.

27. Lazaros G, Vasileiou P, Koutsianas C, et al. Anakinra for the management of resistant idiopathic recurrent pericarditis. Initial experience in 10 adult cases. Ann Rheum Dis 2014;73(12):2215–7.

28. Lazaros G, Imazio M, Brucato A, et al. Anakinra: an emerging option for refractory idiopathic recurrent pericarditis. A systematic review of published evidence. J Cardiovasc Med (Hagerstown) 2016;17: 256–62.

29. Brucato A, Imazio M, Gattorno M, et al. Effect of anakinra on recurrent pericarditis among patients with colchicine resistance and corticosteroid dependence: the AIRTRIP randomized clinical trial. JAMA 2016;316:1906–12.

30. Khandaker MH, Schaff HV, Greason KL, et al. Pericardiectomy vs medical management in patients with relapsing pericarditis. Mayo Clin Proc 2012; 87:1062–70.

31. Imazio M, Brucato A, Adler Y, et al. Prognosis of idiopathic recurrent pericarditis as determined from previously published reports. Am J Cardiol 2007;100: 1026–8.

32. Imazio M, Brucato A, Maestroni S, et al. Risk of constrictive pericarditis after acute pericarditis. Circulation 2011;124:1270–5.

33. Imazio M, Hoit BD. Post-cardiac injury syndromes. An emerging cause of pericardial diseases. Int J Cardiol 2013;168(2):648–52.

Pericardial Effusion

Amir Azarbal, MD, Martin M. LeWinter, MD*

KEYWORDS

• Pericardial effusion • Pericarditis • Cardiac tamponade • Echocardiography • Pericardiocentesis

KEY POINTS

- The normal pericardial sac contains up to 50 mL of a plasma ultrafiltrate. Anything greater constitutes a pathologic effusion.
- The hemodynamic consequences of a pericardial effusion depend on the pressure-volume properties of the pericardial sac.
- As little as 150 mL to 200 mL of rapidly accumulating effusion can cause tamponade, whereas much larger amounts of slowly accumulating fluid are well tolerated.
- Almost any disease that affects the pericardium can cause an effusion.
- Pericardial effusions that are most likely to cause cardiac tamponade include those due to hemorrhage, malignancies, and bacterial infections.

INTRODUCTION: PHYSIOLOGY OF THE PERICARDIUM IN RELATION TO PERICARDIAL EFFUSION

The pericardial sac space is contained between the visceral and parietal layers (see Brian D. Hoit's article, "Anatomy and Physiology of the Pericardium," in this issue) and normally contains up to 50 mL of serous fluid. Accumulation of additional fluid constitutes a pathologic pericardial effusion. The pressure-volume relation (PVR) of the pericardial sac determines the hemodynamic effects of a pericardial effusion. Normally, the PVR is flat (reflecting the high compliance of the pericardium) until the total pericardial volume approximates that of the upper limit of normal pericardial reserve volume, which occurs at a total cardiac volume corresponding to about the upper limit of normal filling. At this point, pericardial compliance decreases and the PVR abruptly becomes steep. The implication of these features is that modest amounts of fluid are well tolerated, but there is little reserve to accommodate additional volume. Thus, once the total volume within the pericardial sac reaches the point at which the

PVR becomes steep, small additional increments in volume result in large increases in intrapericardial pressure with resulting cardiac tamponade (**Fig. 1**). Large but gradual increases in cardiac volume due to chamber dilatation are associated with a rightward shift and flattening of the pericardial PVR. The same phenomenon presumably occurs with a gradually accumulating pericardial effusion. This accounts for the fact that as little as 150 to 200 mL of rapidly accumulating pericardial effusion can cause life-threatening cardiac tamponade whereas large amounts of very slowly accumulating fluid are well tolerated.[1,2]

ETIOLOGY OF PERICARDIAL EFFUSION

Any disease that can cause pericarditis, indeed virtually any disease that can involve the pericardium, can cause an effusion (**Box 1**). Thus, idiopathic pericarditis and numerous infections, neoplasms, autoimmune diseases, radiation, post-ST segment elevation myocardial infarction (STEMI) pericarditis, and noxious substances, for example, blood, may be responsible.[3,4] Acute idiopathic pericarditis is common and usually

Disclosures: None.
Cardiology Unit, The University of Vermont Medical Center, The University of Vermont, 111 Colchester Avenue, Burlington, VT 05401, USA
* Corresponding author.
E-mail address: Martin.lewinter@uvmhealth.org

Cardiol Clin 35 (2017) 515–524
http://dx.doi.org/10.1016/j.ccl.2017.07.005
0733-8651/17/© 2017 Elsevier Inc. All rights reserved.

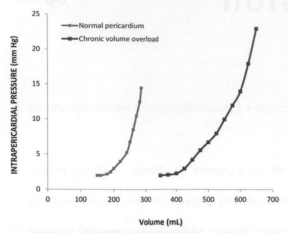

Fig. 1. PVR of the pericardial sac. (*Left*) normal; (*right*) after chronic cardiac dilatation. See text for discussion.

presumed to have a viral etiology. Associated small effusions are not uncommon, but large effusions are less frequent. Some reports have suggested that as many as 20% of pericardial effusions without an obvious cause after routine evaluation constitute the initial manifestation of a cancer.[5] Other, less common causes of pericardial effusion include the early postoperative period after routine cardiac surgery, severe circulatory congestion, and procedural complications of percutaneous cardiac procedures.[6] Finally, a small number of large, chronic, asymptomatic effusions are identified by chance, for example, when chest radiography obtained for an unrelated problem reveals an enlarged cardiac silhouette.

The main clinical significance of pericardial effusion of course is progression to cardiac tamponade and circulatory collapse. The risk of tamponade is highest in patients with bacterial, fungal and HIV-associated infections, neoplastic involvement, and hemorrhagic effusions.[1,7,8]

Following is a more detailed discussion of pericardial effusion in relation to specific etiologic categories.

Idiopathic Pericarditis

The term, *idiopathic*, is used to denote an effusion occurring in association with acute pericarditis for which no specific cause can be found with routine diagnostic testing. As previously, most idiopathic cases are presumed to be viral, but delineation of a specific viral cause is rarely undertaken because of the associated cost and lack of impact on management. Small effusions are common in these cases. Although large effusions are less frequently encountered (less than 1% of idiopathic pericardial effusions in 1

Box 1
Selected causes of pericardial effusion

Idiopathic

Infectious

  Viral (echovirus, coxsackievirus, adenovirus, HIV/AIDS, and so forth)

  Bacterial (*Pneumococcus, Staphylococcus, Streptococcus*, and so forth)

  Fungal (histoplasmosis and coccidiomycosis)

  Protozoal (*Echinococcus* and *Toxoplasma*)

Inflammatory

  Connective tissue disease (systemic lupus erythematosus, rheumatoid arthritis, or scleroderma)

  Vasculitis (polyarteritis nodosa, temporal arteritis, or Churg-Strauss disease)

  Drug induced (procainamide, hydralazine, or isoniazid)

  Postcardiotomy/thoracotomy

  Miscellaneous (sarcoidosis, familial Mediterranean fever, or inflammatory bowel disease)

Postmyocardial infarction

  Early

  Late (Dressler syndrome)

Hemopericardium

  Trauma

  Post–myocardial infarction complications (free wall rupture)

  Dissecting aortic aneurysm

  Iatrogenic (endomyocardial biopsy, post–percutaneous coronary intervention/pacemaker or automated implantable cardioverter-defibrillator placement/ablation/valve repair or replacement/atrial septal defect or ventricular septal defect closure)

  Anticoagulants

Malignancy

Miscellaneous

  Radiation therapy

  Chronic renal failure

  Chylopericardium

  Stress-induced cardiomyopathy

  Hyperthyroidism or hypothyrodisim

---

series),[9] because acute idiopathic pericarditis is such a common form of pericardial disease, the absolute number of patients with large effusions is not trivial. As discussed previously, up to

20% of significant effusions occurring in the setting of a first episode of acute pericarditis ultimately turn out to have a neoplastic etiology on further investigation.[3,10]

Infections

The infections category includes viral, bacterial, mycobacterial, and HIV-associated infections and fungal and protozoal disease. Patients with bacterial effusions are generally critically ill with infection evident elsewhere, for example, pneumonia and/or sepsis. Other components of their illness often dominate the clinical picture; as a result, pericardial effusion and tamponade can be missed.[10]

Postmyocardial Infarction

Small effusions can occur as a result of transient, localized bleeding and inflammation associated with early post-STEMI pericarditis, typically occurring 2 days to 4 days after onset of symptoms. Over a similar time frame, STEMI can also cause larger effusions due to rupture of the left ventricular free wall. Effusions may also occur due to a delayed post-STEMI inflammatory response, also known as Dressler syndrome, which occurs from 1 week to as long as 2 months after the index event. The incidence of all these post-STEMI pericardial effusions has been markedly reduced since the advent of early revascularization for STEMI.[11,12]

Malignancy

Rarely, effusions can occur with primary cardiac malignancies but much more commonly they are due to metastatic tumors, often lung and breast carcinoma, as well as melanoma, Hodgkin disease, and various other lymphomas. It is not unusual for metastatic involvement of the pericardium to present as effusive-constrictive pericarditis, in which features of both effusion and constriction coexist. Rarely, lymphomas can cause an effusion due to interference with lymphatic drainage of the pericardial sac.

Radiation

Radiation can cause both pericardial inflammation and pericardial effusion. Typically, radiation pericarditis occurs weeks to a few months after exposure and improves spontaneously or with anti-inflammatory treatment. Constrictive pericarditis is a much later complication, usually without an effusion.

Cardiac Surgery

Pericardial effusions are common early after any cardiac surgery as well as orthotropic heart transplantation. These generally resolve spontaneously. Postpericardiotomy syndrome, an immune-mediated pericarditis syndrome analogous to Dressler syndrome, occurs within weeks to a few months after surgery. This syndrome typically includes fever, pericarditis, and pleuritis with the chest radiograph often showing bilateral pleural effusions. The incidence has been reported to be between 10% and 40% after cardiac surgery.[11] A small to moderate pericardial effusion is common in postpericardiotomy syndrome and usually resolves spontaneously. Rare complications occurring in less than 1% of patients include cardiac tamponade and constrictive pericarditis.

Hemopericardium

Due to their proliferation, procedural complications of percutaneous cardiac procedures, including coronary interventions, implantable defibrillators, pacemakers, arrhythmia ablation, interatrial shunt closures, and valve replacement/repair, have become common causes of hemopericardium.

Other causes of hemopericardium are trauma and post-STEMI free wall rupture. Hemorrhagic pericardial effusions can also occur in the setting of ascending aortic dissection involving its intrapericardial segment. The latter are typically lethal.

Asymptomatic Effusions

The etiology of these typically large effusions is unknown.[4] They are usually discovered when chest imaging is performed for unrelated reasons. They are well tolerated because of gradual changes in the pericardial PVR (discussed previously) but can unexpectedly progress to tamponade.

Miscellaneous

As discussed previously, pericardial effusions can occur in a wide variety of diseases too numerous to list. Some more notable causes are connective tissue diseases, cardiac amyloidosis, and hypothyroidism and hyperthyroidism. Pericardial effusions in the setting of chronic renal failure and dialysis have been recognized for decades but are now uncommon as a result of advances in the treatment of chronic kidney disease.

Chylous effusions (chylopericardium) are characterized by pericardial fluid that is rich in triglycerides and microscopic fat droplets. They are a rare complication (<1%) after cardiothoracic surgery and also can result from chest trauma, malignancy, tuberculosis, and subclavian vein occlusion or thrombosis. They are usually the result of interruption of small branches of the thoracic duct.[12] The diagnosis can be confirmed by analysis of pericardial fluid. A single pericardiocentesis rarely prevents recurrence. Treatment includes surgical ligation of the thoracic duct and creation of a pericardial window for total drainage. An example of the appearance of a chylous effusion is shown in **Fig. 2**.

In patients with advanced pulmonary hypertension (PH) complicated by right-sided heart failure, a transudative chronic pericardial effusion may develop as a result of impaired reabsorption of pericardial fluid. The presence of a large pericardial effusion carries a poor prognosis. In PH, high right-sided chamber pressures can resist the development of cardiac tamponade. There is a delicate balance between pericardial pressure and right-sided pressures in PH. Therefore, routine drainage of pericardial effusions in the absence of cardiac tamponade should be avoided.[13]

Pericardial effusion is also seen in patients with stress-induced (Takotsubo) cardiomyopathy and was reported to be present in as many as 62% in a series of patients who underwent cardiac MRI (CMR).[14] The presence of pericardial effusion in the setting of stress-induced cardiomyopathy has been attributed to an inflammatory process involving the myocardium. Cardiac tamponade has rarely been reported.[15]

CLINICAL PRESENTATION

Pericardial effusions per se are asymptomatic unless they cause cardiac tamponade (discussed in more detail elsewhere in this issue), which causes dyspnea, tachypnea, tachycardia and symptoms and signs of hypoperfusion along with muffled heart sounds, pulsus paradoxus, and an elevated jugular venous pressure. Patients are more comfortable sitting forward. Many patients with tamponade also have coexistent pericarditis,

with typical pain and a friction rub. Not infrequently, patients experience right upper quadrant abdominal discomfort due to hepatic congestion. Patients may also have symptoms and signs of one of the many underlying diseases that can cause pericardial effusion. In the absence of tamponade, the cardiovascular examination is normal except that in the case of large effusions it is difficult to palpate the cardiac impulse and the heart sounds may be muffled.

LABORATORY EVALUATION
Electrocardiogram

The main abnormalities are reduced voltage and electrical alternans (**Fig. 3**),[1,3,16,17] both of which occur with large effusions. Reduced voltage is nonspecific because it can be seen in infiltrative myocardial disease, pneumothorax, and emphysema. Electrical alternans, that is, alternating QRS voltage, is a specific but insensitive sign of a large effusion, almost always with cardiac tamponade. Electrical alternans is caused by anterior-posterior swinging of the heart with each contraction. If pericardial effusion is accompanied by pericarditis the usual electrocardiographic findings may be present.

Chest Radiograph

The chest radiograph reveals a normal cardiac silhouette until an effusion is at least moderate in size. With larger effusions, the anteroposterior cardiac silhouette assumes a rounded, flask-like appearance (**Fig. 4**). A similar chest radiographic finding can be seen in patients with Ebstein anomaly. The fat pad sign, a linear lucency between the chest wall and the anterior surface of the heart caused by separation of parietal pericardial fat from the epicardium, may be seen on lateral views. In patients with cardiac tamponade, the lungs may appear oligemic. The lungs may also reveal important associated pathology, such as infections and masses.

Echocardiogram

2-D transthoracic echocardiography (TTE) is the imaging modality of choice for evaluation of pericardial effusion as well as tamponade physiology (**Fig. 5**). TTE should also be used to guide periocardiocentesis. Transesophageal echocardiography is more accurate than TTE for delineating the extent and localization of effusions, for example, loculated posterior effusions, which may be difficult to detect with TTE.[4]

Circumferential pericardial effusions appear as an echolucent space between the parietal and

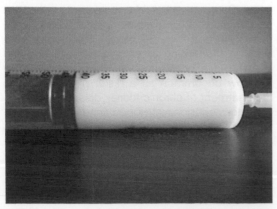

Fig. 2. Milky appearance of a chylous pericardial effusion.

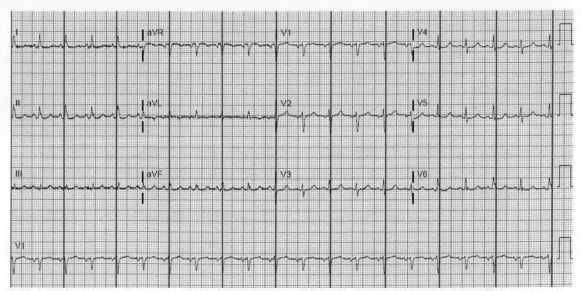

Fig. 3. Electrocardiogram in cardiac tamponade demonstrating electrical alternans and borderline reduced voltage.

visceral pericardium. Circumferential effusions are graded as small (echo-free space in diastole <10 mm), moderate (10–20 mm space), and large (more than 20-mm space). As discussed previously, the hemodynamic significance of an effusion does not always correlate closely with its size and also depends on the rapidity of accumulation. Although tamponade usually occurs in the setting of a circumferential effusion, loculated effusions can also cause regional tamponade, particularly in the postoperative setting.[8,18,19]

TTE can assist in defining some additional characteristics pertinent to pericardial effusion. For instance, fibrinous strands can form within a long-standing effusion adjacent to the epicardial surface of the heart. A nodular and irregular appearance of the effusion with extension into the myocardium suggests a malignant etiology. Coagulum in the pericardial sac due to bloody effusion displays a characteristic snake-like motion reflecting its soft-tissue mass-like structure. A fluid-filled sac adjacent to the right heart may be a congenital pericardial cyst, which is much

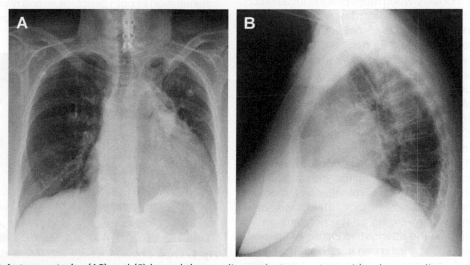

Fig. 4. (A) Anteroposterior (AP) and (B) lateral chest radiographs in a patient with a large malignant pericardial effusion from recurrent squamous cell carcinoma. Note the rounded, flask-like appearance of the cardiac silhouette in the AP view. A left upper lobe mass with left hilar adenopathy is also demonstrated (*asterisk*).

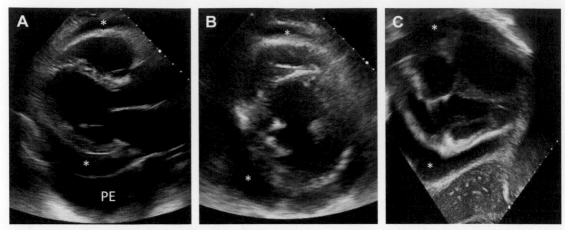

Fig. 5. 2-D echocardiogram in a patient post–atrial fibrillation ablation complicated by hemopericardium. Note the moderate to large effusion (*asterisks*) circumferential to the heart in parasternal long axis (*A*), parasternal short axis (*B*), and subcostal (*C*) views. A left pleural effusion (PE) is also present.

better evaluated with CT or CMR. Rarely, the entry site of a dissecting aortic aneurysm into the pericardium is detected by TTE.

Loculated pericardial effusions mainly occur after surgical or percutaneous procedures or in patients with recurrent pericardial disease. They are particularly important because, depending on their location, they can lead to chamber collapse and hemodynamic compromise despite a small size. Also, depending on their location, percutaneous drainage may not be feasible.

CT

Although 2-D echocardiography is the diagnostic imaging modality of choice for the initial evaluation of pericardial effusion, CT can be an important additional modality when more precise localization and quantification of pericardial fluid are important, when an effusion is complex or loculated, or when a clot is present (**Fig. 6**).[20–22] CT also reliably identifies epicardial fat and differentiates pericardial thickening from pericardial effusion. Pericardial effusions that are accompanied by pericardial thickening (>4 mm) and mediastinal lymphadenopathy are highly suggestive of malignancy.[23] CT scans also better define regions that are more difficult to image with echocardiography. Finally, CT can also distinguish pericardial effusion from conditions that can mimic pericardial disease, such as complex pleural effusions, mediastinal abnormalities, lower lobe atelectasis, and external masses impinging on the pericardium.

Depending on the attenuation values of the pericardial fluid, CT scanning can assist in defining the etiology of pericardial effusions. Attenuation values less than 10 Hounsfield units indicate transudative effusions; low attenuation values close to

that of fat (−60 to −80 Hounsfield units) are seen in chylopericardium. Attenuation values in the range of 20 Hounsfield units to 60 Hounsfield units are usually due to purulent, malignant, or myxedematous pericardial effusions. Finally, effusions with attenuation values greater than 60 Hounsfield units are suggestive of hemorrhage.

Cardiac MRI

CMR is rarely used as a primary imaging modality for evaluation of pericardial effusion (**Fig. 7**). Like CT, however, it demonstrates the localization and amount of pericardial effusion more precisely than the echocardiogram[20,22,24] and also identifies clot and complex or loculated effusions. Importantly, CMR can be used to identify concurrent inflammation of both pericardium and myocardium manifested as late gadolinium enhancement of

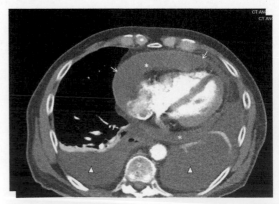

Fig. 6. Chest CT showing large circumferential pericardial effusion (*asterisks*) with mild enhancement of the pericardium (*arrows*). Note the large bilateral pericardial effusions (*triangles*).

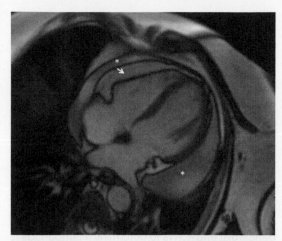

Fig. 7. CMR in a patient with rheumatoid arthritis showing a large circumferential pericardial effusion (*asterisks*). Late gadolinium phase images did not demonstrate late enhancement to suggest active pericardial inflammation. Also note the significant amount of epicardial fat (*arrow*).

these structures (see Bo Xu and colleagues' article, "Imaging of the Pericardium: A Multimodality Cardiovascular Imaging Update," in this issue). Similar to CT, CMR is a useful method for tissue characterization based on signal intensity and quantitation of pericardial thickening.

PERICARDIOCENTESIS AND ANALYSIS OF PERICARDIAL FLUID
Procedural Considerations

In clinical settings where pericardiocentesis is necessary for diagnostic and/or therapeutic purposes, a percutaneous approach is recommended, unless contraindications are present and/or the effusion is thought to not be approachable percutaneously. Immediately prior to pericardiocentesis, it is important to confirm that the effusion is large enough to be drained safely. It is especially important to define loculated effusions or effusions containing clots or fibrinous material that may be difficult to drain percutaneously.

A percutaneous approach should be specifically avoided in the setting of known or suspected major bleeding into the pericardial sac, for example, due to trauma, rupture of the free wall of the left ventricle after an STEMI, or a type A aortic dissection. A recent report suggested, however, that carefully titrated closed pericardiocentesis in patients with aortic dissection is useful in stabilization before definitive surgical repair.[25] Percutaneous pericardiocentesis is reported to be safe in patients with lower bleeding rates, such as those caused by procedural coronary perforation or puncture of a cardiac chamber.

Closed percutaneous pericardiocentesis is usually performed under echocardiographic guidance, which assists in locating the best site for drainage and angulating the pericardiocentesis needle. Although the subxiphoid approach is most commonly used, data from the Mayo Clinic suggested that a para-apical site may be safer and has a success rate greater than 95%.[19,20] Hemodynamic monitoring, including arterial pressure, right atrial and pulmonary capillary wedge pressures, intra-pericardial pressure, and cardiac output prior to, during, and after pericardiocentesis is valuable when feasible, but placement of intravascular catheters should not be allowed to excessively delay drainage. Finally, postprocedure hemodynamic measurements are useful in diagnosing effusive-constrictive pericarditis, with constriction manifested as a persistently elevated right atrial or systemic venous pressure along with the typical venous pressure morphology of constriction after complete drainage. After closed pericardiocentesis, the catheter should preferably be left in the pericardial space under drainage for several days, because this has been shown to reduce recurrences. Intermittent heparin flushes to maintain patency and meticulous care of the entry site are also recommended.[26]

Open surgical pericardiocentesis is rarely the initial method for removal of fluid. It is mainly reserved for bleeding due to trauma or rupture of the left ventricular free wall, loculated effusions, and recurrent effusions severe enough to cause tamponade that require establishment of a pericardial window for therapeutic purposes and tissue sampling for diagnosis.

Other techniques for pericardiocentesis include percutaneous balloon pericardiotomy, particularly in malignant or recurrent effusions,[27] and video-pericardioscopy performed through a small subxiphoid incision both for biopsy and drainage of effusions.[28]

Pericardial Fluid Analysis

Normal pericardial fluid has the features of a plasma ultrafiltrate, with lymphocytes the predominant cell type. The gross appearance of pericardial fluid occasionally has diagnostic utility. Normal pericardial fluid is clear and pale yellow. Serosanguinous-appearing fluid is common, is nonspecific, and does not necessarily indicate active bleeding. Turbid fluid may suggest infection or malignancy, whereas grossly bloody fluid can be seen in malignant and tuberculous effusions. Chylous effusions have been discussed previously (see **Fig. 2**). Cholesterol-rich (gold paint) effusions occur in severe hypothyroidism.

Most pericardial effusions are exudates. Transudative pericardial effusions reduce the diagnostic possibilities and occur with heart failure, hypoalbuminemia, and renal insufficiency, whereas exudative effusions can occur with a wide spectrum of inflammatory, infectious, malignant, or autoimmune processes. Although Light criteria used in differentiation of transudative versus exudative pleural effusions are not fully evaluated and validated for pericardial effusions, in 1 prospective study they had a sensitivity of 98% and specificity of 72% in diagnosis of exudative effusions.[29] Useful criteria in favor of exudative pericardial effusions include a pericardial fluid to serum protein ratio greater than or equal to 0.5 and/or pericardial fluid to serum lactate dehydrogenase ratio greater than or equal to 0.6 and/or pericardial fluid lactate dehydrogenase greater than or equal to 200 U/L. Other measures suggestive of exudative effusions are serum effusion albumin gradient less than 12 g/L and pericardial fluid to serum cholesterol ratio greater than 0.3.[30]

Routine measurements on pericardial fluid should include white blood cell count and differential, hematocrit, and lucose and protein content. Pericardial fluid should be routinely stained and cultured for bacteria, including *Mycobacterium tuberculosis* and fungi. A low glucose concentration points to bacterial pericarditis. If there is any suspicion of tuberculous pericarditis, testing for adenosine deaminase and/or polymerase chain reaction should be routine because waiting for pericardial fluid culture can markedly delay the diagnosis.[23] In cases of suspected malignancy, as much fluid as possible should be submitted for detection of malignant cells because the diagnostic yield is reasonably high. There also may be a role for testing for tumor-specific markers in pericardial fluid.[3]

Pericardial biopsy

The value of open or percutaneous pericardial biopsy to determine the etiology of pericardial effusion is somewhat controversial. Its use has been suggested in neoplastic and tuberculous pericardial effusions and occasionally in instances of no specific cause for pericardial effusion identified. Percutaneous pericardial biopsy via pericardioscopy with extensive sampling has been advocated to improve diagnostic yield,[31] but this has not been thoroughly validated.

MANAGEMENT

Pericardiocentesis (percutaneous or open with biopsy) is by no means always necessary for diagnosis of the cause of pericardial effusion. The cause in many instances is evident or suggested from the history (eg, neoplastic disease, radiation, or severe circulatory congestion) and/or previously obtained diagnostic tests. In instances where the etiology is not clear, additional diagnostic testing should be performed. This may include skin testing for tuberculosis, screening for neoplasms, an autoimmune laboratory panel, work-up for other relevant infections, and screening for thyroid disease. With the exception of bacterial and metastatic effusions, analysis of pericardial fluid in general has a low yield in providing a specific diagnosis, especially if the initial routine work-up has been inconclusive.[10,23]

The most important first step in management of pericardial effusion is to determine if tamponade is present or if there are features suggesting a high chance of development of tamponade in the near term (see Christopher Appleton and colleagues' article, "Cardiac Tamponade," in this issue). If evidence of tamponade is not present initially, features that characterize a high risk for development of tamponade include suspected bacterial, fungal or tuberculous pericarditis; intrapericardial bleeding, and any moderate-to-large pericardial effusion that is not believed chronic or that is increasing in size. It has also been suggested that large, asymptomatic, idiopathic effusions that persist for more than 3 months despite therapy with anti-inflammatory regimens (providing there is evidence of pericardial inflammation) warrant pericardiocentesis.[4,26] The latter effusions have been reported to have a 30% to 35% risk of progression to cardiac tamponade over time and this can occur with little warning.[32]

In cases of tamponade present or threatened, clinical decision making requires urgency, and the threshold for performing pericardiocentesis should be very low. An exception is the occasional patient with acute, idiopathic pericarditis and no more than mild tamponade, especially if the effusion is small. Selected patients can be treated with a nonsteroidal anti-inflammatory agent and colchicine under careful clinical and echocardiographic surveillance to ensure that prompt shrinkage of the effusion occurs without the need for pericardiocentesis.

In the absence of actual tamponade or a high-risk effusion, management should be individualized. The next steps are based on the clinical setting. As discussed previously, attention should be paid to a patient's history and clinical presentation as well as diagnostic laboratory and imaging relevant to the individual presentation rather than routine drainage of the effusion. Moreover, drainage of pericardial effusions in the absence of actual tamponade or high-risk features has low diagnostic yield (7%) and little therapeutic benefit.[26,27]

Medical treatment of nonthreatening effusions should be based on clinical judgment and tailored to the suspected underlying cause. Many of these effusions resolve spontaneously, for example, early post–cardiac surgery. If the effusion is associated with acute, idiopathic pericarditis it almost always decreases in size with conventional treatment with a nonsteroidal anti-inflammatory drug and colchicine. In this setting, there is no need to use corticosteroids initially, especially because their use may encourage recurrences of pericarditis. If the effusion is thought to be caused by an associated disease (eg, connective tissue diseases, cancer, hypothyroidism, or familial Mediterranean fever), the most appropriate treatment of that disease is also the most appropriate treatment of the effusion. In patients with effusive-constrictive pericarditis, imaging the pericardium using CMR with gadolinium or CT scanning to detect evidence of active inflammation is especially useful because these patients may have marked improvement with anti-inflammatory regimens.[33]

PROGNOSIS

The prognosis of pericardial effusion is determined by its etiology. Bacterial and fungal pericarditis is associated with a high mortality rate. Neoplastic effusions are in general seen with advanced disease. Similarly, the prognosis of effusions associated with connective tissue diseases is dictated by the overall prognosis of those diseases. Pericardial effusions secondary to acute idiopathic pericarditis, especially when small, have an excellent prognosis and rarely progress to constrictive pericarditis.[34] As discussed previously, moderate to large, asymptomatic idiopathic effusions carry a risk of tamponade during follow-up but have a good prognosis with elective pericardiocentesis and careful monitoring.

REFERENCES

1. Shabetai R. The pericardium. Norwell (MA): Kluwer; 2003.
2. LeWinter MM, Myhre ESP, Slinker BK. Influence of the pericardium and ventricular interaction on diastolic function. Philadelphia: Lea & Febiger; 1993. p. 103–17.
3. Dudzinski DM, Mak GS, Hung JW. Pericardial diseases. Curr Probl Cardiol 2012;37(3):75–118.
4. Adler Y, Charron P, Imazio M, et al. 2015 ESC guidelines for the diagnosis and management of pericardial diseases: the Task Force for the Diagnosis and Management of Pericardial Diseases of the European Society of Cardiology (ESC) Endorsed by: the European Association for Cardio-Thoracic Surgery (EACTS). Eur Heart J 2015;36(42):2921–64.
5. Ben-Horin S, Bank I, Guetta V, et al. Large symptomatic pericardial effusion as the presentation of unrecognized cancer: a study in 173 consecutive patients undergoing pericardiocentesis. Medicine 2006; 85(1):49–53.
6. Al-Dadah AS, Guthrie TJ, Pasque MK, et al. Clinical course and predictors of pericardial effusion following cardiac transplantation. Transplant Proc 2007;39(5):1589–92.
7. Ditchey R, Engler R, LeWinter M, et al. The role of the right heart in acute cardiac tamponade in dogs. Circ Res 1981;48(5):701–10.
8. Singh S, Wann LS, Schuchard GH, et al. Right ventricular and right atrial collapse in patients with cardiac tamponade–a combined echocardiographic and hemodynamic study. Circulation 1984;70(6):966–71.
9. Imazio M, Cecchi E, Demichelis B, et al. Indicators of poor prognosis of acute pericarditis. Circulation 2007;115(21):2739–44.
10. Abu Fanne R, Banai S, Chorin U, et al. Diagnostic yield of extensive infectious panel testing in acute pericarditis. Cardiology 2011;119(3):134–9.
11. Imazio M, Brucato A, Rovere ME, et al. Contemporary features, risk factors, and prognosis of the post-pericardiotomy syndrome. Am J Cardiol 2011; 108(8):1183–7.
12. Dib C, Tajik AJ, Park S, et al. Chylopericardium in adults: a literature review over the past decade (1996-2006). J Thorac Cardiovasc Surg 2008; 136(3):650–6.
13. Khan MU, Khouzam RN. Protective effect of pulmonary hypertension against right-sided tamponade in pericardial effusion. South Med J 2015;108(1):46–8.
14. Eitel I, Lucke C, Grothoff M, et al. Inflammation in takotsubo cardiomyopathy: insights from cardiovascular magnetic resonance imaging. Eur Radiol 2010;20(2):422–31.
15. Yeh RW, Yu PB, Drachman DE. Takotsubo cardiomyopathy complicated by cardiac tamponade: classic hemodynamic findings with a new disease. Circulation 2010;122(12):1239–41.
16. Maisch B, Seferovic PM, Ristic AD, et al. Guidelines on the diagnosis and management of pericardial diseases executive summary; the Task force on the diagnosis and management of pericardial diseases of the European society of cardiology. Eur Heart J 2004;25(7):587–610.
17. Seferovic PM, Ristic AD, Maksimovic R, et al. Pericardial syndromes: an update after the ESC guidelines 2004. Heart Fail Rev 2013;18(3):255–66.
18. Oh JK, Seward JB, Tajik AJ. The echo manual. 3rd edition. Philadelphia: Lippincott, Williams & Wilkins; 2006.

19. Veress G, Feng D, Oh JK. Echocardiography in pericardial diseases: new developments. Heart Fail Rev 2013;18(3):267–75.

20. Klein AL, Abbara S, Agler DA, et al. American Society of Echocardiography clinical recommendations for multimodality cardiovascular imaging of patients with pericardial disease: endorsed by the Society for Cardiovascular Magnetic Resonance and Society of Cardiovascular Computed Tomography. J Am Soc Echocardiogr 2013;26(9):965–1012.e5.

21. Yared K, Baggish AL, Picard MH, et al. Multimodality imaging of pericardial diseases. JACC Cardiovasc Imaging 2010;3(6):650–60.

22. Bogaert J, Francone M. Pericardial disease: value of CT and MR imaging. Radiology 2013;267(2):340–56.

23. Sagrista-Sauleda J, Merce AS, Soler-Soler J. Diagnosis and management of pericardial effusion. World J Cardiol 2011;3(5):135–43.

24. Bogaert J, Francone M. Cardiovascular magnetic resonance in pericardial diseases. J Cardiovasc Magn Reson 2009;11:14.

25. Cruz I, Stuart B, Caldeira D, et al. Controlled pericardiocentesis in patients with cardiac tamponade complicating aortic dissection: experience of a centre without cardiothoracic surgery. Eur Heart J Acute Cardiovasc Care 2015;4(2):124–8.

26. Gluer R, Murdoch D, Haqqani HM, et al. Pericardiocentesis - How to do it. Heart Lung Circ 2015;24(6):621–5.

27. Swanson N, Mirza I, Wijesinghe N, et al. Primary percutaneous balloon pericardiotomy for malignant pericardial effusion. Catheter Cardiovasc Interv 2008;71(4):504–7.

28. Pego-Fernandes PM, Mariani AW, Fernandes F, et al. The role of videopericardioscopy in evaluating indeterminate pericardial effusions. Heart Surg Forum 2008;11(1):E62–5.

29. Meyers DG, Meyers RE, Prendergast TW. The usefulness of diagnostic tests on pericardial fluid. Chest 1997;111(5):1213–21.

30. Kopcinovic LM, Culej J. Pleural, peritoneal and pericardial effusions - a biochemical approach. Biochem Med (Zagreb) 2014;24(1):123–37.

31. Seferovic PM, Ristic AD, Maksimovic R, et al. Diagnostic value of pericardial biopsy: improvement with extensive sampling enabled by pericardioscopy. Circulation 2003;107(7):978–83.

32. Sagrista-Sauleda J, Angel J, Permanyer-Miralda G, et al. Long-term follow-up of idiopathic chronic pericardial effusion. N Engl J Med 1999;341(27):2054–9.

33. Syed FF, Ntsekhe M, Mayosi BM, et al. Effusive-constrictive pericarditis. Heart Fail Rev 2013;18(3):277–87.

34. Imazio M, Brucato A, Maestroni S, et al. Risk of constrictive pericarditis after acute pericarditis. Circulation 2011;124(11):1270–5.

Cardiac Tamponade

Christopher Appleton, MD[a], Linda Gillam, MD, MPH[b],*,
Konstantinos Koulogiannis, MD[b]

KEYWORDS

- Pericardial effusion • Cardiac compression • Cardiac tamponade • Echo-Doppler findings

KEY POINTS

- Cardiac tamponade is caused by an abnormal increase in fluid accumulation in the pericardial sac, which, by raising intracardiac pressures, impedes normal cardiac filling and reduces cardiac output.
- The clinical manifestations typically reflect elevated right-sided filling pressures, reduced cardiac output, pulsus paradoxus, and imaging evidence of dynamic chamber compression.
- Treatment consists of needle pericardiocentesis, preferably guided by echocardiography, or surgical drainage.

 Video content accompanies this article at http://www.cardiology.theclinics.com.

INTRODUCTION

Cardiac tamponade is caused by an abnormal increase in fluid accumulation in the pericardial sac, which, by raising intracardiac pressures, impedes normal cardiac filling. When the fluid accumulation is rapid, a marked increase in intrapericardial pressure can reduce inflow gradients to such low levels that compensatory reflexes that are activated to maintain cardiac output and blood pressure are overwhelmed and cardiogenic shock and death can occur. Less frequently, cardiac tamponade occurs due to localized, severe compression of cardiac chambers due to a mass, or a localized hematoma after cardiac or thoracic surgery.

In both instances, patients present with tachypnea, tachycardia, and hemodynamic instability with an elevated systemic venous pressure. A clinical hallmark of cardiac tamponade is pulsus paradoxus, or an abnormal decrease in systolic blood pressure with inspiration. Emergency echocardiography using both imaging and Doppler techniques is the primary method for rapid diagnosis and assessing the severity of tamponade. When possible, pericardiocentesis using echo guidance is used to drain pericardial effusions because of its high success rate and low procedural morbidity.

PATHOPHYSIOLOGY
Normal Pericardial Layers and Function

As discussed in other articles in this issue, a small amount of fluid (15–35 mL) exists in the pericardial sac between the smooth surfaced visceral and parietal pericardial layers to facilitate lubrication in the ever-beating heart.[1,2] The serosal visceral pericardium, which is the outermost layer of the myocardium, is thin, elastic, and translucent; and the fibrous parietal pericardium is thicker and inelastic. The visceral pericardium appears to aid diastolic elastic recoil and suction, whereas the parietal pericardium, with attachments to the sternum, diaphragm, vertebrae, and pleura, holds the heart in optimal

Conflicts of Interest: None.
[a] Division of Cardiovascular Diseases, Mayo Clinic Arizona, 13400 East Shea Boulevard, Scottsdale, AZ 85259, USA; [b] Department of Cardiovascular Medicine, Morristown Medical Center/Atlantic Health System, 100 Madison Avenue, Morristown, NJ 07960, USA
* Corresponding author.
E-mail address: ldgillam@gmail.com

Cardiol Clin 35 (2017) 525–537
http://dx.doi.org/10.1016/j.ccl.2017.07.006
0733-8651/17/© 2017 Elsevier Inc. All rights reserved.

orientation for filling and ejection, limits excessive motion, and prevents excessive dilation from acute adverse events, such as mitral chordal rupture or right ventricular (RV) infarction. The parietal pericardium also provides a barrier to contiguous pulmonary infection or cancers.

The parietal pericardium envelopes the heart snugly, contributing more than 50% resting right atrial (RA) pressure and distributes this effect variably over the cardiac chamber pressures. Yet, due to pericardial reflections, irregular spaces between the pericardial layers exist, like the transverse and oblique sinuses (**Fig. 1**), that provide a pericardial reserve volume, which allows for modest changes in cardiac volume with inspiration and changes in body position to occur without the parietal pericardium raising intracardiac pressures (**Fig. 2**). When this reserve volume is exceeded by markedly increased right heart filling on inspiration (chronic obstructive pulmonary disease exacerbation or acute respiratory distress), or acute cardiac chamber dilation, both intrapericardial and intracardiac pressures rise due to the steep nature of the pericardial pressure-volume relation (see **Fig. 2**). This pericardial restraint increases all diastolic intracardiac pressures and results in enhanced and competitive filling between the right and left heart that alternates with the phase of respiration. This is why pulsus paradoxus can be observed in conditions such as status asthmaticus.

Pericardial Effusions

These exist when there is an increased volume of pericardial fluid of any type in the pericardial space. They can present acutely with symptoms or, when chronic, are more likely to be found incidentally after computerized tomography or MRI of the heart or chest or echocardiography ordered for a separate indication. A general rule is that any patient with unexplained jugular venous distension should have an echocardiogram to exclude pericardial effusion. Idiopathic asymptomatic small, medium, and even large pericardial effusions can be seen without tamponade (**Fig. 3**). When these are present, it can be assumed that they have accumulated slowly enough that the fibrous parietal pericardium added additional cells (stretched) so that pericardial pressure is normal or minimally raised.[1,2] The initial focus in idiopathic effusions, if there is no obvious systemic disease, is on ruling out malignancy such as lymphoma, breast, lung, or another type of cancer. Although the diagnostic yield of needle pericardiocentesis for malignancy is low, it can usually been done safely under echo guidance.[3] Alternatively, the pericardium can be biopsied as part of surgical pericardial window creation.

Pericardial fluid can be serous as seen in idiopathic pericarditis, serosanguineous as seen in other inflammatory or malignant conditions, purulent due to infections, or bloody as seen after inadvertent cardiac perforation from an invasive

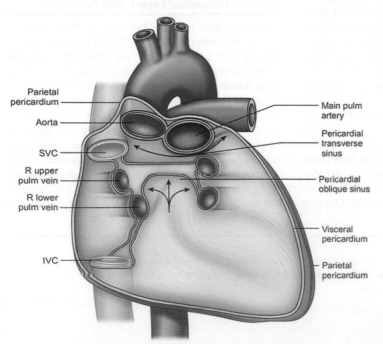

Fig. 1. Anatomic drawing of pericardial space with the heart removed showing the pericardial attachments to the great vessels and pericardial reflections, or transitions from parietal to visceral pericardium. The latter create irregular spaces between the pericardial layers such as the transverse and oblique sinuses as shown. IVC, inferior vena cava; SVC, superior vena cava.

Parietal pericardium

Aorta

SVC

R upper pulm vein

R lower pulm vein

IVC

Main pulm artery

Pericardial transverse sinus

Pericardial oblique sinus

Visceral pericardium

Parietal pericardium

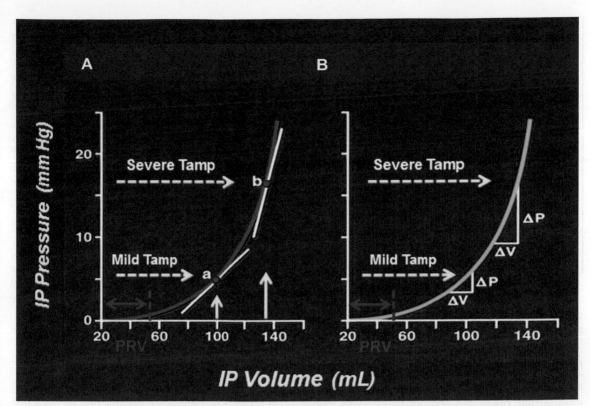

Fig. 2. Schematic drawings (*A, B*) of the intra pericardial pressure (IPP) – volume (P-V) relation at rest and with an *acute* pericardial effusion of increasing volume. Under normal conditions an increase in cardiac size with inspiration, or small increase in pericardial fluid, causes little change in IPP due to the pericardial reserve volume (PRV) provided by the pericardial sinuses (see **Fig. 1**). However, when pericardial fluid exceeds the pericardial reserve volume IPP increases rapidly because of the restraining effect of the parietal pericardium causing cardiac compression and mild cardiac tamponade (point a). As the pressure-volume relation progressively steepens small increases in fluid result in large increases in IPP and severe tamponade occurs (point b); the increasing stiffness illustrated in (*A*) by the tangent to the P-V curve and in (*B*) by the smaller $\Delta V/\Delta P$ ratio.

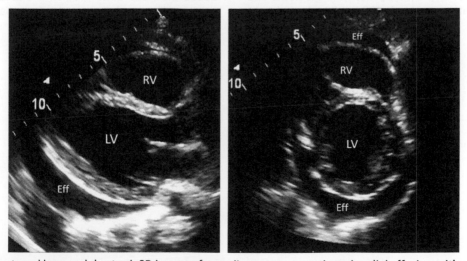

Fig. 3. Parasternal long and short axis 2D images of a medium asymptomatic pericardial effusion without signs of cardiac tamponade. The size of the effusion and lack of 2D and Doppler abnormalities indicate that it has accumulated slowly enough that the parietal pericardium added additional cells (stretched) so that intrapericardial pressure is normal. Eff, pericardial effusion.

the pericardial sac as a complication of an invasive procedure will produce a rapid rise in IPP, being on the very steep portion of the pericardial P-V curve (see **Fig. 2**). At this level, even a small additional increment of fluid will result in a large increase in IPP and possibly lead to hemodynamic collapse and death if not promptly recognized and drained.

Conversely, the fibrous parietal pericardium is stiff but has ability to add new cells (stretch), so if fluid accumulates slowly, chronic effusions of more than 1 L can occasionally be seen without elevation of IPP, or decrease in cardiac size or output as the pericardial P-V relation shifts rightward.[1] A chest radiograph of a large asymptomatic pericardial effusion contrasted with a normal radiograph is shown in **Fig. 4**. However, because the pericardial P-V relation, although shifted to be more compliant, retains the same shape, if pericardial fluid accumulation should increase more rapidly, IPP may suddenly increase with adverse hemodynamic effects on cardiac filling.

Box 1
Common causes of pericardial effusion

Malignancy

Idiopathic (postviral) pericarditis

Interventional procedures with cardiac perforation

Post-pericardiotomy syndrome

Uremia

Myocarditis with pericardial involvement

Transmural myocardial infarction

Bacterial or tuberculous pericarditis

Rheumatologic diseases

Miscellaneous (eg, myxedema, radiation, hypothyroidism)

---

cardiac procedure. **Box 1** shows the most common causes of pericardial effusions.

Intrapericardial Pressure

Normal intrapericardial pressure (IPP) is below intracardiac pressures and phasic changes follow changes in intracardiac volume. With respiration, IPP changes to the same degree as intrathoracic and intracardiac pressures.[2] Therefore, IPP exerts no influence on cardiac filling under normal circumstances. *When a pericardial effusion is present, its hemodynamic effect does not depend on its size, but on its pressure, which is determined by its relation to the pericardial pressure-volume (P-V) relationship* that is *present*. In the acute situation, an effusion of only 100 to 200 mL of blood in

Pathophysiology of Cardiac Tamponade

Cardiac tamponade is present when fluid accumulation in the intrapericardial space is rapid enough in relation to pericardial compliance to raise IPP above resting values.[1,4] The increased pressure is then transmitted to the cardiac chambers; the most important in terms of adverse consequences is the right atrium. Because it is thin walled, has the lowest intracardiac pressure, and is virtually completely surrounded by a pericardial effusion, the right atrium is not only the most vulnerable to compression, but an increase in its pressure reduces the veno-atrial gradients that determine cardiac filling and the maximal cardiac output

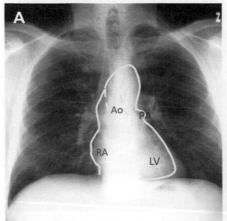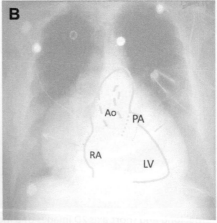

Fig. 4. A chest radiograph of a healthy patient (left) and patient with a very large asymptomatic pericardial effusion (right) with the classic "water bottle shape" heart (*arrows*). Selective underlying cardiac structures and great vessels are labeled. Ao, ascending aorta; LV, left ventricle; PA, pulmonary artery; RA, right atrium.

that can be achieved.[5,6] Systemic venous pressure becomes elevated in concert with the rise in RA pressure, but seldom to a level that maintains normal right heart filling, even with the compensatory mechanisms of venoconstriction and fluid retention.

The reduction in RA filling is mild when IPP is raised only slightly, but with a progressive increase in IPP, cardiac filling continues to decline, and total cardiac volume decreases so the heart becomes smaller, with smaller diastolic ventricular dimensions and the accompanying illusion by imaging of thick-walled, hypertrophied ventricles ("pseudohypertrophy") with increased contractility and ejection fraction. As reduced cardiac inflow worsens, severe cardiac tamponade occurs, compressing all cardiac chambers and reducing their diastolic compliance so that equalization of IPP and mean diastolic intracardiac pressures occurs.[7] Blood is transferred from atrium to ventricle without a change in total cardiac volume. With no blood leaving the heart to lower pressures there is no filling of the right atrium during diastole (loss of y descent) and diastolic filling of the left atrium is also reduced, but to a lesser degree. It is only during ventricular ejection that cardiac volume decreases, lowering atrial pressure (as seen by a dominant atrial X descent) and filling occurs. *The most important concept in understanding cardiac tamponade is that fatal consequences occur when increased IPP reduces the systemic venous-RA pressure gradient (cardiac filling) to a level in which cardiac output can no longer maintain coronary artery and systemic perfusion so that cardiovascular collapse occurs, often abruptly with a vagal component in a phenomenon referred to as the "last drop."*[1]

Cardiac Tamponade as a Continuum

Cardiac tamponade can be mild, moderate, or severe depending on IPP level and its effect on reducing right heart filling, RV stroke volume, and hence left heart cardiac output. The "continuum" concept of the effect of tamponade was elegantly formulated by Reddy[8] based on data in both experimental animals[9–11] and patients.[5–7,12–14] It has been verified and related to the effects of IPP on RA inflow gradients in our own experiments.[15] Abnormal changes in transvalvular flow velocities appear to be very sensitive to only mild increases in IPP and occur before either RA chamber collapse or significant reduction in cardiac output. Systemic blood pressure is often maintained by alpha adrenergic tone until very late in cardiac tamponade so that it is not a

good clinical indicator of severity.[1,14] More reliable clinical indicators of severity of tamponade are tachycardia, tachypnea, and an elevated jugular venous pulse with absence of Y descent and pulsus paradoxus.[7] Because cardiac tamponade kills by interfering with right heart filling and reducing cardiac output, echo-Doppler recordings of hepatic venous flow velocity indicates how compromised the systemic veno-RA pressure gradient is, whereas calculation of stroke volume and cardiac output indicate the degree to which cardiac output has been compromised.[16]

Low Pressure Cardiac Tamponade

In rapidly developing cardiac tamponade, especially hemorrhagic such as is seen as a result of cardiac perforation during an invasive procedure, cardiogenic shock may occur rapidly with relatively small pericardial effusions. This is due to both a rapid rise in IPP and a lack of the normal increase in systemic venous pressure due to the hemorrhage. Such "low systemic venous pressure" tamponade may also occur after dialysis in patients with end-stage renal disease who have uremic pericarditis and a chronic pericardial effusion.[17] In patients who have a low or normal systemic venous pressure, giving fluid or blood will improve RA filling and cardiac output, and at least temporarily lessen their tamponade severity. Giving additional fluid to patients with severe cardiac tamponade who already have an elevated systemic venous pressure rarely improves their hemodynamics and prompt drainage is indicated.

Compensatory Mechanisms

When cardiac tamponade is present, adrenergic tone increases acutely to maintain cardiac filling, cardiac output, and systemic blood pressure.[1,2] This response is mediated through autonomic nervous system reflexes and adrenal catecholamine release. Effects on the heart include increases in heart rate, ventricular contractility, and ejection fraction (stroke volume). At the same time, arterial vasoconstriction helps maintain blood pressure and venoconstriction raises systemic venous pressure. Slower neurohumoral responses are also activated in tamponade that result in salt and water retention, which also raise systemic venous pressure and maintain a more normal veno-atrial pressure gradient.

Clinical Presentation

Patients with significant cardiac tamponade are restless and may complain of dyspnea and chest pain.[1] Sinus tachycardia should be present with blood pressure remaining in the normal range until tamponade is very advanced due to an increase in systemic vascular resistance. Tachypnea is typically present, more likely due to increased CO_2 or lactate production from reduced tissue perfusion, rather than pulmonary venous congestion, as with acute severe tamponade from cardiac perforation mean left atrial pressure may not exceed 15 mm Hg, a level that would be unlikely to cause pulmonary venous congestion and tachypnea. With inspiration, pulsus paradoxus (see the next section) is present. The heart sounds are soft and may vary in intensity with respiration. An occasional S4 gallop may be heard. Increased central venous pressure is seen as jugular venous distension with a dominant X decent during ventricular systole and a diastolic Y descent that is markedly reduced or absent.

Pulsus Paradoxus

During normal inspiration, a decrease in intrathoracic and consequently aortic blood pressure of 3 to 5 mm Hg is typical. Right heart filling increases, but left ventricular (LV) filling decreases by <5% so aortic pulse pressure remains nearly constant even as peak aortic pressure falls (**Fig. 5**). A hallmark of cardiac tamponade is an exaggerated inspiratory decrease in systolic blood pressure known as pulsus paradoxus.

This is generally defined as a >10 mm Hg decrease in systolic arterial pressure during inspiration, and in severe cases can approach 30 mm Hg.[1,7,13,14] The inspiratory decline in blood pressure is due to a combination of a decrease in intrathoracic pressure and more importantly a reduced LV stroke volume and pulse pressure (see **Fig. 5**). Alternative definitions, such as "percent" pulsus paradoxus have also been proposed, such as dividing the absolute inspiratory systolic pressure decrease by the expiratory systolic pressure, to correct for low systolic blood pressure and changes in stroke volume and heart rate.[18] With expiration, LV filling predominates and RV filling decreases, with aortic pressure reaching its zenith due to both the increase in intrathoracic pressure and LV stroke volume, which increases pulse pressure and LV ejection time.

Pulsus paradoxus in cardiac tamponade has fascinated physicians and physiologists for decades, and yet the exact mechanism and hemodynamic determinants of this phenomenon remain incompletely explained. Experimental and clinical evidence have established that pulsus paradoxus in cardiac tamponade is respiratory, driven by reciprocal changes in left and right heart filling and output.[1,4,7–9,12,13,16,19–21] What remains controversial is the fundamental mechanism that causes these reciprocal alterations in ventricular filling and output.

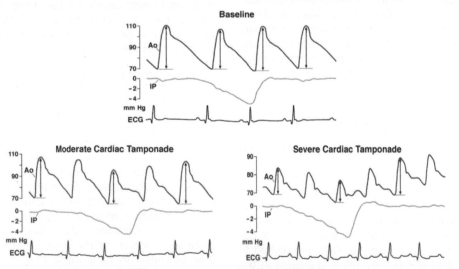

Fig. 5. Aortic (Ao) and intrapleural (IP) pressures recorded with high-fidelity micromanometer catheters during baseline, moderate cardiac tamponade, and then severe tamponade in an experimental animal model.[21] The downward deflection in IP pressure represents inspiration. During baseline with inspiration there is a minimal decrease in aortic pulse pressure (*arrows*) and stroke volume seen on the second beat. With moderate cardiac tamponade, there is a larger drop in inspiratory pressure due to a combination on both intrathoracic pressure and pulse pressure decrease, with borderline pulsus paradoxus. With severe tamponade the heart rate is faster, and blood pressure is lower and the change in inspiratory to expiratory Ao peak and pulse pressures more marked. Ao, aortic pressure; IP, intrapleural pressure.

Two theories remain popular and plausible.[1,22,23] The most popular, first proposed more 60 years ago by Dornhorst and colleagues,[24] suggests that pericardial volume is "fixed" in cardiac tamponade, and that the ventricles compete for space in a "rigid box" surrounded by incompressible fluid, such that an inspiratory increase in right heart filling through ventricular interaction raises left atrial (LA) pressure and impedes left heart filling. Proponents cite experimental [9,21,24] and clinical studies[19,20,25–27] in which increased filling in one ventricle results in an immediate, and opposite decrease in the filling of the other ventricle. Similar respiratory driven reciprocal changes have also been reported for peak RV and LV systolic pressures,[7,21] RV and LV stroke volumes,[25] and peak early diastolic mitral and tricuspid flow velocities.[20,26,27]

An alternative theory regarding pulsus paradoxus is less frequently mentioned and proposes that on inspiration when right heart filling dominates, pulmonary venous pressure falls below LA and pericardial pressure, so that the primary cause of pulsus paradoxus is underfilling of the LV due to a reduction of the upstream pressure that fills the LV, rather than a rise in LV minimum pressure.[8,28] A reduced or reversed pressure gradient between the pulmonary veins and LV during inspiration was suggested nearly a century ago[29] and has been observed in clinical studies.[30] Reddy[8] theorized that the 2 theories described previously may be complementary; with RV and LV filling competitive in cardiac tamponade as determined by their respective filling pressure gradients with changes in both "upstream" and "downstream" pressures contributing to reciprocal increased and decreased ventricular filling and output. However, without measuring all filling pressure gradients simultaneously, it remains uncertain how much the reciprocal RV and LV inflow gradients with respiration that result in pulsus paradoxus are related to ventricular interaction versus changes in the "upstream" venous pressures.

Pulsus paradoxus may be <10 mm Hg on inspiration despite severe cardiac tamponade in several conditions. With severe hypotension or cardiogenic shock, blood pressure and stroke volume may be so low that pulsus paradoxus will be recognized only by using % inspiratory change in systolic blood pressure.[2] Other conditions in which pulsus paradoxus is reduced or absent include a marked elevation in LV filling pressures, significant aortic regurgitation, or an atrial septal defect. In these cases, the inspiratory increase in right heart filling is less able to affect the LV inflow pressure gradients.[1,14,23,31]

Conditions that result in pulsus paradoxus also can occur without pericardial effusion. These vary from the pericardial restraint discussed previously, as seen with respiratory distress and inspiratory overfilling of the right heart, acute chamber dilatation due to severe valvular regurgitation or infarction (especially RV), and even localized tamponade from a postsurgical mediastinal hematoma or tension pneumothorax that compresses some of the cardiac chambers.

Abnormal Cardiac Chamber Invagination (Collapse)

The surface shape of the cardiac chambers is determined by their transmural pressure gradient (chamber pressure – intrathoracic pressure), which exerts an outward force toward the parietal pericardium. As the atria and ventricles contract and relax, phasic pressure changes occur but pressures remain above the normal negative IPP. This situation changes with a pericardial effusion that raises IPP, which has a less phasic and more constant pressure. Being the thinnest wall chamber with the lowest pressure, the right atrium is the first chamber whose pressure can fall below pericardial pressure resulting in invagination. In general, the longer the atrium remains collapsed the more severe the tamponade.[32]

The RV is the next chamber to indent or collapse in cardiac tamponade but this occurs at a different time than RA collapse, as RV minimum pressure occurs in early diastole. In early tamponade, the indentation of the RV free wall or conus may be seen only during expiration, which lowers minimum pressure below pericardial pressure. With higher IPP, RV collapse is seen throughout the respiratory cycle but is shorter with inspiration due to increased filling and longer during expiration when filling is decreased. Unlike the RA, RV collapse can occur only during diastole, although again the longer duration of collapse is associated with more advanced tamponade.

When tamponade is severe, the intrapericardial portion of the LA can sometimes be seen to collapse with timing similar to that of the RA. LV diastolic collapse is rare because IPP must not only exceed LV pressure but overcome the outward force associated with the thick-walled ventricle. The echocardiographic appearance of these findings is discussed later in this article.

An important point about abnormal cardiac chamber collapse is that it simply reflects the relation of IPP to intracardiac pressures and its presence or absence alone should not be used to assess the severity of cardiac tamponade. *To reiterate, it is the reduction of the systemic venous-RA pressure gradient that reduces cardiac filling, and hence RV and LV output, and therefore determines the level of hemodynamic compromise in cardiac tamponade.* Chamber collapse will occur earlier with lower intracardiac pressures, as in hemorrhage or volume depletion, and later or not at all with elevated right heart pressures, as seen in RV infarction[8] or decompensated pulmonary hypertension with right heart failure.[31]

DIAGNOSIS: ROLE OF ECHOCARDIOGRAPHY

When the diagnosis of tamponade is clinically suspected, echocardiography is the test of choice to document the presence, size, and distribution of the pericardial fluid collection as well as to evaluate for evidence of loculation or intrapericardial tissue (hematoma, tumor) that may influence the approach to treatment. Additionally, there are echocardiographic markers of tamponade that can confirm the hemodynamic impact of the effusion and, in some instances, may help establish the diagnosis of tamponade when it has not been suspected clinically. The physiologic underpinnings of these signs have been elucidated in the preceding paragraphs.

CHAMBER COMPRESSION
Right Atrial Inversion

RA inversion (RAI) may be appreciated in any view that shows the RA free wall: parasternal short axis at the level of the great vessels, apical 4-chamber, or their subcostal counterparts (**Fig. 6**). Ordinarily, the contour of the RA is rounded and is never inverted; that is, convex toward the center of the RA. In the context of tamponade, however, abrupt RA inversion is observed, a dynamic phenomenon that is initiated when the atrial volume and pressure are lowest as the atrium relaxes after active contraction (following the P wave on the electrocardiogram). It continues through a variable portion of systole with the curve of the atrial free wall normalizing as the RA fills and intra-atrial pressure rises (Video 1).

In the original report of this finding,[32] RAI was shown to be highly sensitive (100%), but less specific (82%) with a predictive value of 50%. Although the predictive value is not improved through consideration of the degree of inversion as measured by indices of curvature, it is considerably improved by assessing the relative duration of inversion, easily calculated as the ratio of the number of imaging frames in which the atrium is inverted over the number of imaging frames per cardiac cycle (the RA inversion time index). Using an empirically derived cutoff of 0.34 for this index was reported to improve the specificity and predictive value to 100%, maintaining a sensitivity of 94%. RAI is most prominent in early expiration.[32]

Right Ventricular Inversion

RV inversion (RVI) is an equally dynamic phenomenon that can be appreciated in the parasternal long or short axis view that shows the RV outflow tract as well as in views of the RV free wall (apical 4 chamber and its subcostal counterpart) (**Fig. 7**). It may also be appreciated with M-mode echocardiography, particularly one derived from the parasternal long-axis view that shows the most compliant RV outflow tract (**Fig. 8**). It onsets during isovolumic relaxation (early diastole) and continues through a variable portion of diastole.[33] It has been reported to have a sensitivity of 92%, specificity of 100%, and predictive value of

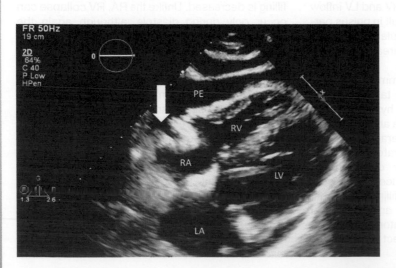

Fig. 6. Early systolic subcostal 4-chamber 2D echocardiogram showing right atrial inversion (*arrow*). PE, pericardial effusion. The dynamic nature of this finding is better appreciated in Video 1 in which there is also RV inversion. LA, left atrium; LV, left ventricle; PE, pericardial effusion; RA, right atrium; RV, right ventricle.

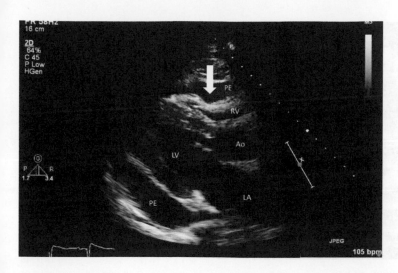

Fig. 7. Diastolic parasternal long-axis 2D echocardiogram showing RV inversion (*arrow*). Ao, aorta; PE, pericardial effusion. The dynamic nature of this finding is better appreciated in Video 2 in which there is also LA inversion.

100%.[33] RVI has been shown to onset when the tamponade has resulted in a fall in cardiac output but before systemic blood pressure falls and is less sensitive than RAI, which occurs when there are subtle hemodynamic changes consistent with tamponade (equilibration of RA, IPP, and pulmonary capillary wedge pressure with obliteration of the y descent).[34]

The presence of RA and RV inversion are dependent on the intrinsic right heart pressures,[35,36] and thus, these signs may be false negatively absent in the presence of RV and/or right atrial hypertension as may occur with pulmonary hypertension and/or tricuspid regurgitation.

Left-Sided Inversion

Because of its relatively higher pressures and variability to which it is enclosed by the pericardium, the LA is less frequently seen to invert.[37] When present, LA inversion (LAI) is best seen in the parasternal long-axis view and has timing similar to that of RAI (**Fig. 9**). Rarer still is LV inversion (**Fig. 10**) that occurs only when the IPP is locally elevated to a point that it exceeds LV pressure. This may occur with loculated effusions but is most often observed as a static phenomenon in the presence of an intrapericardial mass or hematoma.

ECHOCARDIOGRAPHIC MARKERS OF PULSUS PARADOXUS

In addition to the more sensitive and specific findings of chamber inversion, there are echocardiographic manifestations of the exaggerated respiratory changes that form the basis of pulsus paradoxus.[38] These include M-mode findings of enhanced reciprocal changes in ventricular dimensions[12,19,39] and Doppler demonstration of exaggerated respiratory changes in mitral/tricuspid inflow (**Fig. 11**) and

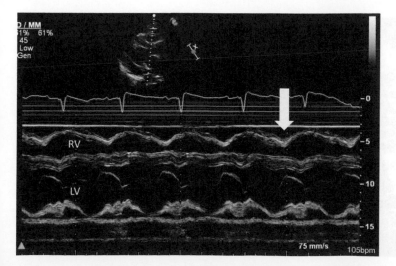

Fig. 8. Parasternal M-mode echocardiogram showing RV inversion (*arrow*). PE, pericardial effusion.

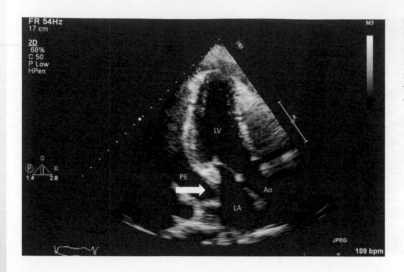

Fig. 9. Early systolic apical 3-chamber 2D echocardiogram showing LA inversion (*arrow*). Ao, aorta; PE, pericardial effusion. The dynamic nature of this finding is better appreciated in Video 2 in which there is also RV inversion.

aortic/pulmonic outflow with changes in right-sided flows being larger than those for left-sided flows.[20,26] According to the current American Society of Echocardiography Guidelines,[40] in the presence of tamponade, the maximal drop in the peak mitral E wave usually exceeds 30% respiratory variation (expiration-inspiration/expiration). For peak tricuspid E inflow, the maximal drop is on the first beat in expiration and usually exceeds greater than 60% respiratory variation. The calculated % will be a negative value. Because the heart has increased contractility and may be "swinging" in the pericardial fluid, a stationary pulsed-wave (PW) sample volume may have difficulty recording adequate inflow signals for interpretation. Therefore, starting with continuous-wave mitral recordings to verify respiratory mitral E-wave changes is helpful, with PW Doppler after. Importantly, recordings showing a longer isovolumic relaxation times (IVRT) with smaller peak mitral velocities and a shorter IVRT on

expiration help confirm that abnormal respiratory mitral velocity changes are present. Although the respiratory changes in transvalvular flow velocities are well recognized, the reduction in their time velocity integrals (TVI) is less well appreciated but is as important. Regurgitation of the A-V valves is rare due to cardiac compression and increased valve coaptation, so the mitral and tricuspid TVIs reflect the amount that ventricular filling is decreased. This is then reflected in the stroke volume and cardiac output calculated by the LV outflow tract diameter, TVI, and heart rate. Predictably, echocardiographic markers of pulsus paradoxus are less sensitive and specific for the diagnosis of tamponade than is chamber inversion.[41,42]

TREATMENT OF CARDIAC TAMPONADE

As the etiology, size, and effect of a pericardial effusion are variable with a continuum of

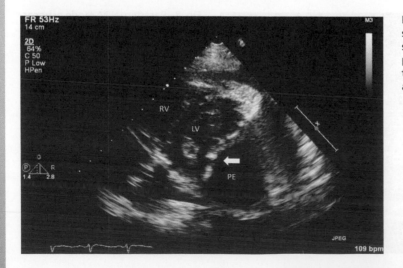

Fig. 10. Early diastolic parasternal short axis 2D echocardiogram showing LV inversion (*arrow*). PE, pericardial effusion. The dynamic nature of this finding is better appreciated in Video 3.

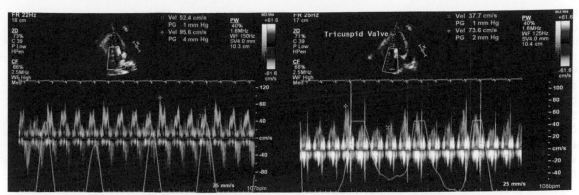

Fig. 11. Pulsed Doppler spectra of mitral (*left panel*) and tricuspid (*right panel*) inflow recorded from an apical 4-chamber view. Note the exaggerated respirophasic changes. The respirometer tracing is the green line on the bottom with a rise corresponding to inspiration. In inspiration, there is an exaggerated increase in transtricuspid velocities with a reciprocal decrease in transmitral flow. This pattern corresponds to pulsus paradoxus and is not specific to tamponade.

hemodynamic effect, multiple factors are important when considering treatment. These include (1) the medical history of the patient; (2) confirming a pericardial effusion is present, whether it is circumferential or loculated and estimating its size; (3) determining an etiology if possible; (4) estimating the effusion's chronicity by the size of the effusion relative to its hemodynamic effect; (5) evaluating whether IPP is elevated, and if so what is the systemic venous pressure and severity of cardiac tamponade; and 6) determining whether pericardiocentesis or open drainage is indicated and what is its urgency.

Regardless of pericardial effusion size, the presence of tachycardia, tachypnea, pulsus paradoxus, and echo-Doppler features of cardiac tamponade (cardiac chamber collapse and increased respiratory variation of transvalvular flow velocities) indicate a potentially life-threatening situation that needs immediate and thorough evaluation. With increasing numbers of invasive cardiac procedures and surgery, any patient with unexplained postoperative hypotension should have an emergency echo to rule out low pericardial volume hemorrhagic cardiac tamponade.

If a patient with a pericardial effusion is in the intensive care unit with hemodynamic monitoring, several useful hemodynamic variables may be available to assess tamponade severity. An arterial pressure line can confirm pulsus paradoxus and show the magnitude of the decrease and increase in pulse pressure and LV ejection time with inspiration and expiration; the more variation usually the more severe hemodynamic compromise. If a pulmonary artery catheter is in place, comparison of mean RA, mean pulmonary wedge, and RV end-diastolic pressure is useful, with equalization and a reduced cardiac output by

thermodilution technique indicating severe tamponade. At heart rates greater than 110 beats per minute, pulmonary artery diastolic pressure may be higher and not equalized with the other end-diastolic pressures because of insufficient time for the pressure to fall to this pressure. An RA or central venous catheter recording that shows only an X descent and absent Y descent with elevated pressure also suggests severe cardiac tamponade. If a mixed venous O2 is available with cardiac output estimation, falling values suggest worsening tamponade regardless of systemic blood pressure.

In patients who are not in the intensive care unit, the previously discussed echo-Doppler techniques may be used to gauge the severity of tamponade. If systemic venous pressure is low by 2D imaging of the inferior vena cava, fluid or blood should be given until the inferior vena cava no longer collapses, which will at least temporarily improve RA filling and cardiac output.

We believe the most specific signs of urgency of drainage in cardiac tamponade are found in PW recordings of hepatic vein flow velocities. This is because it is the reduction in right heart filling that reduces cardiac output and, when critically reduced, leads to cardiovascular collapse and death. In healthy individuals, hepatic venous flow into the heart as recorded by PW Doppler shows that systolic flow predominates over diastolic flow but both augment with inspiration.[43] As IPP increases with a pericardial effusion, RA pressure rises faster than systemic venous pressure so the veno-atrial gradient decreases and hepatic venous velocities and their TVIs decrease. With more severe tamponade, blood can only enter the right heart when cardiac volume is decreasing during systolic ejection so that the diastolic component decreases and then disappears. Typically at this point, systolic hepatic flow velocities have decreased to approximately 20 cm/s and diastolic forward flow velocities are seen only with inspiration, where a blunted increase in both velocities is seen because of rapid equilibration of venous and atrial pressure. As the veno-RA gradient becomes further compromised, diastolic filling disappears all together, and systolic forward flow velocity and TVI fall further, signifying severe tamponade that needs immediate drainage.

A final preterminal stage of cardiac tamponade seen in hepatic venous flow is observed when there is no right heart inflow during expiration and apnea signifying that there is no pressure gradient between the systemic veins and RA at these times. Flow into the heart is seen only with inspiration, which reduces right heart pressures, and, in effect, inspiration and tachypnea are keeping the patient alive. This is an unstable stage that usually deteriorates rapidly into "the final drop" of cardiovascular collapse and death. In our experience, this is a vagal-like reflex with bradycardia and vasodilation from which the patients cannot be resuscitated, even if pericardial drainage is performed.

The therapeutic approach to all forms of tamponade that exhibit a low cardiac output and loss of hepatic venous diastolic filling is to arrange echo-guided pericardiocentesis emergently. Because the terminal event of tamponade appears to be partially vagal in nature with marked systemic vasodilation, we prophylactically administer 2 mg of intravenous atropine to patients who have no diastolic flow in the hepatic veins even with inspiration, or no forward flow at all except with inspiration. The latter patients are in a true medical emergency and may need an urgent pericardiocentesis at bedside, without trying to transport them to the catheterization laboratory. As in all severe cardiac tamponade, even the removal of a small amount of pericardial fluid results in a large decrease in IPP (see **Fig. 2**) and improvement in patient hemodynamics, cardiac output, and symptoms.

Pericardiocentesis should be performed preferably using echocardiographic guidance[44] that includes confirming the presence of the pericardiocentesis needle in the pericardial space with the injection of a small amount of agitated saline and noting the reduction in the pericardial effusion and resolution of echocardiographic markers of tamponade as fluid is withdrawn. A detailed discussion of pericardiocentesis techniques is beyond the scope of this article (see Bernhard Maisch and colleagues' "Percutaneous Therapy in Pericardial Diseases," in this issue). In some patients, surgical creation of a pericardial window may be more appropriate.

SUPPLEMENTARY DATA

Supplementary data related to this article can be found online at http://dx.doi.org/10.1016/j.ccl. 2017.07.006.

REFERENCES

1. Spodick DH. The pericardium. A comprehensive textbook. New York: Mercel Dekker; 1997.
2. Shabetai RF, Mangiardi LF, Bhargava VF, et al. The pericardium and cardiac function. Prog Cardiovasc Dis 1979;22(2):107–34.
3. Tsang TSM, Enriquez-Sarano M, Freeman WK, et al. Consecutive 1127 therapeutic echocardiographically guided pericardiocenteses: clinical profile, practice patterns, and outcomes spanning 21 Years. Mayo Clin Proc 2002;77(5):429–36.
4. Shabetai R. Cardiac tamponade. In: Shabetai R, editor. The pericardium. New York: Grune and Stratton; 1981. p. 121–66.
5. Gabe IT, Mason DT, Gault JH, et al. Effect of respiration on venous return and stroke volume in cardiac tamponade. Br Heart J 1970;32(5):592.
6. Fowler NO, Gabel M. The hemodynamic effects of cardiac tamponade: mainly the result of atrial, not ventricular, compression. Circulation 1985; 71(1):154.
7. Reddy PS, Curtiss EI, Toole JD, et al. Cardiac tamponade: hemodynamic observations in man. Circulation 1978;58(2):265.
8. Reddy PS. Hemodynamics of cardiac tamponade in man. In: Reddy PS, editor. Pericardial disease. New York: Raven Press; 1982. p. 161–82.
9. Shabetai R, Fowler NO, Fenton JC, et al. Pulsus paradoxus. J Clin Invest 1965;44(11):1882–98.
10. Guntheroth WG, Morgan BC, Mullins GL, et al. Effect of respiration on venous return and stroke volume in cardiac tamponade. Circ Res 1967;20(4):381.
11. Ditchey R, Engler R, LeWinter M, et al. The role of the right heart in acute cardiac tamponade in dogs. Circ Res 1981;48(5):701.
12. D'Cruz IA, Cohen HC, Prabhu R, et al. Diagnosis of cardiac tamponade by echocardiography: changes in mitral valve motion and ventricular dimensions, with special reference to paradoxical pulse. Circulation 1975;52(3):460.
13. Reddy PS, Curtiss EI, Uretsky BF. Spectrum of hemodynamic changes in cardiac tamponade. Am J Cardiol 1990;66(20):1487–91.
14. Shabetai R. Pericardial effusion: haemodynamic spectrum. Heart 2004;90(3):255.
15. Gonzalez MS, Basnight MA, Appleton CP. Experimental pericardial effusion: relation of abnormal respiratory variation in mitral flow velocity to hemodynamics and diastolic right heart collapse. J Am Coll Cardiol 1991;17(1):239–48.

16. Candell-Riera J. Tamponade and constriction: an appraisal of echocardiography and external pulse recordings. In: Soler-Soler J, editor. Pericardial disease. Boston: Kluwer Academic Publishers; 1990. p. 17–28.
17. Antman EM, Cargill V, Grossman W. Low-pressure cardiac tamponade. Ann Intern Med 1979;91(3):403–6.
18. Curtiss EI, Reddy PS, Uretsky BF, et al. Pulsus paradoxus: definition and relation to the severity of cardiac tamponade. Am Heart J 1988;115(2):391–8.
19. Settle HP, Adolph RJ, Fowler NO, et al. Echocardiographic study of cardiac tamponade. Circulation 1977;56(6):951.
20. Appleton CP, Hatle LK, Popp RL. Cardiac tamponade and pericardial effusion: respiratory variation in transvalvular flow velocities studied by Doppler echocardiography. J Am Coll Cardiol 1988;11(5):1020–30.
21. Gonzalez MS, Basnight MA, Appleton CP. Experimental cardiac tamponade: a hemodynamic and Doppler echocardiographic reexamination of the relation of right and left heart ejection dynamics to the phase of respiration. J Am Coll Cardiol 1991;18(1):243–52.
22. Shabetai R, Fowler NO, Guntheroth WG. The hemodynamics of cardiac tamponade and constrictive pericarditis. Am J Cardiol 1970;26(5):480–9.
23. Shabetai R. The pathophysiology of pulsus paradoxus in cardiac tamponade. In: Reddy PS, editor. Pericardial disease. New York: Raven Press; 1982. p. 215–30.
24. Dornhorst AC, Howard P, Laethart GL. Pulsus paradoxus. Lancet 1952;259(6711):746–8.
25. Murgo JP, Uhl GS, Felter HG. Right and left heart ejection dynamics during pericardial tamponade in man. In: Reddy PS, editor. Pericardial disease. New York: Raven Press; 1982. p. 189–201.
26. Leeman DE, Levine MJ, Come PC. Doppler echocardiography in cardiac tamponade: exaggerated respiratory variation in transvalvular blood flow velocity integrals. J Am Coll Cardiol 1988;11(3):572–8.
27. Burstow DJ, Oh JK, Bailey KR, et al. Cardiac tamponade: characteristic Doppler observations. Mayo Clin Proc 1989;64(3):312–24.
28. Ruskin J, Bache R, Rembert J, et al. Pressure-flow studies in man: effect of respiration on left ventricular stroke volume. Circulation 1973;48(1):79.
29. Katz L, Gauchat HW. Observations on pulsus paradoxus with special reference to pericardial effusions. II. Experimental. Arch Intern Med 1924;33:371–93.
30. Fitchett DH, Sniderman AD. Inspiratory reduction in left heart filling as a mechanism of pulsus paradoxus in cardiac tamponade. Can J Cardiol 1990;6(8):348–54.
31. Hoit BD, Gabel M, Fowler NO. Cardiac tamponade in left ventricular dysfunction. Circulation 1990;82(4):1370.
32. Gillam LD, Guyer DE, Gibson TC, et al. Hydrodynamic compression of the right atrium: a new echocardiographic sign of cardiac tamponade. Circulation 1983;68(2):294–301.
33. Armstrong WF, Schilt BF, Helper DJ, et al. Diastolic collapse of the right ventricle with cardiac tamponade: an echocardiographic study. Circulation 1982;65(7):1491–6.
34. Singh S, Wann LS, Schuchard GH, et al. Right ventricular and right atrial collapse in patients with cardiac tamponade–a combined echocardiographic and hemodynamic study. Circulation 1984;70(6):966–71.
35. Klopfenstein HS, Cogswell TL, Bernath GA, et al. Alterations in intravascular volume affect the relation between right ventricular diastolic collapse and the hemodynamic severity of cardiac tamponade. J Am Coll Cardiol 1985;6(5):1057–63.
36. Leimgruber PP, Klopfenstein HS, Wann LS, et al. The hemodynamic derangement associated with right ventricular diastolic collapse in cardiac tamponade: an experimental echocardiographic study. Circulation 1983;68(3):612.
37. Kronzon I, Cohen ML, Winer HE. Diastolic atrial compression: a sensitive echocardiographic sign of cardiac tamponade. J Am Coll Cardiol 1983;2(4):770–5.
38. Hoit BD, Shaw D. The paradoxical pulse in tamponade: mechanisms and echocardiography correlates. Echocardiography 1994;11(5):477–87.
39. Schiller NB, Botvinick EH. Right ventricular compression as a sign of cardiac tamponade: an analysis of echocardiographic ventricular dimensions and their clinical implications. Circulation 1977;56(5):774.
40. Klein AL, Abbara S, Agler DA, et al. American Society of Echocardiography Clinical Recommendations for multimodality cardiovascular imaging of patients with pericardial disease: endorsed by the Society for Cardiovascular Magnetic Resonance and Society of Cardiovascular Computed Tomography. J Am Soc Echocardiogr 2013;26(9):965–1012.
41. Singh S, Wann LS, Klopfenstein HS, et al. Usefulness of right ventricular diastolic collapse in diagnosing cardiac tamponade and comparison to pulsus paradoxus. Am J Cardiol 1986;57(8):652–6.
42. Klopfenstein HS, Schuchard GH, Wann LS, et al. The relative merits of pulsus paradoxus and right ventricular diastolic collapse in the early detection of cardiac tamponade: an experimental echocardiographic study. Circulation 1985;71(4):829.
43. Appleton CP, Hatle LK, Popp RL. Superior vena cava and hepatic vein Doppler echocardiography in healthy adults. J Am Coll Cardiol 1987;10(5):1032–9.
44. Tsang TSM, Freeman WK, Sinak LJ, et al. Echocardiographically guided pericardiocentesis: evolution and state-of-the-art technique. Mayo Clin Proc 1998;73(7):647–52.

Constrictive Pericarditis

Terrence D. Welch, MD[a,b,*], Jae K. Oh, MD[c]

KEYWORDS

- Constrictive pericarditis • Heart failure • Cardiac MR • Echocradiography

KEY POINTS

- Constrictive pericarditis is a disorder of cardiac filling caused by a diseased, inelastic pericardium that restricts cardiac chamber expansion.
- Patients present with heart failure symptoms and signs, including dyspnea on exertion, increased venous pressure, and edema.
- Key pathophysiologic features include dissociation of intrathoracic and intracardiac pressures and enhanced ventricular interaction.
- Key echocardiographic features include respiration-related changes in the position of the ventricular septum and Doppler velocities; the myocardium exhibits unique diastolic properties and systolic strain.
- Invasive hemodynamic assessment is the gold standard diagnostic test and requires careful simultaneous recordings of right and left ventricular pressures, ideally with high-fidelity manometer-tipped catheters.

INTRODUCTION

Constrictive pericarditis masquerades as diastolic heart failure, but is distinct in terms of its cause and treatment. A diseased, inelastic pericardium restricts cardiac filling and leads to unique hemodynamic derangements. Recognizing this disorder requires an index of suspicion, a careful history and physical examination, meticulous cardiac imaging, and often invasive hemodynamic assessment. Accurate identification of constrictive pericarditis markedly changes the therapeutic plan for the affected patient. A minority may find relief through antiinflammatory therapies. Others require and benefit from surgical pericardiectomy.

ETIOLOGIES

Tuberculosis was historically the most common cause for constrictive pericarditis in North America; a report from 1962 cited tuberculosis as the cause of 48% of cases of constrictive pericarditis.[1]

Worldwide, this likely remains the case, particularly in areas where human immunodeficiency virus and AIDS are most prevalent. A South African institution reported 121 cases of constrictive pericarditis over 22 years (1990–2012) and of these, tuberculosis was confirmed as the cause in 29.8% of cases and suspected in an additional 61.2% of cases.[2]

In North America and Europe, tuberculosis is now a relatively rare cause of constrictive pericarditis, with reports ranging from less than 1% to 5.6% of cases.[3–6]

- The 3 dominant etiologies reported now in North America and Europe are idiopathic, prior cardiac surgery, and radiation therapy.

For example, the Mayo Clinic reported 135 cases over 10 years (1985–1995) and classified 80% as being idiopathic or owing to prior cardiac surgery, acute pericarditis, or radiation therapy.[3] Also noted was an increase in frequency of cases

Disclosure Statement: The author has no disclosures to make.
[a] Section of Cardiology, Dartmouth-Hitchcock Medical Center, One Medical Center Drive, Lebanon, NH 03756, USA; [b] Department of Internal Medicine, Geisel School of Medicine at Dartmouth, 1 Rope Ferry Road, Hanover, NH 03755, USA; [c] Cardiovascular Diseases, Mayo Clinic, 200 1st Street SW, Rochester, MN 55905, USA
* Corresponding author. Dartmouth-Hitchcock Medical Center, One Medical Center Drive, Lebanon, NH 03756.
E-mail address: Terrence.D.Welch@hitchcock.org

Cardiol Clin 35 (2017) 539–549
http://dx.doi.org/10.1016/j.ccl.2017.07.007
0733-8651/17/© 2017 Elsevier Inc. All rights reserved.

cardiology.theclinics.com

owing to prior cardiac surgery or radiation therapy compared with an historic cohort. The remaining cases were due to rheumatologic disease, infection, malignancy, trauma, asbestosis, drug-induced causes, and complicated pacemaker lead replacement. Other presumably rare causes of constrictive pericarditis include immunoglobulin G4-related disease and Whipple's disease.[7,8]

EPIDEMIOLOGY

Constrictive pericarditis seems to be a relatively rare disorder. Neither the prevalence nor overall incidence of constrictive pericarditis is known. A specific etiologic type, constrictive pericarditis occurring after an episode of acute pericarditis, has been studied and has a low incidence of 1.8%.[9] Constrictive pericarditis is less common after idiopathic or viral pericarditis than after pericarditis owing to connective tissue disease, pericardial injury syndrome, neoplasm, or bacterial infection.

PATHOLOGY

Pathologic changes in constriction most commonly affect the parietal pericardium, but may also affect the visceral pericardium and even the underlying epicardium. In chronic constrictive pericarditis, which develops over months to years, the pericardium is typically fibrotic and calcified. Thickening of the pericardium is often found, but is not required for the disorder to occur. In fact, the thickness of surgically removed constrictive pericardium has been reported to be normal in 18% of cases.[10] In subacute constrictive pericarditis, which develops over days to weeks, inflammation seems to be the dominant pathologic abnormality. These cases of

constrictive pericarditis are more likely to be transient and medically treatable.

PATHOPHYSIOLOGY

The diseased pericardium loses its reserve volume and begins to restrict cardiac chamber expansion. Two fundamental pathophysiologic principles are recognized when this occurs:

1. Dissociation of intrapleural and intracardiac pressures, and
2. Enhanced ventricular interaction.[11]

The principle of dissociation of intrapleural and intracardiac pressures is due to the insulating effects of the diseased pericardium on the cardiac chambers, such that intracardiac pressures no longer change to the same degree as intrapleural pressures during the respiratory cycle.

- In inspiration, intrapleural pressure decreases, but left atrial pressure decreases more modestly, if at all. This reduces the pressure gradient from pulmonary veins (which are intrapleural) to the left atrium, which in turn reduces left heart filling. The interventricular septum shifts toward the left ventricle and right heart filling is favored, which illustrates the principle of enhanced ventricular interaction (Fig. 1).
- During expiration, these phenomena are reversed: intrapleural pressure increases, the pressure gradient between the pulmonary veins and the left atrium is restored, left heart filling increases, the interventricular septum shifts to the right, and right heart filling decreases. The principles of dissociation of intrapleural and intracardiac pressures and

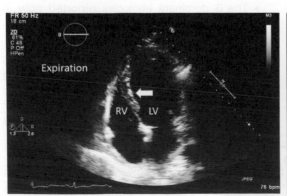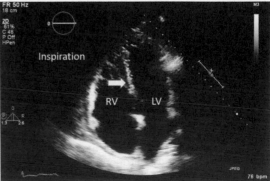

Fig. 1. Enhanced ventricular interaction in constrictive pericarditis. Note the respiration-related shift in the position of the interventricular septum (and relative sizes of the right and left ventricles) in these apical 4-chamber images. The septum shifts (*arrows*) toward the right during expiration (*left panel*) and toward the left during inspiration (*right panel*). LV, left ventricle; RV, right ventricle.

enhanced ventricular interaction are unique to constriction and serve as the foundation for the echocardiographic and invasive hemodynamic evaluation in suspected cases.

As it advances, constrictive pericarditis leads to progressively restricted ventricular filling. Atrial pressures increase and drive rapid early diastolic filling, which abruptly terminates when the ventricle reaches the volume limit imposed by the constrictive pericardium. Diastolic pressures equalize in the cardiac chambers. Cardiac output is compromised and venous pressure increases.

CLINICAL MANIFESTATIONS
Symptoms and Signs

Patients with constrictive pericarditis typically develop an insidious heart failure syndrome with dyspnea on exertion and edema as the most common symptoms.[3] Less commonly, patients may present with chest discomfort, abdominal symptoms, tamponade, an atrial arrhythmia, a recurrent pleural effusion, or liver disease.

Physical Examination

- Almost all patients with constrictive pericarditis have increased venous pressure, making evaluation of the jugular venous waveform the most important component of the physical examination. Aside from being elevated, the pressure waveform is notable because of the steep, deep, y-descent that corresponds with rapid (owing to elevated atrial pressure) and abbreviated (owing to the volume constraint imposed by the abnormal pericardium) early diastolic ventricular filling. The jugular venous pressure may increase with inspiration, which has been termed a Kussmaul sign. Occasionally, patients with constrictive pericarditis may not have an increased jugular venous pressure. This may occur if the constrictive process is mild or if the patient is hypovolemic. Volume loading may be required to reveal constrictive hemodynamics in these cases of occult constriction.[12]
- Lung auscultation may be normal or suggest a pleural effusion.
- On cardiac auscultation, an extra sound may be heard in early diastole and is termed a pericardial knock. The sound corresponds to the abrupt cessation of ventricular filling and occurs at the nadir of the y-descent, or slightly earlier than a typical third heart sound (S3).
- A pulsus paradoxus, defined as a significant (>10 mm Hg) decrease in the systolic arterial

blood pressure from expiration to inspiration, may be noted in constrictive pericarditis. This phenomenon relates to the concepts of dissociation of intrapleural and intracardiac pressures and enhanced ventricular interaction that were described previously.
- Examination of the abdomen may reveal an enlarged and sometimes pulsatile liver along with ascites.
- When constrictive pericarditis is in an advanced stage, cachexia may also be noted.

DIAGNOSIS

Constrictive pericarditis may be difficult to differentiate from other causes of diastolic heart failure or right-sided heart failure. Restrictive cardiomyopathy manifests almost identically and is the classic contending diagnosis. Other diagnostic entities to consider include right ventricular infarction, severe pulmonary hypertension, and severe tricuspid regurgitation. Because diagnosis is challenging, many patients may be undiagnosed or misdiagnosed for some time before constrictive pericarditis is identified accurately. Constrictive pericarditis should, therefore, be considered in all patients presenting with unexplained jugular venous pressure elevation, edema, pleural effusion, or liver disease, particularly if there are risk factors such as prior cardiac surgery or chest irradiation.

Diagnostic workup requires careful integration of historical features, examination findings, laboratory results, and cardiac testing. The initial evaluation includes an electrocardiogram, laboratory workup, chest radiograph, and echocardiogram.

Electrocardiogram

There are no electrocardiographic features that can be relied on to diagnose constrictive pericarditis. Findings could include sinus tachycardia or nonspecific ST-segment and T-wave changes. A minority of patients with constriction have been reported to have low voltage or atrial fibrillation.[10]

Laboratory Data

The initial laboratory workup generally yields nonspecific results. In some cases, liver function tests may be abnormal because of hepatic congestion.

- The plasma brain natriuretic peptide level may be useful in diagnosis, because it tends to be more elevated in restrictive cardiomyopathy and may actually be low in constrictive pericarditis.[13]

Chest Radiograph

Chest radiographic abnormalities, if present, are also typically nonspecific, with pulmonary vascular congestion or pleural effusion being demonstrated in many cases.[10]

- Pericardial calcification is a very helpful finding, because it strongly suggests the diagnosis of chronic constrictive pericarditis (most commonly idiopathic; see **Fig. 3**). This finding was reported in 27% of patients in a large case series.[14]

Comprehensive Echocardiography with Doppler Evaluation

A standard echocardiogram is indicated for all patients suspected to have heart failure, and allows exclusion of common causes such as ventricular systolic dysfunction, valvular heart disease, and pulmonary hypertension. Evidence for constrictive physiology may be present but overlooked if a pericardial disease protocol is not included as part of the study. The examination should include extended clips with simultaneous recording of

respiration to most accurately confirm the presence of constriction and exclude restriction.

- Special attention should be given to the 5 principal echocardiographic findings that were evaluated in the largest and only blinded comparison of patients with constriction (n = 130) versus patients with restriction or severe tricuspid regurgitation (n = 36) at the Mayo Clinic[15] (**Fig. 2**).
- Myocardial strain imaging has also emerged as a helpful adjunct in the diagnosis.

The previously described principles of dissociation of intrapleural and intracardiac pressures and enhanced ventricular interaction underlie many of the echocardiographic features of constrictive pericarditis.

Respiration-Related Ventricular Septal Shift

With inspiration, left heart filling decreases and the interventricular septum shifts to the left (see **Figs. 1** and **2**). With expiration, left heart filling increases and the interventricular septum shifts to the right. This phenomenon may range from subtle to obvious and is best assessed with a combination of 2-dimensional (with extended clips) and M-mode echocardiographic assessment. With a reported sensitivity of 93%, a respiration-related

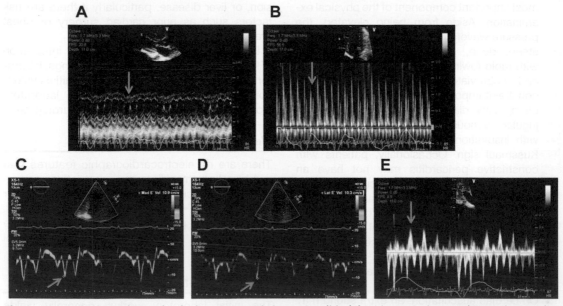

Fig. 2. Principal echocardiographic findings in constrictive pericarditis. (*A*) Mid-ventricular septal M-mode recording (parasternal long axis). Note leftward ventricular septal shift in inspiration (*arrow*). (*B*) Pulsed-wave Doppler recording (apical window) of mitral inflow. Note inspiratory decrease in early (*E*) inflow velocity (*arrow*). (*C*) Medial and (*D*) lateral mitral annular tissue Doppler recordings (apical window). Early (*e'*) diastolic tissue velocities are marked by arrows. Note normal to increased early relaxation velocity (*e'*), with medial velocity slightly greater than lateral. (*E*) Pulsed-wave Doppler recording (subcostal window) within the hepatic vein. Note prominent end-diastolic flow reversals with expiration (*arrow*). (*Adapted from* Welch TD, Ling LH, Espinosa RE, et al. Echocardiographic diagnosis of constrictive pericarditis: Mayo Clinic criteria. Circ Cardiovasc Imaging 2014;7(3):526–34.)

ventricular septal shift may be the most important echocardiographic finding for constriction.[15]

There is also a beat-to-beat shudder of the ventricular septum that likely reflects ventricular interdependence on a millisecond time scale (owing to differences in timing of tricuspid and mitral valve opening).[16] The shudder resembles other causes of abnormal ventricular septal motion (eg, conduction abnormalities and postpericardiotomy status) and is therefore thought to be less diagnostic for constriction than the respiration-related septal shift.

Respiration-Related Variation in Hepatic Vein Doppler Profile

With expiration, left heart filling increases at the expense of right heart filling and the interventricular septum shifts to the right. Hepatic vein diastolic forward flow decreases and there is a prominent reversal of flow at the end of diastole (see **Fig. 2**).[11,17] With inspiration, right heart filling is again favored, which leads to increased hepatic vein diastolic forward flow and less prominent or no reversal of flow at the end of diastole. Although probably the most technically difficult finding to show with Doppler echocardiography, prominent hepatic vein diastolic flow reversal during expiration has a high degree of specificity and is independently associated with a diagnosis of constrictive pericarditis.[15]

Respiration-Related Variation in Mitral Inflow Velocities

With inspiration, decreased left heart filling is manifested through a reduction in mitral early (E) velocity (see **Fig. 2**). With expiration, the mitral E velocity increases. The currently recommended method for calculating the percent change in mitral E velocity is as follows: [(expiratory velocity − inspiratory velocity)/expiratory velocity × 100].[18] Variation in E velocity ranges from 15% to 35% in constriction.[11,15,17,19] Variation of 10% to 15% has been found to be sufficient for differentiating constriction from restriction.[15,19] However, variation in mitral E velocity should not be considered essential to the echocardiographic diagnosis of constriction, because it may not be present when left atrial pressure is very high, is unreliable in the setting of atrial arrhythmias, and has not been found to have an independent association with constriction.[15]

Unique Mitral Annular Tissue Doppler Profile

Preserved or elevated early diastolic mitral annular relaxation velocity

Early diastolic mitral annular tissue velocity (e') is a measure of ventricular diastolic relaxation and is typically reduced in restrictive cardiomyopathy and other forms of heart failure owing to myocardial disease. In constrictive pericarditis, however, the myocardium is usually spared and is capable of demonstrating normal to supranormal e' velocities. Accordingly, finding a normal or increased e' velocity in a patient with heart failure strongly suggests a diagnosis of constrictive pericarditis, and has been shown to be independently associated with the diagnosis.[15,20,21] A medial e' velocity of 9 cm/s or greater seems to be an optimal cutpoint for identifying constriction, with a sensitivity of 83% and a sensitivity of 81%.[15] However, it must be remembered that this velocity may be affected by mitral annular calcification or concomitant myocardial disease, such that some patients with constriction (particularly after cardiac surgery or radiation) will have lower e' velocities.[15,22]

Annulus reversus

In contrast with the normal pattern, the medial e' velocity often equals or exceeds the lateral e' velocity in constriction (see **Fig. 2**). Termed annulus reversus, this phenomenon is likely due to tethering of the lateral myocardium by the constricting pericardium, with compensatory exuberant diastolic relaxation of the septal myocardium.[23]

Annulus paradoxus

Because the e' velocity tends to be preserved or increased in constriction, the E/e' ratio, often looked at as a marker of left-sided filling pressure, does not perform as expected. In other words, despite having high filling pressures, patients with constriction will have lower-than-expected E/e' velocity ratios. This phenomenon has been termed annulus paradoxus.[24]

Mayo Clinic Criteria

The Mayo Clinic group evaluated the test performance characteristics of these echocardiographic findings in a group of 130 patients with surgically confirmed constrictive pericarditis compared with 36 patients with restrictive cardiomyopathy or severe tricuspid regurgitation.[15] The 3 most important findings, based on independent association with the diagnosis of constriction, were (1) respiration-related ventricular septal shift, (2) preserved or increased medial mitral e' velocity, and (3) prominent hepatic vein expiratory diastolic flow reversals. These findings performed well even in the setting of atrial fibrillation or flutter. The presence of ventricular septal shift in combination with either a medial e' of 9 cm/s or greater or a hepatic vein expiratory diastolic reversal ratio of 0.79 or greater was 87% sensitive and 91% specific for the diagnosis of constrictive pericarditis.

Myocardial strain imaging

Speckle tracking strain imaging has also emerged as an important tool for differentiating constriction from restriction and other forms of heart failure. Global longitudinal strain is more likely to be preserved in constriction and reduced in restriction.[25] Circumferential strain, in contrast, is more likely to be reduced in constriction. There is also a unique regional longitudinal strain pattern that has been demonstrated in constriction, in which the lateral ventricular strain is reduced as compared with the septal ventricular strain.[26] This is likely due to the tethering effects of the constrictive pericardium.

Other echocardiographic findings

Two additional echocardiographic findings that are expected in constriction are:

1. Plethora of the inferior vena cava, and
2. Superior vena cava velocities that do not vary much with respiration.

These findings do not allow differentiation from restriction, but are expected in the setting of increased venous pressure. The relatively flat Doppler velocity pattern in the superior vena cava is particularly helpful when evaluating patients with severe lung disease, in whom dramatic intrathoracic pressure swings may cause echocardiographic findings that mimic the enhanced ventricular interaction expected in constriction. Significant changes in superior vena cava velocities in this setting provide the clue that constriction is not actually present.[27]

Additional findings that may be helpful in identifying constriction include:

1. Distortion of the ventricular contour by the constrictive pericardium, and
2. Tethering of the right ventricular free wall at its interface with the liver.[15]

In summary, the comprehensive, pericardial protocol echocardiogram with Doppler allows a detailed assessment of cardiac structure and function and in many cases of constriction will provide diagnostic evidence. Additional investigation thereafter will depend on the degree to which the echocardiographic findings are considered to be diagnostic, the clinical suspicion for constriction, and institutional practice patterns. Options include computed tomography (CT) scanning, cardiac MRI, and invasive hemodynamic catheterization.

Computed Tomography Scanning

- CT scanning is useful for assessing thickness of the pericardium and the extent of calcification, if any[28] (**Fig. 3**). Such abnormalities are helpful when present, but are not required for the diagnosis of constriction. In a study of 143 patients with surgically confirmed constriction, 97 underwent preoperative CT scanning; of those, 35% had pericardial calcification and 72% had pericardial thickening.[10]
- Deformation of the ventricular contour on CT, analogous to that sometimes seen with echocardiographic imaging, is suggestive of constrictive pericarditis.
- CT scanning may also be helpful in preoperative planning, such that the relationship of the pericardium to vascular and other important thoracic structures may be delineated.[18]

Cardiac MRI

Gated cardiac MRI has become integral to the diagnosis and management of constrictive pericarditis because of the information that it provides on anatomy, cardiac hemodynamic abnormalities, and tissue characterization.

- Characteristic findings include pericardial thickening and pericardial–myocardial adherence.[18]
- Real-time cine imaging allows detection of the same respiration-related ventricular septal shift that is evident with echocardiography.
- Respiratory variation across the mitral and tricuspid valves may also be examined, although this is more technically difficult.[29]
- Delayed imaging after the administration of gadolinium may reveal enhancement of the pericardium (see **Fig. 3**). Such delayed gadolinium enhancement has been shown to correspond to increased fibroblast proliferation and neovascularization, as well as more prominent chronic inflammation and granulation tissue.[30] Constriction with delayed gadolinium enhancement of the pericardium has also been shown to be more likely to respond to antiinflammatory therapy, making cardiac MRI an important part of treatment planning.[31]

Hemodynamic Catheterization

Still considered to be the gold standard diagnostic test for constrictive pericarditis, cardiac catheterization with hemodynamic assessment is performed when noninvasive studies are nondiagnostic or are considered to be insufficiently

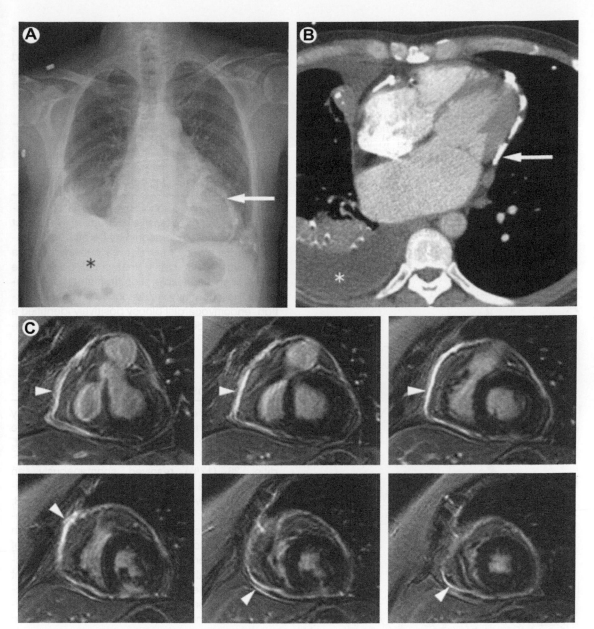

Fig. 3. Radiographic imaging findings in constrictive pericarditis. (*A, B*) Pericardial calcification (*arrows*) and a right pleural effusion (*asterisks*) by chest radiography and computed tomography scanning, respectively. (*C*) Delayed gadolinium enhancement (*arrowheads*) of the circumferential pericardium a patient with constrictive pericarditis. This finding suggests inflammation of the pericardium that may respond to antiinflammatory therapy. (*From* Syed FF, Schaff HV, Oh JK. Constrictive pericarditis–a curable diastolic heart failure. Nat Rev Cardiol 2014;11(9):530–44.)

conclusive.[32] There are several classic hemodynamic features of constrictive pericarditis:

- Increased central venous pressure;
- Near-equalization of right and left heart filling pressures;
- Modest elevation in right ventricular systolic pressure (<50 mm Hg); and

- A right ventricular end-diastolic pressure that is at least one-third of the right ventricular systolic pressure.

These classic features, however, may also be seen in restrictive cardiomyopathy and are therefore insufficient to establish the diagnosis.[33]

- The modern hemodynamic criteria are based on the principle of enhanced ventricular interaction, as discussed elsewhere in this article. The heightened interaction between the ventricles may be detected through simultaneous evaluation of right and left ventricular pressures, ideally using high-fidelity manometer-tipped catheters. The ventricular systolic pressures will be expected to vary discordantly during the respiratory cycle in constrictive pericarditis, as opposed to the concordant variation expected in restrictive cardiomyopathy (**Fig. 4**). An increased ratio of right ventricular to left ventricular systolic area (systolic area index) has been shown to have a sensitivity of 97% and a predictive accuracy of 100% for the identification of

patients with surgically proven constrictive pericarditis.[34] Dissociation of intrapleural and intracardiac pressures may also be detected through careful inspection of simultaneous pulmonary capillary wedge pressure and left ventricular diastolic pressure tracings.

The principal imaging- and catheterization-based findings in constriction are summarized in **Box 1**.

Biopsy and Surgical Exploration

Occasionally, the diagnosis may remain in question, even after extensive evaluation. In select cases, surgical exploration may be offered. Endomyocardial biopsy may also be considered as a less invasive alternative that could obviate the need for surgical exploration. In a study of 54 patients thought to have either constriction or restriction, endomyocardial biopsy positively identified a restrictive cardiomyopathy in approximately one-third of cases.[35]

TREATMENT
Transient Constrictive Pericarditis

In a minority of cases, constrictive pericarditis may be due to an inflammatory process and resolve spontaneously or with antiinflammatory treatment. In a review of 212 cases of constrictive pericarditis, 36 (17%) resolved spontaneously, an average of 8.3 weeks after diagnosis.[36] An effusive–constrictive process (described in William R. Miranda and Jae K. Oh's article, "Effusive-Constrictive Pericarditis," in this issue), in which pericardial fluid accumulates between layers of constrictive pericardium, was identified in the majority (67%) of these cases. Most cases of transient constriction seem to be idiopathic or due to infection, trauma, or malignancy. Identification of pericardial inflammation is best accomplished through the use of cardiac MRI, as previously described, with delayed gadolinium enhancement of the pericardium indicating an inflammatory and potentially reversible process[31] (see **Fig. 3C**). Recent evidence suggests that PET and CT imaging using ^{18}F-labeled fluorodeoxyglucose is an effective alternative imaging modality for assessing pericardial inflammation and predicting response to antiinflammatory therapy.[37]

- When there is evidence for pericardial inflammation, and markers of chronic constriction (eg, cachexia, atrial fibrillation, pericardial calcification, or hepatic dysfunction) are absent, a 2- to 3-month trial of antiinflammatory therapy is therefore appropriate.[32]

A

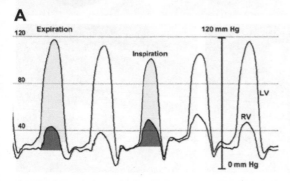

B

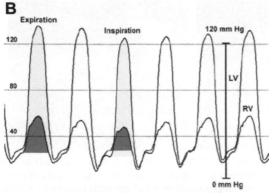

Fig. 4. High-fidelity pressure tracings in a patient with (A) constrictive pericarditis and (B) restrictive cardiomyopathy. (A) In constriction, the area under the right ventricular (RV) systolic pressure curve (*orange shaded area*) increases and the area under the left ventricular (LV) systolic pressure curve (*yellow shaded area*) decreases. This discordance is due to enhanced ventricular interaction. (B) In restriction, the areas under the RV and LV systolic pressure curves decrease concordantly during inspiration. (*From* Talreja DR, Nishimura RA, Oh JK, et al. Constrictive pericarditis in the modern era: novel criteria for diagnosis in the cardiac catheterization laboratory. J Am Coll Cardiol 2008;51:315–9.)

Box 1
Principal diagnostic findings in constrictive pericarditis

Echocardiography

- Two-dimensional: respiration-related ventricular septal shift and plethora of the inferior vena cava
- Hepatic vein Doppler assessment: prominent end-diastolic reversal of flow during expiration
- Mitral annular tissue Doppler: preserved or exaggerated e′ velocities (medial e′ typically ≥9 cm/s), often with medial e′ greater than lateral e′
- Mitral inflow Doppler assessment: exaggerated respiratory variation in E velocity
- Speckle tracking myocardial strain imaging: preserved global longitudinal systolic strain, with relative reduction in lateral longitudinal strain compared with septal longitudinal strain

Computed tomography

- Pericardial thickening
- Pericardial calcification
- Deformation of cardiac contour
- Dilatation of the inferior vena cava

MRI

- Pericardial thickening
- Myocardial tagging sequences: pericardial–myocardial adherence
- Real-time cine imaging: respiration-related ventricular septal shift (as seen with echocardiography)
- Delayed imaging after gadolinium administration: pericardial enhancement, corresponding with inflammation

Hemodynamic catheterization

- Increased venous pressure
- Elevation and near-equalization of right and left heart diastolic pressures
- Relatively dissociated intrathoracic (pulmonary capillary wedge) pressure and left ventricular diastolic pressure (with inspiration, exaggerated decrease in pulmonary capillary wedge pressure compared with left ventricular diastolic pressure)
- Discordance in systolic pressure changes in the right and left ventricles during the respiratory cycle (with inspiration, right ventricular systolic pressure increases and left ventricular systolic pressure decreases)

- Colchicine is typically used in combination with either a nonsteroidal antiinflammatory drug or an oral steroid, depending on clinical circumstances.[31]

Chronic Constrictive Pericarditis

In the majority of cases, constrictive pericarditis is chronic and progressive. With the exception of tuberculous constriction (see Sung-A Chang's article, "Tuberculous and Infectious Pericarditis," in this issue), which responds to antibiotic therapy, chronic constrictive pericarditis has no effective medical treatments. Diuretic therapy may be used to relieve congestion, but is strictly palliative.

- The only effective treatment for symptomatic, chronic constrictive pericarditis is surgical

pericardiectomy.[32] The procedure, described in detail in Pouya Hemmati and colleagues' article, "Contemporary Techniques of Pericardiectomy for Pericardial Disease," in this issue, should include removal of as much pericardium as possible and ideally be performed by an experienced surgeon in a center with special interest in pericardial disease.

- In relatively high-volume centers, pericardiectomy has an average reported perioperative mortality rate of 6.0% to 7.1%.[3–6]
- Longer term survival is inferior to an age- and sex-matched cohort and depends on etiology and patient characteristics.[3]
- Patients with idiopathic constrictive pericarditis have the best outcomes, with reported survival rates of 80% or higher at 5 to 7 years.[4–6]

- Patients with constrictive pericarditis owing to chest radiation have markedly poorer outcomes, with 2 studies reporting approximately 30% survival at 7 to 10 years,[3,4] and 2 others reporting 0% to 11% survival at 5 years.[5,6] The unfavorable outcomes after pericardiectomy for patients with radiation-induced constriction likely relate to the widespread damaging effects of radiation on other parts of the heart (myocardium, valves, coronary arteries) and lungs.
- The prognosis after pericardiectomy also seems to worsen with advanced New York Heart Association functional class, older age, impaired renal function, pulmonary hypertension, decreased left ventricular ejection fraction, and increased Child-Pugh liver disease score.[3,4,7,38]
- Those patients who do survive long term after pericardiectomy generally enjoy significant symptomatic benefit, with more than 80% reporting New York Heart Association class I or II symptoms.

SUMMARY

Constrictive pericarditis should be considered in all cases of unexplained heart failure, particularly when symptoms and signs are predominantly right-sided and when the ejection fraction is preserved. Diagnosis and distinction from restrictive cardiomyopathy remains challenging, and rests primarily on identification of the unique pathophysiologic processes in constriction: dissociation of intrapleural and intracardiac pressures and enhanced ventricular interaction. The most helpful initial diagnostic test is a comprehensive echocardiogram with Doppler imaging. In many cases, further assessment will include cross-sectional imaging with CT, cardiac MRI, and hemodynamic catheterization. Cardiac MRI is particularly helpful in identifying cases of possible "transient" constriction that may respond to antiinflammatory therapy. Complete surgical pericardiectomy remains the only effective treatment for patients with chronic symptomatic constriction. Outcomes after pericardiectomy are best for patients without end-stage disease and who have not received chest radiation.

REFERENCES

1. Robertson R, Arnold CR. Constrictive pericarditis with particular reference to etiology. Circulation 1962;26:525–9.
2. Mutyaba AK, Balkaran S, Cloete R, et al. Constrictive pericarditis requiring pericardiectomy at Groote Schuur Hospital, Cape Town, South Africa: causes and perioperative outcomes in the HIV era (1990-2012). J Thorac Cardiovasc Surg 2014;148(6): 3058–65.e1.
3. Ling LH, Oh JK, Schaff HV, et al. Constrictive pericarditis in the modern era: evolving clinical spectrum and impact on outcome after pericardiectomy. Circulation 1999;100:1380–6.
4. Bertog SC, Thambidorai SK, Parakh K, et al. Constrictive pericarditis: etiology and cause-specific survival after pericardiectomy. J Am Coll Cardiol 2004;43:1445–52.
5. George TJ, Arnaoutakis GJ, Beaty CA, et al. Contemporary etiologies, risk factors, and outcomes after pericardiectomy. Ann Thorac Surg 2012;94: 445–51.
6. Szabo G, Schmack B, Bulut C, et al. Constrictive pericarditis: risks, aetiologies and outcomes after total pericardiectomy: 24 years of experience. Eur J Cardiothorac Surg 2013;44:1023–8 [discussion: 1028].
7. Sekiguchi H, Horie R, Suri RM, et al. Constrictive pericarditis caused by immunoglobulin G4-related disease. Circ Heart Fail 2012;5:e30–1.
8. Stojan G, Melia MT, Khandhar SJ, et al. Constrictive pleuropericarditis: a dominant clinical manifestation in Whipple's disease. BMC Infect Dis 2013;13:579.
9. Imazio M, Brucato A, Maestroni S, et al. Risk of constrictive pericarditis after acute pericarditis. Circulation 2011;124:1270–5.
10. Talreja DR, Edwards WD, Danielson GK, et al. Constrictive pericarditis in 26 patients with histologically normal pericardial thickness. Circulation 2003; 108:1852–7.
11. Hatle LK, Appleton CP, Popp RL. Differentiation of constrictive pericarditis and restrictive cardiomyopathy by Doppler echocardiography. Circulation 1989;79:357–70.
12. Bush CA, Stang JM, Wooley CF, et al. Occult constrictive pericardial disease. Diagnosis by rapid volume expansion and correction by pericardiectomy. Circulation 1977;56:924–30.
13. Babuin L, Alegria JR, Oh JK, et al. Brain natriuretic peptide levels in constrictive pericarditis and restrictive cardiomyopathy. J Am Coll Cardiol 2006;47: 1489–91.
14. Ling LH, Oh JK, Breen JF, et al. Calcific constrictive pericarditis: is it still with us? Ann Intern Med 2000; 132:444–50.
15. Welch TD, Ling LH, Espinosa RE, et al. Echocardiographic diagnosis of constrictive pericarditis: Mayo Clinic criteria. Circ Cardiovasc Imaging 2014;7: 526–34.
16. Coylewright M, Welch TD, Nishimura RA. Mechanism of septal bounce in constrictive pericarditis: a simultaneous cardiac catheterisation and echocardiographic study. Heart 2013;99(18):1376.

17. Oh JK, Hatle LK, Seward JB, et al. Diagnostic role of Doppler echocardiography in constrictive pericarditis. J Am Coll Cardiol 1994;23:154–62.

18. Klein AL, Abbara S, Agler DA, et al. American society of echocardiography clinical recommendations for multimodality cardiovascular imaging of patients with pericardial disease: endorsed by the society for cardiovascular magnetic resonance and society of cardiovascular computed tomography. J Am Soc Echocardiogr 2013;26:965–1012. e15.

19. Rajagopalan N, Garcia MJ, Rodriguez L, et al. Comparison of new Doppler echocardiographic methods to differentiate constrictive pericardial heart disease and restrictive cardiomyopathy. Am J Cardiol 2001; 87:86–94.

20. Garcia MJ, Rodriguez L, Ares M, et al. Differentiation of constrictive pericarditis from restrictive cardiomyopathy: assessment of left ventricular diastolic velocities in longitudinal axis by Doppler tissue imaging. J Am Coll Cardiol 1996;27:108–14.

21. Ha JW, Ommen SR, Tajik AJ, et al. Differentiation of constrictive pericarditis from restrictive cardiomyopathy using mitral annular velocity by tissue Doppler echocardiography. Am J Cardiol 2004; 94:316–9.

22. Sengupta PP, Mohan JC, Mehta V, et al. Accuracy and pitfalls of early diastolic motion of the mitral annulus for diagnosing constrictive pericarditis by tissue Doppler imaging. Am J Cardiol 2004;93: 886–90.

23. Reuss CS, Wilansky SM, Lester SJ, et al. Using mitral 'annulus reversus' to diagnose constrictive pericarditis. Eur J Echocardiogr 2009;10:372–5.

24. Ha JW, Oh JK, Ling LH, et al. Annulus paradoxus: transmitral flow velocity to mitral annular velocity ratio is inversely proportional to pulmonary capillary wedge pressure in patients with constrictive pericarditis. Circulation 2001;104:976–8.

25. Sengupta PP, Krishnamoorthy VK, Abhayaratna WP, et al. Disparate patterns of left ventricular mechanics differentiate constrictive pericarditis from restrictive cardiomyopathy. JACC Cardiovasc Imaging 2008;1:29–38.

26. Kusunose K, Dahiya A, Popovic ZB, et al. Biventricular mechanics in constrictive pericarditis comparison with restrictive cardiomyopathy and impact of pericardiectomy. Circ Cardiovasc Imaging 2013;6: 399–406.

27. Boonyaratavej S, Oh JK, Tajik AJ, et al. Comparison of mitral inflow and superior vena cava Doppler velocities in chronic obstructive pulmonary disease and constrictive pericarditis. J Am Coll Cardiol 1998;32:2043–8.

28. Adler Y, Charron P. The 2015 ESC Guidelines on the diagnosis and management of pericardial diseases. Eur Heart J 2015;36:2873–4.

29. Thavendiranathan P, Verhaert D, Walls MC, et al. Simultaneous right and left heart real-time, free-breathing CMR flow quantification identifies constrictive physiology. JACC Cardiovasc Imaging 2012;5:15–24.

30. Zurick AO, Bolen MA, Kwon DH, et al. Pericardial delayed hyperenhancement with CMR imaging in patients with constrictive pericarditis undergoing surgical pericardiectomy: a case series with histopathological correlation. JACC Cardiovasc Imaging 2011;4:1180–91.

31. Feng D, Glockner J, Kim K, et al. Cardiac magnetic resonance imaging pericardial late gadolinium enhancement and elevated inflammatory markers can predict the reversibility of constrictive pericarditis after antiinflammatory medical therapy: a pilot study. Circulation 2011;124: 1830–7.

32. Adler Y, Charron P, Imazio M, et al. 2015 ESC Guidelines for the diagnosis and management of pericardial diseases: the task force for the diagnosis and management of pericardial diseases of the European society of cardiology (ESC)endorsed by: the European Association for Cardio-Thoracic Surgery (EACTS). Eur Heart J 2015;36:2921–64.

33. Vaitkus PT, Kussmaul WG. Constrictive pericarditis versus restrictive cardiomyopathy: a reappraisal and update of diagnostic criteria. Am Heart J 1991;122:1431–41.

34. Talreja DR, Nishimura RA, Oh JK, et al. Constrictive pericarditis in the modern era: novel criteria for diagnosis in the cardiac catheterization laboratory. J Am Coll Cardiol 2008;51:315–9.

35. Schoenfeld MH, Supple EW, Dec GW Jr, et al. Restrictive cardiomyopathy versus constrictive pericarditis: role of endomyocardial biopsy in avoiding unnecessary thoracotomy. Circulation 1987;75: 1012–7.

36. Haley JH, Tajik AJ, Danielson GK, et al. Transient constrictive pericarditis: causes and natural history. J Am Coll Cardiol 2004;43:271–5.

37. Chang SA, Choi JY, Kim EK, et al. [18F]Fluorodeoxyglucose PET/CT predicts response to steroid therapy in constrictive pericarditis. J Am Coll Cardiol 2017;69:750–2.

38. Komoda T, Frumkin A, Knosalla C, et al. Child-Pugh score predicts survival after radical pericardiectomy for constrictive pericarditis. Ann Thorac Surg 2013; 96:1679–85.

Effusive-Constrictive Pericarditis

William R. Miranda, MD, Jae K. Oh, MD*

KEYWORDS

- Effusive-constrictive pericarditis • Pericardiocentesis • Echocardiography

KEY POINTS

- In effusive-constrictive pericarditis (ECP), a hemodynamically significant pericardial effusion coexists with decreased pericardial compliance.
- The hallmark of ECP is the persistence of elevated right atrial pressure postpericardiocentesis.
- The reported prevalence of ECP has varied significantly, but it seems higher in tuberculous pericarditis and lower in idiopathic cases.
- A diagnosis of ECP is traditionally based on invasive hemodynamics. The presence of echocardiographic features of constrictive pericarditis postpericardiocentesisis, however, can detect ECP.
- Data on the prognosis and optimal treatment of ECP are still limited. Anti-inflammatory therapy should be the first line of treatment. Pericardiectomy should be reserved for refractory cases.

INTRODUCTION

The coexistence of pericardial effusive and constrictive features was first brought to attention more than 50 years ago[1,2] and was also described by Paul Wood in the subacute phase of tuberculous pericarditis.[3] Better characterization of this clinical entity did not occur until the series reported by Hancock[4] and Sagrista-Sauleda and colleagues.[5] Almost 15 years later, the understanding and appreciation of effusive-constrictive pericarditis (ECP) is still incomplete, with data limited to case reports,[6–9] small case series,[4] and only a few prospective studies.[5,10–12] This review summarizes the available data on ECP and describes the authors' own clinical experience.

PATHOPHYSIOLOGY

In ECP, a hemodynamically significant pericardial effusion coexists with decreased pericardial compliance. Consequently, as the cardiac compression is relieved by pericardial fluid drainage and intrapericardial pressure falls, the features of constrictive pericarditis (CP) become predominant. This is manifested by the persistence of elevated right atrial pressure after pericardiocentesis, the hemodynamic hallmark of ECP.[13]

Although cardiac tamponade and CP are both pericardial disorders leading to abnormal cardiac filling, their pathophysiologies are markedly different. In tamponade, early diastolic filling is significantly impaired due to elevated intrapericardial pressures. Systemic venous pressure rises and adrenergic tone increases to overcome the decrease in cardiac output. If tamponade continues to progress and compensatory mechanisms are overwhelmed, shock ensues unless pericardiocentesis is performed. In contrast, in CP early diastolic filling prevails — the increase in filling pressures secondary to the inelastic pericardium promotes increased ventricular filling in early diastole. As the pericardial reserve is exhausted in mid to late diastole, however, ventricular filling markedly decreases. These differences lead to their classic hemodynamic features[14,15]: blunting of the y descent in tamponade

Department of Cardiovascular Diseases, Mayo Clinic, 200 First Street Southwest, Rochester, MN 55905, USA
* Corresponding author.
E-mail address: oh.jae@mayo.edu

Cardiol Clin 35 (2017) 551–558
http://dx.doi.org/10.1016/j.ccl.2017.07.008

and deep, rapid ventricular filling waves in CP (square root sign or dip-and-plateau pattern).

Although ECP is frequently thought of as the conversion from tamponade to constrictive physiology after pericardiocentesis, ECP cases represent a spectrum of patients with pericardial effusions, elevated intrapericardial pressures, and decreased pericardial compliance. Therefore, patients with ECP have hemodynamics that fall on a continuum between pure effusive tamponade on the one hand and chronic CP on the other. This accounts for the clinical variability and for lack of full understanding of the underlying pathophysiology, because ECP is actually part of a clinical spectrum. This spectrum is evident in Sagrista-Sauleda and colleagues' series[5] where, despite all patients having clinical tamponade and documented decreased right atrial transmural pressure, right atrial contours pre-pericardiocentesis were not typical of tamponade. Hence, despite the elevated intrapericardial pressures and low right atrial transmural pressure (as seen in tamponade), ECP has different underlying hemodynamics. This was better exemplified by Hancock,[4] who showed that right atrial contour in ECP differed from both tamponade and CP, with the relationship between x and y descents in ECP intermediate between the 2 entities. Lastly, in the authors' experience, overt tamponade is not a mandatory component of ECP. A similar observation was reported by Ntsekhe and colleagues[16] in a series of 68 patients with tuberculous pericardial effusions; tamponade confirmed by cardiac catheterization was present in only 56% of patients. There was no difference in the prevalence of tamponade between ECP and non-ECP groups in their cohort. Patients with ECP, however, had higher right atrial pressures, suggesting that the hemodynamic effects of the effusion and reduced pericardial compliance are additive.

Bloody effusions are common in patients with ECP[4,5] and it has been postulated that the presence of blood in the pericardial space might promote more exuberant inflammation and decreased pericardial compliance. Patients with tuberculous ECP were found to have higher levels of interleukin 10 and interferon gamma in the pericardial fluid as well as serum interleukin 10 and tissue growth factor β compared with patients with non-ECP tuberculous pericarditis.[16] These cytokines may foster pericardial inflammation/fibrosis and be related to higher prevalence of ECP in tuberculous pericarditis. In a series of patients with nontuberculous pericardial effusions, the authors observed that, although no differences in pericardial total white blood cell count was seen, the percentage of neutrophils was higher in ECP patients. This also suggests more florid inflammation in these patients.[17] Although the hemodynamic derangements in ECP are believed secondary to constriction from the visceral pericardium,[18] findings at time of pericardiectomy are of thickening of both visceral and parietal pericardia, with associated pericardial fluid and adhesions.[4,5,13] Pericardial edema with active inflammation might also be seen, whereas pericardial calcifications are not typical.

EPIDEMIOLOGY

The reported prevalence of ECP among patients with a pericardial effusion has ranged widely, from 1% to 2%[5,19] to more than 50%.[10,11] This variation can be attributed to differences in methodology (diagnosis of ECP based on catheterization vs echocardiography) and the cohorts studied. It is clear, however, that the prevalence with ECP is closely related to the associated etiologies.[13] ECP seems much more prevalent in tuberculous pericarditis than in idiopathic pericarditis. In a series of 68 patients with tuberculous pericardial effusions, 53% were diagnosed with ECP.[13] Similar results have been reported in other groups of patients with tuberculous pericarditis.[11] In contrast, in a single-center European series, ECP was diagnosed in 1.3% of patients undergoing pericardiocentesis, corresponding to 7.9% of tamponade cases.[5] The most common etiologies were idiopathic, neoplastic, and postradiation, in order of frequency. These etiologies are in agreement with observations from a North American center,[18] in which idiopathic cases corresponded to the vast majority of ECP patients identified, followed by radiation-heart disease. This epidemiologic profile would also be akin to the one currently observed for CP in Europe and the United States, where idiopathic and radiation are among leading causes. Compared with CP in developed countries, however, the lack of postoperative/postprocedural cases in these 2 ECP series differentiates the populations and may be related to lower volumes of cardiac surgery and percutaneous interventions during the study periods (4 decades and 2 decades ago, respectively). In a series of 205 consecutive patients undergoing pericardiocentesis at the authors' institution,[17] post–cardiac surgery and percutaneous procedure-related effusions corresponded to more than 50% of cases. The overall prevalence of ECP (diagnosed by echocardiography) in the authors' cohort was 16%. Other causes reported in the literature include ECP secondary to purulent pericarditis, trauma, neoplastic involvement, and end-stage renal disease.[13] Nevertheless, it is conceivable that ECP might occur with any disease leading to pericardial inflammation.

CLINICAL PRESENTATION

The clinical presentation is variable. Although ECP might develop in the setting of acute pericardial effusion (for example, iatrogenic effusions related to cardiac percutaneous procedure), patients generally present with symptoms lasting days or weeks. In acute cases, symptoms of tamponade (in particular hemodynamic instability) may prevail until pericardiocentesis is performed. In subacute cases, fatigue, shortness of breath, and leg edema are the most common complaints. Pleuritic chest pain related to underlying pericarditis can also occur.

Patients might also present with CP-like symptoms or require hospitalization for heart failure weeks after pericardiocentesis, after features of ECP have not been recognized immediately postcentesis. In these cases, the clinical picture is similar to the one seen in transient CP (discussed later) and, in that stage, the distinction between these 2 entities might be impossible, if not artificial.

DIAGNOSIS
Physical Examination

The persistence of elevated jugular venous pressure postpericardiocentesis is often the first sign ECP might be present. It should be ensured, however, that the pericardial effusion has been appropriately drained (thus, that tamponade is no longer present) and that no other explanation for the elevated central venous pressure is present (for example, severe tricuspid regurgitation).

At the bedside, patients show elevated jugular pressure with prominent x and y descents, similar to the pattern seen in CP. This is in contrast to the presence of deep x and blunted y descents seen with tamponade. Admittedly, proper analysis of the venous morphology can be challenging, particularly in the setting of tachycardia. Therefore, the red flag for the clinician should be the persistence of elevated central venous pressure after pericardiocentesis.

Pleural effusions might also be present, particularly in ECP cases after cardiac surgery (postpericardiotomy syndrome). Pericardial knocks are uncommon.[4]

Electrocardiogram and Chest Radiography

There are no pathognomic electrocardiographic features of ECP. Depending on the associated clinical scenario, electrocardiography may show findings similar to tamponade or pericarditis; in subacute cases, nonspecific ST-T wave changes are seen. Prior to pericardiocentesis, enlarged cardiac silhouette might be present on chest radiograph. Pericardial calcification is not typical and suggests chronic pericardial inflammation and fibrosis, as seen in long-standing CP.

Cardiac Catheterization

Diagnosis of ECP is traditionally based on invasive hemodynamic features, suggested to be present if right atrial pressure fails to drop below 10 mm Hg or by 50% or more postpericardiocentesis (**Fig. 1**).[5] Curiously, despite the reliance on catheterization findings for the diagnosis, there are limited data on the expected postpericardiocentesis hemodynamic findings in patients with ECP. In the series of Sagrista-Sauleda and colleagues,[5] median right atrial pressure postpericardiocentesis was 15 mm Hg and left ventricular end-diastolic pressure 20.5 mm Hg; pulmonary artery wedge pressure was not reported. Right atrial tracings showed equal x and y descents or predominance of the y descent in a majority of patients; similar findings were reported in Hancock's[4] original series. Most importantly, all patients showed rapid right ventricular filling waves (dip-and-plateau) supporting prominent early diastolic filling, a hemodynamic feature of CP. There was no equalization of end-diastolic pressures (ie, within 5 mm Hg) in 4 of 10 patients whose right and left end-diastolic pressure were available (with left-sided pressures higher). The prevalence of ventricular interdependence postcentesis was assessed in a group of 16 patients with tuberculous pericarditis diagnosed with ECP.[11] The investigators reported ventricular discordance present in 56% of patients, a much lower prevalence than reported in CP patients (>90%).[20,21]

The prepericardiocentesis features of ECP are also largely unknown. In Sagrista-Sauleda and colleagues' series,[5] despite cardiac tamponade being an inclusion criterion, almost half of the patients had at least similar x and y descents prepericardiocentesis (1 patient had predominance of the y descent), findings not expected in tamponade physiology. This was also highlighted by Hancock,[4] who suggested that right atrial contour in ECP showed intermediate findings compared with tamponade (predominance of systolic filling [ie, x descent]) and CP (predominance of diastolic filling [ie, y descent]). In a series of 68 patients with tuberculous pericarditis, those with ECP had higher right atrial pressures than those with effusive nonconstrictive pericarditis, and prepericardiocentesis right atrial

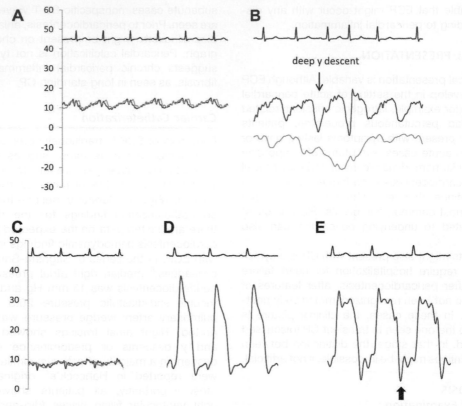

Fig. 1. Cardiac catheterization findings in ECP. Prior to pericardiocentesis (*A*), findings are consistent with tampo-nade with mild elevation in right atrial pressures (*red*), equalization of right filling, and intrapericardial pressures (*blue*). Postpericardiocentesis (*B*), there is normalization of intrapericardial pressures but right atrial pressures remain elevated. Note the development of deep *y* descents after drainage of the pericardial effusion. (*C*) Shows prepericardiocentesis right atrial (*red*) and intrapericardial pressures (*blue*) in a different patient; right ventricular tracings are shown (*D*). Note the rapid ventricular filling waves seen postpericardiocentesis (*E, arrow*).

pressure greater than 15 mm Hg was a predictor of ECP.[16] Not all patients had tamponade confirmed by catheterization in their cohort but there were no differences in the prevalence of tamponade between groups.

Echocardiography

Although the diagnosis of ECP was initially described based on invasive hemodynamics, right heart catheterization at the time of pericardiocent-esis is not routinely performed in most institutions. It has been proposed that the presence of echo-cardiographic features of CP[14,22] (respirophasic septal shift, inspiratory decreases in mitral E velocities greater than 25%, expiratory reversals in the hepatic veins, and dilatation of inferior vena cava) after centesis would be indicative of ECP (**Fig. 2**) (see Terrence D. Welch and Jae K. Oh's article, "Constrictive Pericarditis," in this issue). Minor respirophasic changes in E velocity and mild septal shift are common, however, in

patients postpericardiocentesis and immediately postcardiac surgery. These are typically transient, resolving spontaneously. Thus, in the absence of other clinical or echocardiographic signs of CP (elevated neck veins, dilatation of the inferior vena cava, or restrictive mitral inflow), those find-ings should be interpreted with caution.

The performance of echo-Doppler in the diag-nosis of ECP was reported in a group of 32 pa-tients with tuberculous pericarditis undergoing pericardiocentesis.[11] ECP was defined based on traditional invasive hemodynamic criteria, whereas echocardiographic diagnostic criteria was defined by greater than or equal to 25% respiratory varia-tion in the mitral E wave or clear respirophasic septal shift. The investigators reported a sensitivity of 81% and a specificity of 75% for the echocar-diographic diagnosis of ECP. Data regarding he-patic vein pulsed wave Doppler and tissue Doppler of the mitral annulus were not included in the study. The authors have observed[17] that patients with an echocardiographic diagnosis of

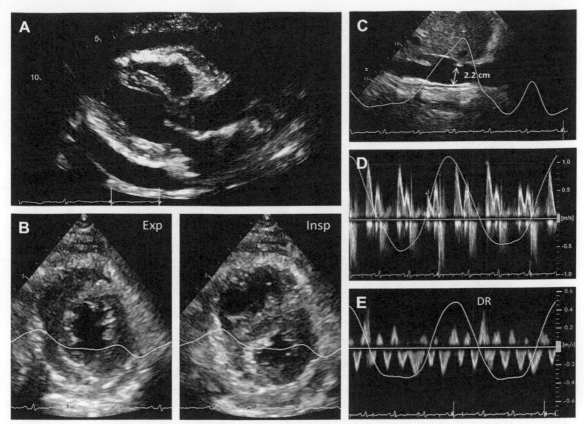

Fig. 2. Echocardiographic findings in a patient with ECP. Prior to pericardiocentesis, 2-D parasternal long-axis view shows a large circumferential pericardial effusion (*A*); echocardiographic features of cardiac tamponade were present. After complete drainage of the pericardial space, marked respirophasic shift (*B*), persistence of inferior vena cava dilatation (*C*), significant respiratory variations in the mitral E velocities (*D*), and expiratory diastolic flow reversals in the hepatic veins (*E*) were seen. The constellation of findings was consistent with ECP.

ECP (defined by respirophasic variation in E velocity greater than 25% and septal shift or hepatic vein/mitral tissue Doppler findings of CP) have higher medial mitral e' velocities and shorter mitral deceleration times as well as higher prevalence of expiratory flow reversals in the hepatic veins compared with patients with effusive pericarditis. Dilatation of the inferior vena cava was present in all patients fulfilling echocardiographic criteria for ECP.

Whether ECP could be diagnosed (or suspected) based on echo-Doppler, even prior to pericardiocentesis, is unclear. In study discussed previously,[17] the authors noted that patients with ECP demonstrated elevated medial mitral e' velocities before pericardiocentesis was performed. In addition, respirophasic septal shift was more common prepericardiocentesis in the ECP group compared with non-ECP patients. In the authors' experience, it also seems that patients with ECP have higher mitral E velocities and E/A ratios prior

to centesis than patients with cardiac tamponade (where E/A ratios are typically ≤1). In Sagrista-Sauleda and colleagues'[5] original description, in 7 of their 15 patients, ECP had been suspected prior to pericardiocentesis based on abnormal septal motion and rapid transmitral diastolic forward flow on echocardiography.

Computerized Tomography and Magnetic Resonance

Cardiac computerized tomography (CT) and magnetic resonance in patients with ECP typically show a combination of pericardial effusion and signs of pericardial inflammation (pericardial thickening or enhancement) prior to pericardiocentesis (**Fig. 3**). These modalities might be particularly helpful in identifying the presence of loculated, complex pericardial effusions, which might occur in postoperative or tuberculosis cases. Pericardial thickening (≥4 mm) might be present, but its

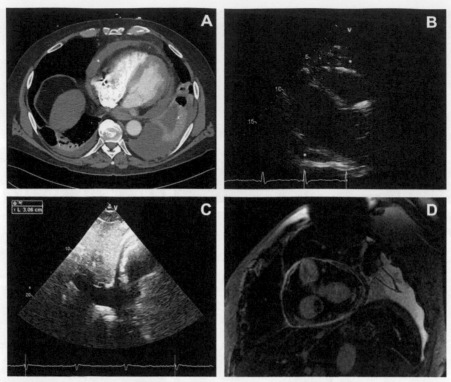

Fig. 3. CT and magnetic resonance findings in patient with ECP. Chest CT (*A*) shows a moderate pericardial effusion (*asterisk*) and associated pericardial enhancement; bilateral pleural effusions are present. The pericardial effusion was confirmed by transthoracic echocardiographic (*B*). Postpericardiocentesis, there was persistence of inferior vena cava dilatation (*C*) and obvious constrictive features; cardiac magnetic resonance (*D*) revealed pericardial thickening and pericardial late gadolinium enhancement; a small residual effusion is also seen.

prevalence in ECP is unknown (pericardial thickening is absent in 20% of patients with surgically proved CP).[23] Dilatation of inferior vena cava, a surrogate for elevated right atrial pressures, is generally present.

TREATMENT AND PROGNOSIS

In cases of a specific cause identified, such as rheumatologic disorder or tuberculosis, therapy should be targeted to the associated disorder (discussion of management of tuberculous ECP is outside the scope of this article). The optimal treatment of ECP in idiopathic, iatrogenic (procedure-related) or even malignant cases is still unclear. Therapeutic options include nonsteroidal anti-inflammatory agents or corticosteroids. Although the superiority of steroid therapy in ECP has not been proved, several members of the authors' group favor initiation of steroids in patients with pericarditis If constrictive features are present. High doses of steroids should be avoided and the doses should be tapered slowly (See Massimo Imazio and Fiorenzo Gaitas' article, "Acute and Recurrent Pericarditis," in this issue). In cases

where only mild constrictive features and symptoms present, the choice of nonsteroidal agents as a first-line therapy is reasonable (regimen similar to the one used in acute pericarditis), but close follow-up is mandatory. Data regarding the benefits of adjuvant colchicine therapy in ECP are lacking, but the authors typically recommend it unless contraindications are present.

Similar to its prevalence, the reported prognosis of ECP has been highly variable in the literature. In Sagrista-Saulda and colleagues' series,[5] more than half of patients required pericardiectomy during follow-up. A systemic review, including data from 20 patients with nonmalignant ECP, reported an overall pericardiectomy rate of 65%.[10] In the authors' experience, the prognosis has been more favorable, particularly in idiopathic cases. For example, in a series of 33 ECP patients diagnosed by echocardiography at the authors' center, only 2 required pericardiectomy for persistent symptoms.[17] It is possible that the prognosis might be better in the current era given the increased awareness and prompt initiation of more aggressive anti-inflammatory treatment of ECP (and transient CP). These results might be reflective, however, of the population seen at the authors' institution. As in malignant pericarditis,[24] patients with ECP secondary to a malignant process tend to have a poor prognosis, usually succumbing from the underlying process.

Pericardiectomy should be reserved for refractory cases, where symptoms of CP persist despite therapy. Mortality rates for pericardiectomy have markedly decreased over the past 30 years, with high-volume centers currently achieving rates between 5% and 10%.[25,26] The perioperative mortality in ECP cases is unknown, however. A radical (complete) rather than anterior pericardiectomy is recommended[27]; thus this surgical procedure should be performed by a surgeon with experience in pericardial disease.

Because the visceral pericardium contributes significantly to constriction in ECP, investigators have suggested that removal of the visceral layer (epicardiectomy) should be performed.[18] The waffle procedure might also be an option in cases of epicardial constriction suspected/present.[28,29]

OTHER CONSTRICTIVE PERICARDITIS–LIKE SYNDROMES

Two other clinical entities are worth discussing in this article because they share similarities with ECP. As ECP, these entities have also been called uncommon patterns CP.[30]

Transient Constrictive Pericarditis

Sagrista-Sauleda and colleagues[31] reported a group of patients presenting with features of CP during the resolving phase of acute pericarditis (not all initially presenting with cardiac tamponade). The prognosis of these patients was good and none of them underwent pericardiectomy. The definition of transient CP has varied in the literature, but, currently, it is accepted as a temporary form of CP that follows an episode of pericarditis and resolves with anti-inflammatory therapy.[31] This definition is arbitrary, however, and patients with transient CP, as well as patients with ECP, are part of a clinical spectrum of patients presenting with pericardial inflammation and decreased pericardial compliance.

Pericardial effusions are commonly seen in transient CP, occurring in two-thirds of cases.[31] Patients typically have signs of ongoing inflammation by serum markers or by cardiac magnetic resonance (ie, gadolinium enhancement) at the time of diagnosis.[32] Therapy should focus on aggressive treatment of the underlying inflammation, with nonsteroidal anti-inflammatory agents or corticosteroids plus colchicine. The optimal medical regimen and duration is still unknown. It

is the authors' experience, however, that patients typically observe clinical improvement within a week but at least 2 to 3 months of therapy are needed for complete and sustained response. Therefore, in the setting of evidence of ongoing inflammation, aggressive medical therapy should be first line of treatment rather than pericardiectomy; surgery should also be reserved for refractory cases.

Occult Constrictive Pericarditis

Occult CP was described in a subset of patients whose features of CP were only evidenced after fluid challenge.[33] Because the invasive hemodynamic findings of CP are load dependent, it is the authors' institution's practice to rapidly infuse normal saline during cardiac catheterization in patients with suspected CP who have been on diuretics and, as a consequence, have low right atrial pressures (<15 mm Hg). This is not performed routinely, however, to diagnose occult cases and it has been shown that rapid infusion of volume can elevate filling pressures even in patients without cardiac disease. Thus, the authors do not recommend diagnosing CP based on hemodynamics post–fluid challenge in the absence of other clinical and diagnostic findings of CP.

SUMMARY

In ECP, a hemodynamically significant pericardial effusion coexists with decreased pericardial compliance. The hallmark of ECP is the persistence of elevated right atrial pressures after pericardiocentesis is performed. Although a diagnosis of ECP has been traditionally based on cardiac catheterization data, the presence of echocardiography features of CP postpericardiocentesis might also be diagnostic. Data on the diagnosis and management of ECP are still limited. Further studies comparing invasive hemodynamics and echocardiographic data are needed for better understanding of its pathophysiology, prevalence, and prognosis.

ACKNOWLEDGMENTS

The author's thank Dr Nandan Anavekar for providing some of the images included in the article.

REFERENCES

1. Burchell HB. Problems in the recognition and treatment of pericarditis. J Lancet 1954;74:465–70.

2. Spodick DH, Kumar S. Subacute constrictive pericarditis with cardiac tamponade. Dis Chest 1968; 54:62–6.

3. Wood P. Chronic constrictive pericarditis. Am J Cardiol 1961;7:48–61.

4. Hancock EW. Subacute effusive-constrictive pericarditis. Circulation 1971;43:183–92.

5. Sagrista-Sauleda J, Angel J, Sanchez A, et al. Effusive-constrictive pericarditis. N Engl J Med 2004; 350:469–75.

6. Steinberg I. Effusive-constrictive radiation pericarditis. Two cases illustrating value of angiocardiography in diagnosis. Am J Cardiol 1967;19:434–9.

7. Nakayama Y, Ohtani Y, Kobayakawa N, et al. A case of early phase dialysis associated effusive constrictive pericarditis with distinct surgical findings. Int Heart J 2009;50:685–91.

8. Plana JC, Iskander SS, Ostrowski ML, et al. Cardiac angiosarcoma: an unusual presentation simulating mitral stenosis and constrictive-effusive pericarditis. J Am Soc Echocardiogr 2003;16:1331–3.

9. Baker CM, Orsinelli DA. Subacute effusive-constrictive pericarditis: diagnosis by serial echocardiography. J Am Soc Echocardiogr 2004;17: 1204–6.

10. Ntsekhe M, Shey Wiysonge C, Commerford PJ, et al. The prevalence and outcome of effusive constrictive pericarditis: a systematic review of the literature. Cardiovasc J Afr 2012;23:281–5.

11. van der Bijl P, Herbst P, Doubell AF. Redefining effusive-constrictive pericarditis with echocardiography. J Cardiovasc Ultrasound 2016;24:317–23.

12. Reuter H, Burgess LJ, Louw VJ, et al. The management of tuberculous pericardial effusion: experience in 233 consecutive patients. Cardiovasc J S Afr 2007;18:20–5.

13. Syed FF, Ntsekhe M, Mayosi BM, et al. Effusive-constrictive pericarditis. Heart Fail Rev 2013;18: 277–87.

14. Miranda WR, Oh JK. Constrictive pericarditis: a practical clinical approach. Prog Cardiovasc Dis 2017;59:369–79.

15. Holmes DR Jr, Nishimura R, Fountain R, et al. Iatrogenic pericardial effusion and tamponade in the percutaneous intracardiac intervention era. JACC Cardiovasc Interv 2009;2:705–17.

16. Ntsekhe M, Matthews K, Syed FF, et al. Prevalence, hemodynamics, and cytokine profile of effusive-constrictive pericarditis in patients with tuberculous pericardial effusion. PLoS One 2013;8:e77532.

17. Kim KH, Miranda WR, Sinak LJ, et al. Effusive-constrictive pericarditis following pericardiocentesis: incidence, associated findings and natural history. JACC Cardiovasc Imag, in press.

18. Hancock EW. A clearer view of effusive-constrictive pericarditis. N Engl J Med 2004;350:435–7.

19. Nugue O, Millaire A, Porte H, et al. Pericardioscopy in the etiologic diagnosis of pericardial effusion in 141 consecutive patients. Circulation 1996;94: 1635–41.

20. Talreja DR, Nishimura RA, Oh JK, et al. Constrictive pericarditis in the modern era: novel criteria for diagnosis in the cardiac catheterization laboratory. J Am Coll Cardiol 2008;51:315–9.

21. Hurrell DG, Nishimura RA, Higano ST, et al. Value of dynamic respiratory changes in left and right ventricular pressures for the diagnosis of constrictive pericarditis. Circulation 1996;93:2007–13.

22. Welch TD, Ling LH, Espinosa RE, et al. Echocardiographic diagnosis of constrictive pericarditis: Mayo Clinic criteria. Circ Cardiovasc Imaging 2014;7: 526–34.

23. Talreja DR, Edwards WD, Danielson GK, et al. Constrictive pericarditis in 26 patients with histologically normal pericardial thickness. Circulation 2003; 108:1852–7.

24. Tsang TS, Seward JB, Barnes ME, et al. Outcomes of primary and secondary treatment of pericardial effusion in patients with malignancy. Mayo Clin Proc 2000;75:248–53.

25. Gillaspie EA, Stulak JM, Daly RC, et al. A 20-year experience with isolated pericardiectomy: analysis of indications and outcomes. J Thorac Cardiovasc Surg 2016;152:448–58.

26. Bertog SC, Thambidorai SK, Parakh K, et al. Constrictive pericarditis: etiology and cause-specific survival after pericardiectomy. J Am Coll Cardiol 2004;43:1445–52.

27. Cho YH, Schaff HV. Surgery for pericardial disease. Heart Fail Rev 2013;18:375–87.

28. Kao CL, Chang JP. Modified method for epicardial constriction: the electric-Waffle procedure. J Cardiovasc Surg (Torino) 2001;42:643–6.

29. Heimbecker RO, Smith D, Shimizu S, et al. Surgical technique for the management of constrictive epicarditis complicating constrictive pericarditis (the waffle procedure). Ann Thorac Surg 1983;36:605–6.

30. Sagrista-Sauleda J. Pericardial constriction: uncommon patterns. Heart 2004;90:257–8.

31. Sagrista-Sauleda J, Permanyer-Miralda G, Candell-Riera J, et al. Transient cardiac constriction: an unrecognized pattern of evolution in effusive acute idiopathic pericarditis. Am J Cardiol 1987;59:961–6.

32. Feng D, Glockner J, Kim K, et al. Cardiac magnetic resonance imaging pericardial late gadolinium enhancement and elevated inflammatory markers can predict the reversibility of constrictive pericarditis after antiinflammatory medical therapy: a pilot study. Circulation 2011;124:1830–7.

33. Bush CA, Stang JM, Wooley CF, et al. Occult constrictive pericardial disease. Diagnosis by rapid volume expansion and correction by pericardiectomy. Circulation 1977;56:924–30.

Contemporary Techniques of Pericardiectomy for Pericardial Disease

Pouya Hemmati, MD, Kevin L. Greason, MD,
Hartzell V. Schaff, MD*

KEYWORDS

- Pericardiectomy • Constrictive pericarditis • Diastolic heart failure

KEY POINTS

- Pericardiectomy is a potentially curative treatment for constrictive pericarditis.
- Adequate pericardial resection is crucial to prevent recurrent or persistent hemodynamic compromise and symptoms owing to residual constrictive physiology.
- The etiology of constrictive pericarditis has an important impact on survival after pericardiectomy and can be associated with additional cardiac disease.
- Survival remains low in those with radiation-induced constrictive pericarditis, predominantly owing to concomitant radiation-induced cardiac pathology.

INTRODUCTION

Constrictive pericarditis is a condition in which the pericardium is fibrotic and stiffened, presumably owing to a prior inflammatory process. The diseased pericardium limits diastolic filling of the heart, producing characteristic signs and symptoms of right-sided heart failure. There are several etiologies of constrictive pericarditis that are observed in varying frequencies in different patient populations. In the United States and other developed nations, the cause of constrictive pericarditis is most commonly thought to be idiopathic in nature, likely secondary to prior viral infection. However, documented preceding inflammatory pericarditis is the exception rather than the rule.[1] The next leading causes are iatrogenic, including mediastinal radiation and, more commonly, previous cardiac surgery. In developing countries, infectious processes are the most common cause, with tuberculous pericarditis being the leading etiology.[2]

Patients may present with signs and symptoms indistinguishable from other cardiac conditions, including those of right-sided heart failure (peripheral edema, ascites, venous congestion, hepatomegaly, or jugular venous pressure elevation) or left-sided heart failure (dyspnea or pleural effusion). One should consider constrictive pericarditis in patients with right-sided heart failure with preserved left ventricular ejection fraction in the absence of tricuspid regurgitation and patients with pericardial calcification on imaging.[1,3] The differential diagnosis also includes restrictive cardiomyopathy, tricuspid valve disease, and chronic liver disease with ascites.

Differentiating constrictive pericarditis is essential because of availability of treatment modalities. Antiinflammatory medications can resolve acute, transient disease, but the take-home point is that symptomatic patients with chronic constriction can only be cured with an operation.[4] Constrictive pericarditis can be classified as transient, effusive–constrictive (where features of constriction and

---

Conflicts of Interest: None.
Department of Cardiovascular Surgery, Mayo Clinic, 200 First Street Southwest, Rochester, MN 55905, USA
* Corresponding author.
E-mail address: schaff@mayo.edu

Cardiol Clin 35 (2017) 559–566
http://dx.doi.org/10.1016/j.ccl.2017.07.009
0733-8651/17/© 2017 Elsevier Inc. All rights reserved.

cardiac tamponade coexist), radiation induced, tuberculous, or calcific.

Echocardiography and adjunct modalities such as cardiac MRI, computed tomography, and, in some patients, cardiac catheterization, can clarify the diagnosis in most cases. Constrictive physiology can present with septal shift with respiratory variation, transmitral velocity anomalies (increased mitral annular e' velocities), and hepatic vein flow variations with respiration.[2]

INDICATIONS

Pericardiectomy is performed most often for patients with chronic constriction, but surgical removal of the pericardium is also useful in atients with relapsing pericarditis refractory to antiinflammatory therapy.[4] Rarely, patients may present signs and symptoms of acute inflammation accompanying evidence of constrictive physiology, and an initial trial of antiinflammatory medical therapy may be appropriate.[5] However, it is important not to delay definitive intervention in patients with chronic constriction, because early surgical intervention may be associated with better outcomes.[6]

CONTRAINDICATIONS

Contraindications to pericardiectomy in patients with chronic constrictive pericarditis are similar to those of other major cardiac operations. The patient needs to be able to tolerate general anesthesia and a cardiac operation with potential need for cardiopulmonary bypass (CPB). Specific contraindications might include hepatic dysfunction with cirrhosis and ascites, uncontrolled infection or sepsis, and other systemic diseases limiting life expectancy. If the anticipated risks of an operation outweigh the potential benefits, patients with mild symptoms can be treated medically and observed for symptomatic progression.

Most patients with chronic constrictive pericarditis experience hemodynamic improvement after pericardiectomy, but the degree of recovery and improvement in physical activities depends on the extent and etiology of disease and comorbid conditions. Procedural risk is increased in patients with end-stage constrictive pericarditis pathophysiology, with manifestations such as a resting cardiac index of 1.2 $L/m^2/min$ or less with signs of cachexia, cardiogenic cirrhosis with subsequent hypoalbuminemia, and protein-losing enteropathy. Patients with mixed constrictive–restrictive disease commonly owing to radiation-induced myocardial damage also have increased

risk in the perioperative period, relatively poor long-term survival, and may have persistent symptoms after pericardiectomy.[7,8]

SURGICAL APPROACH
General

Diagnostic studies to establish the diagnosis of constriction are covered in other articles in this series, but it should be emphasized that findings on clinical examination coupled with detailed Doppler echocardiographic assessment are sufficient to establish the diagnosis of constriction in most patients.[9] Additional imaging to assess pericardial thickness may be useful, but pericardial thickness is normal in 12% to 18% of patients with hemodynamically significant constriction.[10,11]

General preoperative planning for pericardiectomy is similar to other major cardiac procedures, with special attention to associated tricuspid valve regurgitation and adequacy of hepatic function, including vitamin K–dependent coagulation factors. Optimizing preoperative volume status with diuresis may be beneficial in some patients, but often diuretics are ineffective until constriction is relieved and pericardiectomy should not be delayed in patients with advanced heart failure.

Some surgical teams advocate minimal paralysis during anesthesia with use of short-acting muscle blockade agents to facilitate identification of phrenic nerves by stimulation during and after dissection. Inflammatory adhesions may obscure the phrenic nerves and low energy electrocautery settings and adjunct nerve stimulation may be useful in identifying the phrenic nerve to avoid nerve injury. Intraoperative transesophageal echocardiography should be used in all cases of pericardiectomy for chronic constriction to assess cardiac size and function during and after removal of the pericardium[12,13] and, as discussed elsewhere in this article, to examine atrioventricular valve function after release of pericardial constraint.

Incision

A median sternotomy is used for most patients undergoing pericardiectomy for constrictive pericarditis. This approach gives wide access to the pericardium and simplifies cannulation if CPB is necessary for dissection, control of bleeding, or performing other cardiac procedures, such as addressing atrioventricular valve regurgitation.[14,15]

In contrast with other operations where cardiac repair often results in lessening of tricuspid valve regurgitation, pericardiectomy and release of constriction may lead to right ventricular and tricuspid annular dilatation with worsening of functional valve leakage.[14] Furthermore, it has been our experience that the need for tricuspid valve annuloplasty is difficult to predict and, because persistent valve leakage is associated with reduced survival after pericardiectomy, we have a liberal policy for tricuspid valve annuloplasty when regurgitation worsens with pericardiectomy. A similar phenomenon has been reported with worsening of mitral valve regurgitation after pericardiectomy.[15]

Pericardiectomy can be performed through an anterolateral thoracotomy, but we generally reserve that approach for cosmetic considerations and in special situations when midline repeat sternotomy might be hazardous because of previous operations. The anterolateral thoracotomy provides good exposure of the lateral aspect of the pericardium, which is sometimes difficult to visualize through a median sternotomy without CPB. However, it is difficult to access the right heart or perform intracardiac repairs or concomitant procedures through the lateral incision. If additional exposure is required, the anterolateral incision can be extended to a bilateral thoracotomy. Axillary or femoral cannulation is also possible if CPB is necessary.

Cardiopulmonary Bypass

Given the need to manipulate the ventricles for adequate pericardial dissection, CPB may be necessary for cardiac decompression and circulatory support. Extracorporeal circulation is necessary for concomitant procedures such as tricuspid valve repair, and CPB facilitates repair of cardiac injuries secondary to difficult dissection planes, which are common in the setting of previous cardiac operations or mediastinal radiation. CPB can also be used to optimize postpericardiectomy hemodynamics by removing excess intravascular volume to avoid ventricular distension after pericardial constraint is relieved.

Ascending aortic cannulation and 2-stage single venous cannulation without aortic occlusion or cardioplegia are sufficient for most isolated pericardiectomies. In a large sample of more than 800 pericardiectomies performed at Mayo Clinic since 1990, CPB was used in more than 60%, and aortic cross-clamping was performed in one-third of these patients (median aortic cross-clamp time of 35 minutes).

SURGICAL TECHNIQUE

Anterior pericardiectomy is limited to removal of the pericardium between the left and right phrenic nerves. It is relatively simple to perform, and some groups consider this a complete pericardiectomy.[6,16] Anterior pericardiectomy improves hemodynamics in many patients, but this limited procedure may be inadequate in others. The basal, diaphragmatic (inferior), and left posterolateral aspects of the heart can still be tethered by the constrictive pericardium, leading to recurrence or persistence of the constrictive pathophysiology.[17]

We believe it is important to free both ventricles, including releasing the inferior aspect of the heart, from the constricting layers of diaphragmatic pericardium. We remove this portion of pericardium, as well as a portion posterior to the left phrenic nerve.[18–20] What constitutes an adequate pericardiectomy has been debated,[21] but we have had patients referred for reoperation with recurrent symptoms caused by constriction owing to residual diaphragmatic pericardium.[22]

Operation Details

After median sternotomy, the pericardium is incised in the midline (**Fig. 1**). The operation is facilitated by early entry into both pleural spaces so that the phrenic nerves can be identified. If the nerve is easily visualized, we score the pericardium from the pleural side approximately 1 to 1.5 cm anterior to the nerve. This line is followed when the anterior pericardium is removed.

Dissection of the pericardium is performed sharply with scissors and electrocautery, and the fibrous pericardium is removed. It is critically important to identify the correct plane of dissection to prevent residual epicardial constriction. When the dissection is in the correct plane and sufficiently deep, the coronary arteries can be

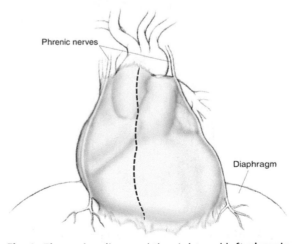

Phrenic nerves

Diaphragm

Fig. 1. The pericardium and the right and left phrenic nerves are shown through a median sternotomy exposure. The pericardium is incised near the midline. (*Courtesy of* Mayo Clinic, Rochester, MN; with permission. Used with permission of Mayo Foundation for Medical Education and Research. All rights reserved.)

seen. Some surgeons favor the harmonic scalpel for additional dissection,[23] and the Cavitational Ultrasonic Surgical Aspiration System can be used for fragmenting calcified deposits.[24] In our experience, electrocautery has been safe and efficacious despite the risk of cardiac electrical stimulation, especially when using CPB.

As mentioned, both pleural spaces are entered to ensure adequate visualization of the phrenic nerves, and dissection from the midline rightward continues to approximately 1 to 1.5 cm anterior to the right phrenic nerve. There is little pericardium between the right phrenic nerve and the pulmonary veins, but it is important to note that the nerve courses anteriorly in the upper mediastinum in the area of the superior vena cava, and the line of excision is more anterior in this cephalad portion of the pericardium.

Next, dissection is carried leftward from the midline to a similar level 1 to 1.5 cm anterior to the left phrenic nerve. We excise the anterior pericardium and extend dissection as far posteriorly as possible so that the entire left ventricle is freed from adhesions (**Fig. 2**). Care should be taken in dissection lateral to the main pulmonary artery to avoid left phrenic nerve injury.

Dissection is then performed between the diaphragmatic pericardium and the inferior surfaces of the right and left ventricles. The left ventricular apex is in close proximity to the left phrenic nerve and is typically associated with a fat pad. We usually excise this fat pad to improve exposure. The diaphragmatic pericardium is easily separated

from the underlying muscular and fibrous portions of the diaphragm, and this dissection is carried posterior to the left phrenic nerve as far as possible (**Fig. 3**). Even in the setting of significant fibrosis and calcification, the inferior pericardium can usually be separated from the underlying fibrous, central diaphragm (**Figs. 4** and **5** for labeled postdissection exposure and intraoperative photographs, respectively).[25] Residual defects in the diaphragm after dissection can be safely closed directly or repaired with a patch of bovine pericardium. Intraoperative transesophageal echocardiography provides valuable assessment of cardiac function, with specific focus on resolution of constrictive physiology and changes in valvular function.

Additional Procedures

In some instances, dense epicardial constriction may be difficult to remove completely. In these areas, constriction can be relieved by incising the fibrous rind, referred to as the Waffle procedure.[26] This technique uses multiple longitudinal and transverse incisions of the epicardium with a 15 blade, taking care to avoid coronary branches.

Another important structural concern is the pre-existing or postpericardiectomy development of tricuspid valve regurgitation. Moderate or severe tricuspid regurgitation is present on preoperative

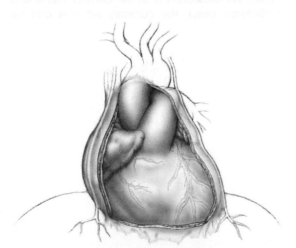

Fig. 2. After sharp dissection toward the left and right phrenic nerves, the anterior pericardium is removed exposing the epicardial coronary arteries. The pericardium beneath each phrenic nerve is preserved to avoid injury. (*Courtesy of* Mayo Clinic, Rochester, MN; with permission. Used with permission of Mayo Foundation for Medical Education and Research. All rights reserved.)

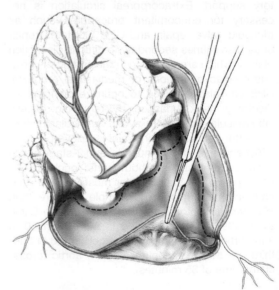

Fig. 3. The heart is freed from the diaphragmatic aspect of the pericardium and the pericardium posterior to the left phrenic nerve. The pericardium is then dissected from the diaphragm as shown. (*Courtesy of* Mayo Clinic, Rochester, MN; with permission. Used with permission of Mayo Foundation for Medical Education and Research. All rights reserved.)

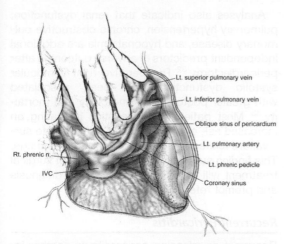

Fig. 4. View of the surgical field after removal of the diaphragmatic pericardium and a portion of pericardium posterior to the left (Lt.) phrenic nerve. Note the small strip of residual pericardium beneath the phrenic nerves and in the oblique sinus posterior to the left atrium. IVC, inferior vena cava; Rt., right. (*Courtesy of* Mayo Clinic, Rochester, MN; with permission. Used with permission of Mayo Foundation for Medical Education and Research. All rights reserved.)

echocardiography in up to 20% of patients with constrictive pericarditis.[14] Indeed, pericardiectomy can exacerbate tricuspid regurgitation, presumably owing to right ventricular expansion and tricuspid valve annular dilation. Preexisting tricuspid regurgitation is a risk factor for late death after pericardiectomy and, thus, we favor concomitant tricuspid valve repair in those patients with moderate or worse regurgitation after pericardiectomy.[14]

Tricuspid valve repair requires bicaval cannulation for CPB to allow entry into the right atrium. A De Vega suture annuloplasty is usually sufficient to repair functional tricuspid regurgitation, but some surgeons favor ring annuloplasty.[27] Overall, concomitant tricuspid valve repair has been performed in more than 12% of patients undergoing pericardiectomy for constrictive pericarditis at Mayo Clinic since 1990.

POSTOPERATIVE MANAGEMENT

Standard postoperative management involves hemodynamic and rhythm monitoring in the intensive care unit and cardiac output optimization with inotropic support. Some degree of low cardiac output is not unusual after pericardiectomy for chronic constriction owing to transient ventricular distention, injury to epicardial coronary arteries, or some degree of underlying myocardial atrophy caused by chronic constraint.[12,28] Others have described more severe degrees of right heart failure after pericardiectomy. Beckmann and colleagues[29] recently reported the early postoperative use of extracorporeal membrane oxygenation in 12% of patients undergoing pericardiectomy for chronic constriction.

OUTCOMES
Mortality

Early as well as overall mortality, as in any other operation, depends on preoperative comorbidities and the extent of disease. In recent publications, perioperative mortality has ranged between 6%

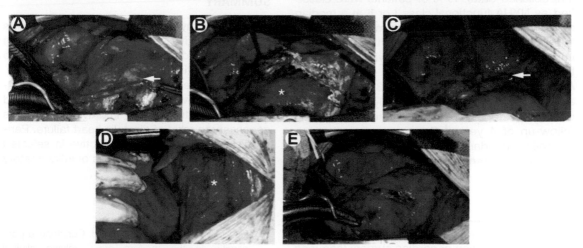

Fig. 5. Intraoperative photographs. (*A*) Initial exposure of the pericardium (*arrow*). (*B*) Anterior surface of the heart (*asterisk*) after anterior pericardium dissection. (*C*) The heart is retracted to the right and the left phrenic nerve pedicle is identified (*arrow*). The pericardium posterior to the nerve will be removed. (*D*) The heart is retracted cephalad and the pericardium has been removed from the muscular and membranous regions of the diaphragm (*asterisk*). (*E*) The heart after radical pericardiectomy. (*Adapted from* Syed FF, Schaff HV, Oh JK. Constrictive pericarditis–a curable diastolic heart failure. Nat Rev Cardiol 2014;11(9):540; with permission.)

and 7%.[16,19,20] Pericardiectomy for constrictive pericarditis has been performed at Mayo Clinic in more than 1066 patients since the first operation in 1936, and operative mortality among 807 patients in the current era (since 1990) is 5.2%. This represents considerable improvement in risk of death early after operation compared with prior eras, during which operative mortality was 12% to 14%.[30,31]

Despite the lower risk of an operation, overall survival of patients after pericardiectomy has not improved in the current era, primarily owing to increased numbers of patients with radiation-induced constriction and patients with concomitant heart disease who developed postoperative constrictive pericarditis. At Mayo Clinic, before 1990, the 5- and 10-year survivals after pericardiectomy were 71% and 59%, respectively, compared with 63% and 46%, respectively, in the contemporary cohort. In addition to different distribution of etiologies of constriction, patients in the contemporary era were older (61 vs 49 years; P<.001), more symptomatic (New York Heart Association [NYHA] functional class III or IV in 79% vs 71%; P<.001), and more frequently underwent concomitant operations (21% vs 5%; P<.001).

Residual diastolic dysfunction may persist in a significant proportion of patients. A previous study from our institution demonstrated that 43% of patients had abnormal diastolic functional parameters on echocardiography beyond 3 months postoperatively.[13] However, abnormal diastolic function detected on Doppler echocardiography does not correlate directly with functional status. As reported by Gillaspie and colleagues (unpublished data), 77% of patients were classified as NYHA functional class I or II at a median of 29 months after pericardiectomy for constrictive pericarditis. This represents substantial improvement as 84% presented with NYHA functional class III or IV symptoms preoperatively. Another analysis showed that 83% of patients are either asymptomatic or mildly symptomatic during postoperative evaluation with mean follow-up of 4 years.[1] Recurrent symptoms are typically secondary to underlying myocardial disease or recurrent versus residual constrictive pericarditis.

Risk Factors

Operative risk factors include older age, prior mediastinal radiation or cardiac surgery (common etiologies of pericarditis in the developed world), concomitant myocardial or valvular disease, need for CPB, and preoperative functional class (NYHA functional class III or IV symptoms, and extent of right and/or left ventricular dysfunction).

Analyses also indicate that renal dysfunction, pulmonary hypertension, chronic obstructive pulmonary disease, and hyponatremia are additional independent predictors of adverse outcomes after pericardiectomy.[32] Preoperative right ventricular systolic dysfunction has been associated with greater postoperative morbidity and mortality.[33] Most patient characteristics indicating an increased risk of operation and reduced late survival are related to advanced symptoms and age. This finding suggests that the outcome of surgical treatment will only improve with early diagnosis and prompt referral for treatment.

Recurrent Pericarditis

Recurrent or relapsing pericarditis is another indication for pericardiectomy, and operation is reserved for patients who fail medical treatment with antiinflammatory medications such as colchicine, corticosteroids, and nonsteroidal antiinflammatory drugs. It is important to perform a complete pericardiectomy in these cases, including removing the diaphragmatic pericardium and the portion posterior to the left phrenic nerve. Removal of pericardium in patients with relapsing pericarditis is extremely safe and effective. In a review of 58 patients undergoing pericardiectomy for relapsing pericarditis, there was no perioperative mortality and minimal morbidity. The rate of recurrent symptoms was markedly reduced in the surgical patients compared with a group of medically treated patients.[4]

SUMMARY

Pericardiectomy can be curative in patients with constrictive pericarditis and operation should not be delayed, especially for those who are symptomatic and/or require diuretic therapy. With adequate extent of resection, pericardiectomy relieves constrictive physiology and diastolic constraint, and improves symptoms secondary to relief of diastolic heart failure. Pericardiectomy is also highly effective in selected patients with recurrent episodes of inflammatory pericarditis.

REFERENCES

1. Ling LH, Oh JK, Schaff HV, et al. Constrictive pericarditis in the modern era: evolving clinical spectrum and impact on outcome after pericardiectomy. Circulation 1999;100(13):1380–6.
2. Syed FF, Schaff HV, Oh JK. Constrictive pericarditis–a curable diastolic heart failure. Nat Rev Cardiol 2014;11(9):530–44.

3. Ling LH, Oh JK, Breen JF, et al. Calcific constrictive pericarditis: is it still with us? Ann Intern Med 2000; 132(6):444–50.

4. Khandaker MH, Schaff HV, Greason KL, et al. Pericardiectomy vs medical management in patients with relapsing pericarditis. Mayo Clin Proc 2012; 87(11):1062–70.

5. Haley JH, Tajik AJ, Danielson GK, et al. Transient constrictive pericarditis: causes and natural history. J Am Coll Cardiol 2004;43(2):271–5.

6. Vistarini N, Chen C, Mazine A, et al. Pericardiectomy for constrictive pericarditis: 20 years of experience at the Montreal Heart Institute. Ann Thorac Surg 2015;100(1):107–13.

7. Ni Y, von Segesser LK, Turina M. Futility of pericardiectomy for postirradiation constrictive pericarditis? Ann Thorac Surg 1990;49(3):445–8.

8. Karram T, Rinkevitch D, Markiewicz W. Poor outcome in radiation-induced constrictive pericarditis. Int J Radiat Oncol Biol Phys 1993;25(2): 329–31.

9. Welch TD, Ling LH, Espinosa RE, et al. Echocardiographic diagnosis of constrictive pericarditis: Mayo Clinic criteria. Circ Cardiovasc Imaging 2014;7(3): 526–34.

10. Seifert FC, Miller DC, Oesterle SN, et al. Surgical treatment of constrictive pericarditis: analysis of outcome and diagnostic error. Circulation 1985; 72(3 Pt 2):II264–73.

11. Talreja DR, Edwards WD, Danielson GK, et al. Constrictive pericarditis in 26 patients with histologically normal pericardial thickness. Circulation 2003; 108(15):1852–7.

12. Ha J-W, Oh JK, Schaff HV, et al. Impact of left ventricular function on immediate and long-term outcomes after pericardiectomy in constrictive pericarditis. J Thorac Cardiovasc Surg 2008; 136(5):1136–41.

13. Senni M, Redfield MM, Ling LH, et al. Left ventricular systolic and diastolic function after pericardiectomy in patients with constrictive pericarditis: Doppler echocardiographic findings and correlation with clinical status. J Am Coll Cardiol 1999;33(5): 1182–8.

14. Góngora E, Dearani JA, Orszulak TA, et al. Tricuspid regurgitation in patients undergoing pericardiectomy for constrictive pericarditis. Ann Thorac Surg 2008;85(1):163–70 [discussion: 170–1].

15. Nakamura T, Masai T, Yamauchi T, et al. Successful surgical management for severe mitral regurgitation unmasked after pericardiectomy for chronic constrictive pericarditis. Ann Thorac Surg 2008; 86(6):1994–6.

16. Bertog SC, Thambidorai SK, Parakh K, et al. Constrictive pericarditis: etiology and cause-specific survival after pericardiectomy. J Am Coll Cardiol 2004;43(8):1445–52.

17. Cho YH, Schaff HV. Extent of pericardial resection for constrictive pericardiectomy. Ann Thorac Surg 2012;94(6):2180.

18. Cho YH, Schaff HV. Surgery for pericardial disease. Heart Fail Rev 2013;18(3):375–87.

19. Szabó G, Schmack B, Bulut C, et al. Constrictive pericarditis: risks, aetiologies and outcomes after total pericardiectomy: 24 years of experience. Eur J Cardiothorac Surg 2013;44(6):1023–8 [discussion: 1028].

20. George TJ, Arnaoutakis GJ, Beaty CA, et al. Contemporary etiologies, risk factors, and outcomes after pericardiectomy. Ann Thorac Surg 2012;94(2): 445–51.

21. Glower D. Invited commentary. Ann Thorac Surg 2012;93(4):1240–1.

22. Cho YH, Schaff HV, Dearani JA, et al. Completion pericardiectomy for recurrent constrictive pericarditis: importance of timing of recurrence on late clinical outcome of operation. Ann Thorac Surg 2012; 93(4):1236–40.

23. Uchida T, Bando K, Minatoya K, et al. Pericardiectomy for constrictive pericarditis using the harmonic scalpel. Ann Thorac Surg 2001;72(3):924–5.

24. Uchino M, Yoshikai M, Sato H, et al. Surgical repair of severely calcific constrictive pericarditis;report of a case. Kyobu Geka 2015;68(6):468–71 [in Japanese].

25. Villavicencio MA, Dearani JA, Sundt TM. Pericardiectomy for constrictive or recurrent inflammatory pericarditis. Oper Tech Thorac Cardiovasc Surg 2008;13(1):2–13.

26. Yamamoto N, Ohara K, Nie M, et al. For what type of constrictive pericarditis is the waffle procedure effective? Asian Cardiovasc Thorac Ann 2011; 19(2):115–8.

27. Shinn SH, Schaff HV. Evidence-based surgical management of acquired tricuspid valve disease. Nat Rev Cardiol 2013;10(4):190–203.

28. Dines DE, Edwards JE, Burchell HB. Myocardial atrophy in constrictive pericarditis. Proc Staff Meet Mayo Clin 1958;33(4):93–9.

29. Beckmann E, Ismail I, Cebotari S, et al. Right-sided heart failure and extracorporeal life support in patients undergoing pericardiectomy for constrictive pericarditis: a risk factor analysis for adverse outcome. Thorac Cardiovasc Surg 2016. http://dx. doi.org/10.1055/s-0036-1593817.

30. McCaughan BC, Schaff HV, Piehler JM, et al. Early and late results of pericardiectomy for constrictive pericarditis. J Thorac Cardiovasc Surg 1985;89(3): 340–50. Available at: https://www.ncbi.nlm.nih.gov/ pubmed/3974269?access_num=3974269&link_type= MED&dopt=Abstract. Accessed January 23, 2017.

31. Cameron J, Oesterle SN, Baldwin JC, et al. The etiologic spectrum of constrictive pericarditis. Am Heart J 1987;113(2 Pt 1):354–60.

32. Busch C, Penov K, Amorim PA, et al. Risk factors for mortality after pericardiectomy for chronic constrictive pericarditis in a large single-centre cohort. Eur J Cardiothorac Surg 2015;48(6): e110–6.

33. Choudhry MW, Homsi M, Mastouri R, et al. Prevalence and prognostic value of right ventricular systolic dysfunction in patients with constrictive pericarditis who underwent pericardiectomy. Am J Cardiol 2015;116(3):469–73.

Percutaneous Therapy in Pericardial Diseases

Bernhard Maisch, MD, FESC[a],*, Arsen D. Ristić, MD, PhD, FESC[b],
Sabine Pankuweit, PhD[c], Petar Seferovic, MD, FESC[b]

KEYWORDS

- Pericardiocentesis • Pericarditis • Pericardial effusion • Cardiac tamponade
- Intrapericardial therapy • Percutaneous balloon pericardiotomy
- Percutaneous intrapericardial left atrial appendage ligation

KEY POINTS

- Echocardiographic and fluoroscopic guidance have greatly increased safety and feasibility for pericardiocentesis, providing current major complication rates of less than 2% and essentially no mortality.
- Devices for pericardiocentesis facilitate access to the pericardium in the absence of effusion, but are not needed routinely for patients with pericardial disease.
- Intrapericardial application of fibrinolytics can facilitate complete drainage of dense pericardial effusion in purulent or tuberculous pericarditis.
- Intrapericardial cytostatic treatment could be useful in preventing recurrences of neoplastic pericardial effusion; intrapericardial steroids can be applied in managing recurrent autoreactive pericardial disease.
- Percutaneous balloon pericardiotomy or percutaneous pericardiostomy can be used for palliative management of patients with recurrent neoplastic and autoreactive pericardial effusions.

INTRODUCTION

Depending on the etiology, clinical presentation, and hemodynamic status, patients with pericardial diseases may require interventional procedures in addition to medical management. In patients with a rapidly accumulating pericardial effusion and cardiac tamponade, urgent drainage of the pericardial effusion is lifesaving.[1] Echocardiographic and/or fluoroscopic guidance for this procedure has greatly increased safety and feasibility.[2] Several devices have been tested to facilitate pericardiocentesis (PerDucer, PeriAttacher, AttachLifter, visual puncture systems, Grasper, Scissors, and Reverse slitter), although these are mainly intended to enable access to the pericardium in the absence of effusion for epicardial ablation or left atrial appendage ligation. Purulent or tuberculous infections are life threatening and require prompt drainage; intrapericardial application of a fibrinolytic agent or surgical management may sometimes be needed.[2,3] In recurrent, large pericardial effusions or cardiac tamponade

Disclosure statement: The authors have no conflicts of interest to declare.
Supported by the German Ministry for Education Research (BMBF) in the German Heart Failure Competence Network, the Cardiac Promotion Society Marburg (VFdK) and individual grants from the UKGM and the Medical Faculty Marburg to B. Maisch and S. Pankuweit.
[a] Faculty of Medicine, Philipps University and Heart and Vessel Center, Feldbergstr. 45, Marburg 35043, Germany; [b] Department of Cardiology, Clinical Centre of Serbia, Belgrade University School of Medicine, Koste Todorovića 8, Belgrade 11000, Serbia; [c] Faculty of Medicine and Cardiology Clinic, UKGM, Baldingerstrasse 1, Marburg 35043, Germany
* Corresponding author.
E-mail address: bermaisch@gmail.com

Cardiol Clin 35 (2017) 567–588
http://dx.doi.org/10.1016/j.ccl.2017.07.010

various medications can be applied intrapericardially to prevent further relapses or perform sclerotherapy. Percutaneous balloon pericardiotomy or percutaneous pericardiostomy are rarely applied alternatives to manage and prevent recurrent pericardial effusion.

PERICARDIOCENTESIS AND PERCUTANEOUS DRAINAGE OF PERICARDIAL EFFUSION

Drainage of a pericardial effusion is indicated in patients with cardiac tamponade, for symptomatic moderate to large pericardial effusions not responsive to medical therapy, and for effusions with suspected bacterial or neoplastic etiologies.[4] Large, chronic effusions have a 30% to 35% risk of progression to cardiac tamponade.[5] Also, subacute, large effusions not responsive to conventional therapy and with collapse of the right chambers have an increased risk of progression with potential benefit of preventive drainage.[6] Halpern and colleagues[7] introduced a scoring index to assist in the selection of patients for pericardiocentesis, based on clinical presentation, laboratory data, echocardiographic assessment, and hemodynamics. In 2014, the European Society of Cardiology Working Group on Myocardial and Pericardial Diseases proposed an alternative triage strategy that incorporated probabilities of progression to cardiac tamponade for different etiologies and clinical symptoms and signs, as well as the parameters obtained by imaging.[1]

The routine part of preparation for the procedure should include a basic laboratory screen, especially taking note of the coagulation status. An International Normalized Ratio of greater than 1.5 and thrombocytopenia of less than 50,000/mL are relative contraindications and should be corrected before the procedure.[4] However, in a recent percutaneous pericardiocentesis study in 212 patients with cancer, no procedure-related deaths were recorded and only 4 patients had major procedure-related bleeding (1.9%), regardless of whether the platelet count was greater than or less than 50,000/mL ($P = .1281$).[8] In a retrospective analysis of 60 echocardiography-guided and fluoroscopy-guided pericardial procedures in patients with cancer with thrombocytopenia, Iliescu and colleagues as well as Tsang and colleagues[9,10] also reported a low rate of major complications (2%) comparable with the rates reported in large series of echocardiography-guided pericardiocenteses in the general population. The complications included 1 entry site hematoma, 1 small pleural effusion, and 1 left hemothorax requiring surgical evacuation. Platelet transfusion did not modify the overall risk of the procedure,

presumably because 15% to 25% of patients with malignancies are refractory to platelet transfusion. Although 25% of the subjects had critical thrombocytopenia (<20,000 platelets/mL) and 40% had 20,000 to 50,000 platelets/mL, the micropuncture technique and a lateral approach for pericardiocentesis with echocardiography and fluoroscopy guidance seemed to be as safe as when performed in the general population.[9] Accordingly, pericardiocentesis can be performed safely in patients with thrombocytopenia, assuming that proper imaging guidance is used.[11]

PERCUTANEOUS PERICARDIOCENTESIS VERSUS SURGICAL PERICARDIOTOMY

Before the advent of echocardiography, clinicians had 2 choices: open surgical drainage or blind pericardiocentesis. At that time, a small subxyphoid incision and drainage of the pericardium under direct vision was safer than the blind puncture, given the risk of cardiac chamber perforation and a periprocedural mortality of up to 4% with the blind approach.[12] A percutaneous approach did, however, have a lower risk of a secondary infection. With echocardiographic guidance, the feasibility and safety of percutaneous pericardiocentesis increased tremendously because the size and distribution of the effusion could be identified at the time of puncture. Pericardiocentesis and percutaneous drainage of pericardial effusion is nowadays feasible and safe in the great majority of patients with pericardial disease. Surgical management remains reserved for hemopericardium owing to trauma, type A aortic dissection, ventricular free wall rupture in acute myocardial infarction, and some patients with purulent pericarditis and rare complications of interventional or electrophysiology procedures. If surgery is not available promptly or the patient is too unstable to survive the transfer, pericardiocentesis and controlled pericardial drainage of very small volumes of a hemorrhagic effusion can be attempted to stabilize the patient (mean total volume drained was 40.1 ± 30.6 mL, in several small portions, just to maintain a systolic blood pressure of approximately 90 mm Hg).[13,14]

ECHOCARDIOGRAPHY-GUIDED PERICARDIOCENTESIS

Pericardiocentesis can be performed in the catheterization laboratory, the echocardiography laboratory, or even as a bedside procedure in emergencies. The needle trajectory should follow the angulation of the imaging transducer. The best spot for pericardiocentesis is the one on the chest wall closest to the greatest amount of the pericardial effusion, avoiding vital structures (liver, lungs, and blood vessels). In most patients this would be from the subxiphoid or apical–intercostal area. ECG, blood pressure monitoring and stringent aseptic and antiseptic measures should be employed during pericardiocentesis. Several pericardiocentesis sets are available (Merit Medical 6F or 8.3 F, Boston Scientific, Marlborough, MA; Peri-Vac 8.3 F, Lock Pericardiocentesis Set and Tray 8F, Cook Medical, Bloomington, IN; and so on). If such a set is not on hand, any needle (eg, Touhy blunt tip), J-tip guidewire and vascular introducer, and a pigtail catheter can be successfully used for the drainage of pericardial effusion. In emergencies, a 16- to 18-gauge polyteflon-sheathed intravenous needle and a pig-tail catheter or a 7-F central venous catheter is sufficient to drain the pericardial effusion safely. The use of a polyteflon-sheathed intravenous needle for entry eliminates the need for electrocardiographic monitoring of the steel needle; this is also more practical than the use of dedicated echo probes with a channel for the needle for continuous echocardiographic monitoring during pericardiocentesis or a bracket mounted on the echocardiographic probe to support the needle.[2,15] Once the pericardial space is entered, and fluid obtained, only the polyteflon sheath is advanced and the steel core is immediately withdrawn. This step provides safe manipulation after entry into the effusion and avoids the hazard of a sharp needle injury to vital structures on the surface of the heart, where most vulnerable are coronary veins and the thin walls of the right atrium and the right ventricle. Critical aspects of the procedure are (1) determination of the optimal entry site and of the puncturing needle trajectory (**Fig. 1** *left*), (2) use of a polyteflon-sheathed needle, (3) advancement of the needle in a straight line without side-to-side manipulation during pericardiocentesis (see **Fig. 1** *right*), and (4) confirmation of the polyteflon sheath position by echocardiographic imaging from a remote window with agitated saline (echo-contrast) (can be skipped if serous effusion is obtained).[16]

The most serious complications of pericardiocentesis are laceration and perforation of the myocardium and the coronary vessels. In addition, patients can experience pneumothorax, arrhythmias (usually vasovagal bradycardia), air embolism, and puncture of the peritoneal cavity or abdominal viscera. Internal mammary artery fistulas, acute pulmonary edema, circulatory collapse, and purulent pericarditis have been rarely reported.[2] Although major complications are rare, packed red blood cells should be typed and cross-matched before the procedure in case transfusion is required urgently. General anesthesia, intubation, and positive pressure ventilation should be avoided before pericardial drainage is begun. A comparative analysis of feasibility and safety of major pericardiocentesis series is presented in **Table 1**.[8,10,12,15,17–24]

In the Mayo Clinic series of 1127 echocardiography-guided pericardiocenteses, 97% of the procedures were successful and associated with only 1.2% major and 3.5% minor complications.[10] Major complications included chamber lacerations requiring surgery (n = 6; 1 fatal), injury to an intercostal vessel (n = 1), pneumothoraces requiring drainage (n = 5), ventricular tachycardia (n = 1), and bacteremia (n = 1). Minor complications included transient chamber entries (n = 11), small pneumothorax (n = 8), vasovagal response (n = 2), nonsustained supraventricular tachycardia (n = 2), pericardial catheter occlusion (n = 8), and pleuro-pericardial fistula (n = 9). Similar safety and efficacy rates for echo-guided pericardiocentesis have been shown in various populations including pediatric patients,[25] iatrogenic cardiac perforations,[26] post-cardiotomy syndrome,[27] malignancies,[8,28] and systemic autoimmune diseases.[29]

Maggiolini and colleagues[15] performed 161 real-time echocardiography-guided pericardiocentesis

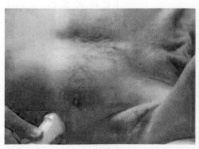
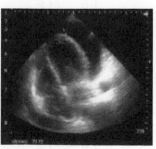
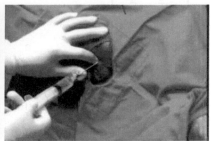

Fig. 1. Echocardiography-guided pericardiocentesis using intercostal approach. Trajectory of the puncturing needle is predetermined by the position and the angle of the echocardiography probe at the point on the chest wall closest to the largest accumulation of pericardial effusion in diastole.

Table 1
Comparative analysis of feasibility and safety of major pericardiocentesis series

Author, (Reference)	Guidance and Approach	Number of Procedures	Most Frequent Etiologies	Feasibility	Mortality	Major Complications	Minor Complications
Tsang et al,[10] 2002	Echo	1127	Malignancy, iatrogenic or postcardiotomy 70%	97%	0.0009% (1 heart chamber laceration)	1.2% (6 heart chamber lacerations requiring surgery, 1 injury to an intercostal vessel, 5 pneumothoraces requiring drainage, 1 ventricular tachycardia, 1 bacteriemia)	3.5% (11 transient chamber entries, 8 small pneumothoraces, 2 vasovagal reactions, 2 NSVT, 8 pericardial catheter occlusions, 9 pleuropericardial fistulas)
Battistoni et al,[17] 2016	Noncontinuous echo guided	478	Malignancy or postcardiotomy 60%	98%	0%	1%	Not reported
Akyuz et al,[18] 2015	Echo (subxiphoid 85%, intercostal 15%)	301	Malignant 28%, viral 7.3%, uremic 7.9%, postcardiotomy 7.9%, tuberculosis 6.6%, idiopathic/ indeterminate 26.3%	97%	0%	1.3% (1 case of pneumothorax, 1 case of right coronary artery perforation, and 2 cases of right ventricular perforation all requiring surgical correction)	1.3% (4 transient arrhythmias, 1 case of sinus bradycardia, 1 case of atrial flutter, and 2 cases of atrial fibrillation)
El Haddad et al,[8] 2015	Echo + fluoroscopy + CT (echo, 93%, echo/ fluoroscopy, 42%, CT - 8%) (subxiphoid 63%, intercostal 37%)	212	Malignant 100%	99%	0%	2.4% (bacteriemia, intercostal artery laceration requiring surgery, pneumothorax requiring drainage, liver laceration)	34% (NSVT -17%, pericardial catheter occlusion - 9%)

Study	Guidance / approach	N	Etiology				
Kolek and Brat,[19] 2017	Echo (subxiphoid 85%, intercostal 15%)	208	Postcardiotomy 100%	98.6%	0%	1%	Not reported
Jaussaud et al,[20] 2012	Echo (subxiphoid 91.9%, left parasternal 8.1%)	197	Postcardiotomy 100%	80.2%	0%	1.5% (right ventricular puncture requiring surgery)	2.5% (spontaneously healed right ventricular puncture)
Maggiolini et al,[15] 2016	Real-time echo in ICU[a] (intercostal 69%, subxiphoid 26.7%, left parasternal 1.2%)	161	Malignant 34%, infectious 11.2%, postcardiotomy 9.9%, idiopathic 15.5%, iatrogenic 4.9%, uremic 4.9%	99%	0%	1.2% (1 mediastinal hematoma, 1 pleuropericardial shunt requiring thoracocentesis)	4.3% (1 small pleuropericardial shunt, 1 transient complete AV block, 3 vasovagal reactions, 2 acute pulmonary edemas)
Lindenberger et al,[21] 2003	Echo in the cath lab (subxiphoid 97%, intercostal 3%)	135	Malignant 25%, infectious/inflammatory 13%, postcardiotomy 41%, idiopathic/indeterminate 18%	98%	0%	0.7% (1 ventricular puncture leading to a cardiac tamponade and reintervention)	7% (transient arrhythmia 6, vasovagal reaction 2, dyspnea 1)
Vayre et al,[22] 2000	Continuous echo (subxiphoid 99%, intercostal 1%)	110	Idiopathic 14.5%, malignant 45.5%, miscellaneous 40%	91.7%	5.4% (postinfarction rupture 4.5%, sudden death in malignant disease 0.9%)	0.9% (accidental puncture of the right ventricle requiring volume loading)	20.1% (accidental puncture of the right ventricle 10%, arrhythmias 5.4%, vasovagal hypotension 5.4%)

(continued on next page)

Table 1
(continued)

Author, Reference	Guidance and Approach	Number of Procedures	Most Frequent Etiologies	Feasibility	Mortality	Major Complications	Minor Complications
Duvernoy et al,[23] 1992	Fluoroscopy (subxiphoid 100%)	352 (303 patients)	Postcardiotomy 59.1%, malignant 19.3%, idiopathic pericarditis 14.2%	95.7%	0.6% (1 aortic aneurysm, and 1 postinfarction rupture)	3.7% (3 cardiac perforations, 2 cardiac arrhythmias, 4 cases of arterial bleeding, 2 cases of pneumothorax, 1 infection, and 1 major vagal reaction)	26.1% (accidental cardiac perforation not requiring surgery 20 cases, abdominal pain 4, pneumothorax 2, pain 55, fever/leukocytosis 9, arrhythmia 2)
Maisch et al,[2] 2011; Maisch et al,[24] 2013	Echo + fluoroscopy (subxiphoid 100%)	259	Viral 12%, malignant 28%, autoreactive or lymphocytic 35%	93.3%	0%	0%	1.3% (3 cardiac perforations resolved with autotransfusion with no need for surgery, 1 major vagal reaction (0.4%)
Krikorian and Hancock,[12] 1978	No imaging available, ECG monitoring from the needle tip (subxiphoid 97.6%, intercostal 2.4%)	165 (123 patients)	Idiopathic 13.5%, indeterminate 18%, rheumatic disease 12%, malignant 16%, traumatic 9%, radiation 7.5%, uremic 5%	86.2%	4% (1 perforation of the right ventricle, 2 ongoing hemorrhage, 1 sudden death in a patient with scleroderma and pulmonary hypertension, 1 iatrogenic purulent pericarditis	4% (hemopericardium with new or increased tamponade, requiring surgery in 4/5 patients)	NSVT 0.8%, several patients with vasovagal hypotension

Abbreviations: AV, atrioventricular; cath lab, cardiac catheterization laboratory; CT, computed tomography; ECG, electrocardiogram; Echo, echocardiography; ICU, intensive care unit; NSVT, Nonsustained supraventricular tachycardia (paroxysmal atrial fibrillation in 60%).

[a] Real-time echo-guided procedure was enabled by a multiangle bracket mounted on the echocardiographic probe to support the needle and enable its continuous visualization during the puncture.

procedures with 99% success. A multiangle bracket mounted on the echocardiographic probe to support the needle used for pericardiocentesis enabled its continuous visualization during the puncture. No lacerations or punctures of cardiac chambers occurred. Major complications (1.2%) included 1 mediastinal hematoma managed surgically in an anticoagulated patient and 1 pleuropericardial shunt requiring thoracocentesis. Using the subxiphoid approach, Vayre and colleagues[22] observed a much higher complication rate with 10% perforations of the right ventricle in 110 pericardiocentesis procedures for tamponade guided by contrast 2-dimensional echocardiography.

MULTIMODALITY IMAGING FOR PERICARDIOCENTESIS GUIDANCE

In several studies, 2 imaging modalities have been combined for pericardiocentesis guidance. After using echocardiography for selection of the approach and the trajectory of the needle, "real-time" fluoroscopy guidance can be used in the cardiac catheterization laboratory[8,23,24]; computed tomography[30,31] or MRI guidance[32] are alternative approaches, used only rarely. In 212 patients with cancer, pericardiocentesis guided by echocardiography (93%), combined echocardiography and fluoroscopy (42%), and computed tomography (8%) was successful in 99%, and there were no procedure-related deaths, while major complications occurred in 2.4% of the cases.[8] In patients with a higher risk of bleeding, a 5-F micropuncture kit (Cook Medical) was used in this study. Systems for computer guidance of pericardiocentesis have been also developed, but are not routinely used in clinical practice.[33]

FLUOROSCOPY-GUIDED PERICARDIOCENTESIS

Depending on the size and distribution of the effusion, its etiology, the personal experience of the operator, and the available facilities, a preferable setting for pericardiocentesis would be the cardiac catheterization laboratory, where fluoroscopic guidance can be added to echocardiography orientation. This approach may offer real-time control of potentially superior quality in comparison to echocardiographic imaging only, because echocardiography-guided pericardiocentesis without a probe-mounted needle does not allow visualization of the needle in 56% to 75% of cases.[15] The epicardial halo phenomenon can be used for the guidance of the procedure.[34] It reliably detects the "epicardial border zone," thus enabling a safe access even to small pericardial

effusions. The sensitivity of the sign is 92% in the lateral view and is associated with the size of the pericardial effusion and the body mass index. Hemodynamic assessment to exclude effusive-constrictive pericarditis and pericardial biopsies can be performed during the same session. However, radiation exposure for the patient and operators and the higher costs of the procedure are potential drawbacks.

Electrocardiogram and systemic blood pressure monitoring, aseptic conditions, selection of the appropriate needle, and drainage catheters apply for echocardiography-guided and fluoroscopy-guided procedures alike. Before and at the end of drainage, intrapericardial pressure should be recorded.

The subxiphoid route is extrapleural and avoids the coronary and internal mammary arteries. The operator intermittently attempts to aspirate fluid and injects small amounts of contrast. The lateral angiographic view provides the best visualization of the puncturing needle and its relation to the diaphragm and the pericardium (**Fig. 2**). If hemorrhagic fluid is freely aspirated, a few milliliters of the contrast medium may be injected under fluoroscopic observation. The appearance of a sluggish layering of the contrast medium inferiorly indicates that the needle is correctly positioned.

A soft J-tip guidewire is introduced and after dilatation exchanged for a multihole pigtail catheter. It is essential to check the position of the guidewire in at least 2 angiographic projections. If the guidewire was placed erroneously in an intracardiac position, this should be recognized before insertion of the dilator and drainage catheter. If, despite the caution, the introducer set or the catheter have perforated the heart and are laying intracardially, the catheter should be secured and emergent cardiac surgical assistance should be obtained. Alternatively, a second puncture can be attempted. If successful, surgery may be avoided using autotransfusion of pericardial blood to the femoral vein. The successful use of angioseal has been reported for management of a perforation after epicardial ablation.[35]

In a series of 352 fluoroscopy-guided percutaneous pericardiocentesis, only 13 major complications occurred: 3 cardiac perforations (0.9%), 2 cardiac arrhythmias (0.6%), 4 cases of arterial bleeding (1.1%), 2 cases of pneumothorax (0.6%), 1 infection (0.3%), and 1 major vagal reaction (0.3%).[23] No difference in complications was found between pericardiocenteses for pericardial effusions after cardiac surgery (208 patients) and those for effusions of nonsurgical (144 patients) origin. In the Marburg experience

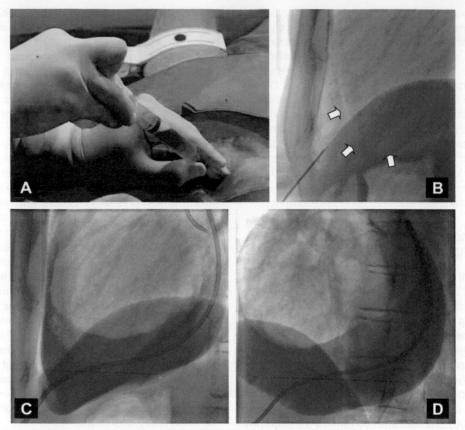

Fig. 2. Pericardiocentesis guided by fluoroscopy using the subxiphoid approach in a lateral angiographic view. (*A*) Puncturing needle is slowly approaching the heart shadow and the epicardial halo phenomenon (*white arrows* in *B*). The position of the needle was checked by injection of the angiographic contrast media (*white arrow*) and the needle exchanged for a 0,038″ J-tip guide wire. (*C*) Lateral view. The guidewire was exchanged for an 8.3-F pig-tail catheter (Merit Medical, Boston Scientific, Marlborough, MA) and after taking the 100-mL effusion samples for laboratory analyses the position of the catheter, size and distribution of the effusion was confirmed by intrapericardial injection of 40 mL of the contrast media (*black area* in *C* and *D*). (*D*) Anteroposterior view. The pericardial drainage catheter is in a proper position, injection of the contrast media demonstrates a large, circular pericardial effusion.

with fluoroscopic control of pericardiocentesis, there was no mortality and the incidence of major complications was significantly reduced by using the epicardial halo phenomenon in the lateral view. Major complications (1.3%) included 3 cases of cardiac perforation or arterial bleeding (all resolved with autotransfusion with no need for surgery) and 1 major vagal reaction (0.4%).[24]

PROLONGED CATHETER DRAINAGE OF PERICARDIAL EFFUSION

Brain natriuretic peptide plasma levels are suppressed in the presence of severe pericardial effusion, and may increase after pericardiocentesis.[36] To prevent pulmonary edema, rapid drainage of more than 1 L effusion should be avoided and prolonged catheter drainage should be provided for

the remaining effusion, especially in patients with concomitant heart failure.

The recurrence of pericardial effusion within 6 months of the initial procedure was 27% for patients who underwent simple pericardiocentesis and 14% for those who had extended drainage using a pigtail catheter.[10] In the recent series of 212 patients with cancer with catheter drainage for 3 to 5 days, a low recurrence rate (10%) was achieved.[8] The ongoing DROP trial (DRainage or Pericardiocentesis alone for recurrent nonmalignant, nonbacterial pericardial effusions requiring intervention) is the first multicenter randomized trial evaluating the efficacy and safety of pericardiocentesis alone versus pericardiocentesis plus extended pericardial drainage for recurrent nonmalignant, nonbacterial pericardial effusions refractory to medical therapy. This study is intended to provide appropriate evidence to support or discourage the further routine use of extended pericardial drainage.[37]

AMBULATORY PERICARDIAL DRAINAGE USING A PERMANENT PORT SYSTEM

Using video-assisted thoracoscopy under general anesthesia, a port system was implanted through the subxiphoid window into the pericardial space of 40 patients, thereby enabling home management of recurrent pericardial effusion in advanced malignancy.[38] The reservoir body was placed in a subcutaneous pocket and the outlet catheter inserted into the pleural cavity. The patients have used the system 1 to 5 times a week (mean, 3 ± 1). No infections or recurrent effusions were noted and the device was easily controlled at home in all cases.

CARDIAC CATHETERIZATION DURING PERICARDIOCENTESIS

Right heart catheterization can be performed simultaneously with pericardiocentesis. This allows monitoring for hemodynamic improvement as the effusion is drained, and also identification of hemodynamic abnormalities that persist in cases of effusive–constrictive pericarditis. Invasive hemodynamics and measurement of pericardial pressures are useful for diagnosis and for guidance of the procedure, particularly in complex cases.[2] After successful pericardiocentesis, if the intrapericardial pressure decreases to zero or becomes negative, and the right atrial pressure remains elevated, the differential diagnosis includes effusive–constrictive pericarditis (especially in patients with tuberculosis or prior irradiation for neoplastic disease), preexisting left ventricular dysfunction with heart failure, tricuspid valve disease, and restrictive cardiomyopathy. Sagrista-Sauleda and coworkers[5] identified 15 patients with effusive–constrictive pericarditis among 190 individuals who underwent combined pericardiocentesis and catheterization. Before catheterization, concomitant constriction was recognized in only 7 patients. Therefore, without cardiac catheterization the diagnosis would have be missed in 8 of the 15 patients (53.3%). It is also possible to make the diagnosis of effusive–constrictive pericarditis by echocardiography if constrictive echocardiographic features persist after complete drainage of the pericardial effusion.

PERICARDIOSCOPY, AND EPICARDIAL AND PERICARDIAL BIOPSIES

Biochemical pericardial fluid analyses are mostly nonspecific. However, high levels of unstimulated interferon-gamma, adenosine

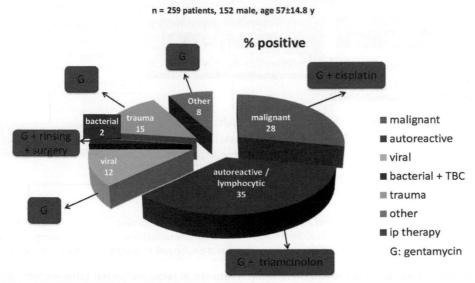

Etiology and Intrapericardial Treatment in Pericardial Effusions

n = 259 patients, 152 male, age 57±14.8 y

% positive

malignant
autoreactive
viral
bacterial + TBC
trauma
other
ip therapy
G: gentamycin

Fig. 3. Diagnosis and treatment of pericardial effusions over 21 years in the Marburg tertiary referral center for pericardial diseases. TBC, tuberculosis. (*From* Maisch B, Rupp H, Ristic A, et al. Pericardioscopy and epi- and pericardial biopsy - a new window to the heart improving etiological diagnoses and permitting targeted intrapericardial therapy. Heart Fail Rev 2013;18(3):320; with permission.)

deaminase, or lysozymes may indicate tuberculous infection. In cases of sepsis, of tuberculosis, or in positive patients with human immunodeficiency virus, bacterial cultures can be diagnostic. If promptly performed, fluid cytology can separate malignant from nonmalignant effusions, but additional histologic, immunohistochemistry and molecular analysis (polymerase chain reaction for microbial agents) will typically be required for definitive.[24]

Pericardioscopy permits the visualization of the pericardial space with its epicardial and pericardial layers and allows targeted biopsies from both, avoiding epicardial vessels and increasing the probability of uncovering the underlying etiology. Endoscopic inspection may show protrusions, hemorrhagic areas, or neovascularization. Pericardial biopsy can also be performed under radiologic guidance alone, but the diagnostic value of biopsies taken under pericardioscopy is higher (**Fig. 3**).[24,39]

INTRAPERICARDIAL TREATMENT

Intrapericardial treatment may be considered in selected patients with recurrent pericardial diseases according to the algorithm outlined in **Fig. 4** after a complete diagnostic workup and failure to respond to standard medical therapy and prolonged effusion drainage.

In neoplastic pericardial effusion (most frequently owing to lung or breast cancer), intrapericardial cytostatic therapy has been proposed in combination with systemic antineoplastic treatment, which should be tailored in collaboration with the oncologist.[40–47] In our experience, neoplastic pericardial effusion caused by lung cancer (22/42), breast cancer (8/42), or other metastatic disorders (12/42) was treated with intrapericardial cisplatin: 30 mg/m² cisplatin in 100 mL of 0.9% saline were given in a single slow injection through the intrapericardially located pigtail catheter.[47] It was kept there for 24 hours and then evacuated. Cisplatin is an alkylating agent with additional antitelomerase activity. In

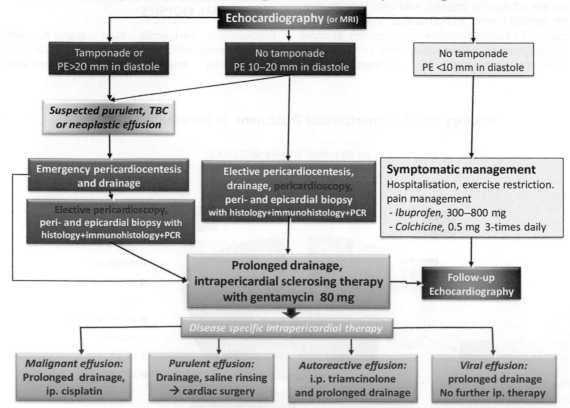

Fig. 4. Flow chart from diagnosis to intrapericardial treatment in large pericardial effusions with and without tamponade. Ip, intrapericardial; PCR, polymerase chain reaction; PE, pericardial effusion. (*From* Maisch B, Rupp H, Ristic A, et al. Pericardioscopy and epi- and pericardial biopsy - a new window to the heart improving etiological diagnoses and permitting targeted intrapericardial therapy. Heart Fail Rev 2013;18(3):319; with permission.)

our study,[47,48] 41 of the 42 patients could be promptly discharged. In the mean follow-up of 8.5 ± 3.2 months, none of the patients treated with cisplatin died owing to cardiac tamponade. Relapses within the 6-month follow-up were recorded in 8 patients (3 breast cancers, 1 lung cancer, 4 other tumors). The success rate of intrapericardial cisplatin corresponds with similar data reported in patients with lung cancer.[49,50] Cisplatin was highly effective immediately together with pericardiocentesis but less successful after 6 months in the prevention of a recurring effusion in 3 of our 8 patients with breast cancer, who had to undergo a second pericardial puncture.[47] Colleoni and colleagues[41] reported on the installation of thiotepa (15 mg on days 1, 3, and 5), which is also an alkylating agent with sclerosing and cytostatic activity, an immediate response to the treatment of 9 patients with breast cancer and 11 patients with lunch cancer, but also a recurrence in 3 patients during follow-up. Their data correspond with work by Girardi and colleagues[42] and Martioni and colleagues.[51]

Chen and colleagues[52] evaluated the safety and efficacy of the intrapericardial application of bevacizumab (100 or 200 mg every 2 weeks), a monoclonal antibody against the vascular endothelial growth factor receptor, which inhibits angiogenesis, for treating symptomatic malignant pericardial effusion in 7 patients with advanced cancer. Systemic oncologic treatment continued for all patients. The median survival was 168 days (range, 22–224). In 6 of 7 patients, effusion did not recur. Toxicity associated with bevacizumab intrapericardial treatment was mild and manageable in all patients. In lung cancer, however, the US Food and Drug Administration withdrew permission for treatment owing to reported serious side effects in 2011.

Numico and colleagues[53] treated 22 consecutive patients with malignant pericardial effusion with intrapericardial instillation of 10 mg of bleomycin. The pericardial catheter was then clamped for 48 hours, and removed only when the drainage was less than 25 mL daily. Twelve patients (54%) achieved complete response and 9 (41%) a partial response. Only 1 (5%) had a treatment failure and underwent surgery. Mild side effects (thoracic pain and supraventricular arrhythmias) occurred in 7 patients (32%). The 1-year pericardial effusion–free and progression-free survival rate was 74.0% (95% CI, 51.0–97.3). At a median follow-up of 75 months, a relapse was detected in 4 patients (18%). The 1- and 2-year overall survival rates were 33.9% (95% CI, 13.6–54.2) and 14.5% (95% CI, 0.0–29.5), respectively, with patients with lung cancer having a shorter survival

than patients with breast cancer. These and other agents applied so far intrapericardially for the treatment of neoplastic pericardial effusion are listed in **Table 2**.

The intrapericardial treatment for autoreactive and lymphocytic pericarditis with crystalloid triamcinolone is an optional antiinflammatory treatment in patients with recurrent pericarditis and negative polymerase chain reactions on cardiotropic viral genomes in biopsy and pericardial fluid. It avoids the systemic side effects of corticoid treatment in many cases and allows a high local dose. Two treatment regimens have been tested in 84 patients with 600 and 300 mg/m^2 body surface area.[89] Both showed comparable high success rates: recurrence was prevented in 92.6% of the patient group treated with 600 mg/m^2 and 86.7% of those treated with 300 mg/m^2 after 3 months and 86 versus 82.1%, respectively, after 1 year. The instillation was retained in the pericardium, and owing to the crystalloid suspension, triamcinolone stays active for 3 to 4 weeks. Nevertheless, it was well-tolerated. It was accompanied by 0.5 mg colchicine twice daily after drainage of the effusion. Transient iatrogenic Cushing syndrome was observed more frequently in patients receiving the higher intrapericardial dose (29.6% vs 13.3%). In rare cases of refractory uremic pericarditis, evacuation of the effusion and triamcinolone instillation has also been effective.[90–92]

Purulent pericarditis is a rare, acute, and fulminant illness that is fatal if untreated. Despite prompt percutaneous pericardiocentesis and extensive rinsing of the pericardial cavity, or even surgical drainage with saline irrigation and maximal systemic antibiotic treatment, the prognosis remains poor. Intrapericardial antibiotic instillation is not enough,[4] and the mortality rate is about 40% to 50%.[93] Instead of surgery, pericardiocentesis and frequent irrigation of the pericardial cavity with urokinase, streptokinase, or recombinant tissue plasminogen activator was successfully attempted in small series of patients.[93–97] Intrapericardial urokinase has been also reported to prevent later constriction by Cui and colleagues.[98] Intrapericardial application of fibrinolytics is under evaluation in a large, prospective, randomized trial for the potential to facilitate complete drainage of dense pericardial effusion, mainly owing to tuberculous pericarditis.[99]

DEVICES FOR PERICARDIOCENTESIS
Pericardial Effusion Access Using the PerDUCER Device

The PerDUCER instrument for pericardiocentesis (Comedicus Inc., Columbia Heights, MN)

Table 2
Intrapericardial treatment in patients with neoplastic pericardial effusion

Intrapericardial Treatment (Reference)	Number of Patients Treated	Treatment Success (%)	Follow-up (mo)	Side Effects and Complications
Cisplatin[43,47–51,54–61]	107	83.3–100	4–24	• Nausea (6.7%) • Atrial arrhythmias (4.4%) • Constriction (1.1%) • Myocardial ischemia (1%)
Thiotepa[40–43,51]	112	79–83	6–24	• Thrombocytopenia (0.9%) • Leucopoenia (0.9%)
Antitumor antibiotics • Bleomycin[53,62–66] • Mitomycin C[67–70] • Aclarubicin[67]	96	70–100	3–12	• Constriction (2.4%) for mito-mycin C treatment
Tetracycline[63,71–76]	222	73–75	3–25	• Severe pain (15%–70%) • Atrial arrhythmias (9%) • Fever (7.5%–9%) • Infection (0.5%)
Mitoxantrone[77–80]	48	60–100	5–15	• Mild leukopenia in 2 patients • Lack of appetite
Radioactive chromic phosphate[44,81,82]	75	71–95	8–24	• None
Autologous tumor infiltrating lymphocytes activated with IL-2[83]	4	100	3–15	• Low-grade fever (100%) • Tachycardia (25%)
OK-432[84–88]	10	70	1–11	• Fever (60%) • Pain (50%)
Bevacizumab[52]	7	71.4%	1–7	• Proteinuria • Thrombus formation • Nausea and vomiting

Abbreviations: IL, interleukin; OK-432, penicillin-treated and heat-treated lyophilized powder of the substrain of *Streptococcus pyogenes* A3.

Adapted from Maisch B, Ristić AD, Seferović M, et al. Interventional pericardiology: pericardiocentesis, pericardioscopy, pericardial biopsy, balloon pericardiotomy, and intrapericardial therapy. Heidelberg (Germany): Springer; 2011. p. 137; with permission of Springer Nature.

was developed to enable percutaneous pericardial access in the absence of pericardial effusion. The concept of the PerDUCER includes a combination of vacuum suction and tangential puncture of the parietal pericardium.[100,101] It contains a 21-gauge introducer needle located inside a stainless steel sheath, which ends with a plastic view tube and a hemispheric side hole cavity, where the pericardium is captured by a vacuum and tangentially punctured by an introducer needle. The size of the side hole determines the maximum thickness of the pericardium that can be captured (2 mm). The procedure includes 2 major steps: (1) subxiphoid access to the anterior mediastinum, and (2) pericardial capture, puncture, insertion of the guidewire, and catheter for sampling of pericardial fluid or delivery of intrapericardial treatment.

In addition to the favorable experimental, cadaver, and animal experience regarding the feasibility and safety of the procedure, clinical experience in accessing normal pericardium with the PerDUCER comprises semiclosed chest attempts (direct vision) performed in 8 patients before an elective surgical intervention requiring a sternotomy.[101] An additional 4 patients underwent a closed chest, fluoroscopy-assisted procedure. Guidewire insertion was successful in 10 of 12 patients (7 on first attempt, 3 on second) without adverse hemodynamic effects or arrhythmia.

The PerDUCER was successful in 2 of 6 patients with myopericarditis participating in the study of intrapericardial treatment with triamcinolone (pericardial effusion in all of <180 mL). The selection of the pericardial site for the application of the PerDUCER was facilitated by flexible endoscopy (AF 1101 BI, Karl Storz, Tuttlingen, Germany) that enabled detection of an area of pericardium free of adipose tissue and adhesions to successfully apply the PerDUCER.[102] There were no acute or late complications in any of the procedures.

Similarly, in a previously reported series of 5 patients with large to moderate pericardial effusions, the procedure was not successful despite good mediastinal access and capture of the pericardium.[103] In the study performed in patients who had undergone bypass surgery with a normal pericardium, the PerDUCER procedure in patients with moderate or large pericardial effusions procedure was accomplished successfully in all 8 patients studied in the open chest setting.[100] However, in an additional 4 patients studied before sternotomy for aortocoronary bypass, pericardial access with the PerDUCER in patients with moderate or large pericardial effusions could be achieved only in 2. Although the addition of flexible endoscopy improves the feasibility, it certainly complicates and increases the costs of the procedure. The introduction of a large introducer set into the mediastinal space is often painful despite local anesthesia, analgesia, and sedation.

If the pericardium is thin enough so that part of the pericardial space is also within the suction head, the needle reaches the underlying pericardial space. Although such a device has been used successfully in pigs, it failed in 4 of 6 patients with myopericarditis and a small (132 ± 49 mL) pericardial effusion.[102] The reason could be loss of vacuum, tissue detachment, and thus failure of accessing the pericardial space.

The PeriAttacher for Accessing the Pericardial Space

After the very limited success of PerDUCER, a modification was developed and patented (the PeriAttacher).[2] The device body features a continuous bore, and the distal end features several jaws that can be opened and closed. A needle for the tissue puncture is located in the jaws and is moveable within the continuous bore. The guide tube features a deflection mechanism on its distal end for deflecting the distal end of the penetrating needle. The addition of a multitude of suction channels in the suction head could be expected to better fill the suction head itself. The vacuum channels within the capture mechanism are provided to help hold a captured body duct and open the duct interior to facilitate introduction of a fluid into the lumen of the duct. Also in this device, a

needle is disposed within an axial passage in the shaft and punctures the duct within the suction head. In the case of a thickened pericardium, the pericardium would be captured and held by the vacuum channels within the suction head. When the needle is advanced, it might only travel into the thickened pericardium and not into the underlying sac.[2]

The AttachGuider

An AttachGuider device allows fixation of the device within the pericardial space. The device features at least 2 means of attachment separated from each other in the direction of the desired movement (eg, forward or backward)m which could be activated one after another for the guidance of the forward movement. After activation of the first means of attachment and activation of the means of forward movement, a part of the device that is not attached is moved in the direction of the desired movement. These steps can be repeated as desired, whereby the direction of the bending is adjustable. The device can be used for epicardial lead implantation or epicardial ablation.[2]

The AttachLifter

The rationale of the AttachLifter is to create separation of the pericardium from the epicardium, allowing safe pericardial access in the absence of pericardial effusion.[104] The pericardial attachment results in an increased negative pressure that is monitored and displayed by various means (as in the PeriAttacher). A pressure recording can monitor the negative pressure upon attachment. In contrast with the PerDUCER, the pericardium is lifted away from the epicardium and punctured outside the suction head. The suction head has flexible clamps that grab the tissue more effectively and also provide a seal when a negative pressure is applied. The opening of the suction head ("attacher") is narrowed by flexible clamps that grab the tissue and improve the vacuum seal in the case of uneven tissue. The suction head is turned by approximately 90° to the right and the needle, which is outside the vacuum channel, is pushed forward into the "tent," thereby entering the pericardial space. Therefore, a "safety ridge" for needle guidance is present and prevents injury to the epicardium. In case of markedly thickened tissue, the forwarded needle is left in the tissue, the suction head is turned further to the right, and a stiff guidewire is pushed through a guide tube (at a 90° angle relative to the longitudinal suction head) through the firmly attached pericardium into the pericardial space. A flexible endoscope can be used to inspect the pericardium before puncture.[2,104]

Visual Puncture Systems

The visual puncture system was designed to integrate a microimaging fiber into an 18-guage needle to facilitate visual guidance during pericardiocentesis.[105] The device was tested in an experimental model (balloon-in-balloon structure, inner 10″ red balloon, filled with 240 mL red ink and the outer 10″ white balloon filled with 360 mL or 480 mL saline to simulate pericardial effusions of 1–2 cm or >2 cm). Under visual guidance, the 18-guage needle successfully entered into the pericardial sac with proper positioning. By further advancing the microimaging fiber beyond the needle tip, clear anatomy of the epicardium and the inner surface could be acquired.

The Grasper, Scissors, and Reverse Slitter

Three novel devices were developed to enable pericardial access in patients with no pericardial effusion, all of which can be deployed "over-the-wire" after percutaneous puncture.[106] The grasper permits to seize the parietal pericardium providing leverage for incision. The scissors enable antegrade cutting maneuvers. The reverse slitter allows retrograde incisions and has a deflectable tip that increases the potential cutting area. The base of the scissors and reverse slitter are blunt, ensuring that the cutting element is always away from the myocardium. These devices have been tested in animal studies with excellent feasibility and safety.

PERCUTANEOUS BALLOON PERICARDIOTOMY

Percutaneous balloon pericardiotomy may be performed for the management of recurring, mainly neoplastic pericardial effusion (class IIb recommendation).[2–4] It decreases the risk of the neoplastic effusion relapses, which can be up to 62%.[107] The success rate is low in malignant mesothelioma.[108] The procedure has also been performed in nonmalignant, noninfectious, large pericardial effusion or cardiac tamponade if prolonged pericardial drainage was not successful,[3,109] and in a septic patient with purulent effusion.[110] Spread of neoplastic cells or infection from the pericardial to the pleural cavity or the peritoneum remains a possible concern and is one of the reasons why this procedure is not widely applied.[3] Other contraindications include major coagulation disorders, effusive–constrictive pericarditis, loculated pericardial effusions, large left pleural effusion, advanced respiratory insufficiency, and a history of pneumonectomy.[111]

The procedure is performed under local anesthesia and fluoroscopic guidance in the cardiac catheterization laboratory, immediately after pericardiocentesis or in the next session. The pericardium is predilated with fascial dilators (7- to 11-F) and through the corresponding sheath a large balloon is introduced over the guidewire. To position the balloon at the pericardial margin, angiographic contrast is injected intrapericardially. Several balloon inflations (6 ATM, 1–2 minutes each) are usually necessary for the central indentation to disappear (**Fig. 5**), creating a window at the parietal pericardium

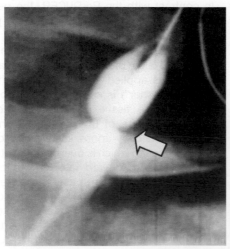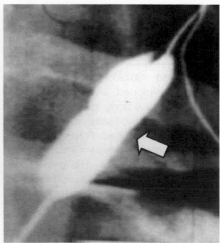

Fig. 5. Percutaneous balloon pericardiotomy using a triple balloon catheter (Schneider Trefoil-Meier). Inflated balloon with indentation (*left*), fully inflated balloon and indentation disappears (*right*). (*From* Maisch B, Ristic AD, Seferovic M, et al. Interventional pericardiology: pericardiocentesis, pericardioscopy, pericardial biopsy, balloon pericardiotomy, and intrapericardial therapy. Heidelberg (Germany): Springer; 2011. p. 157; with permission.)

Table 3
Major studies on percutaneous balloon pericardiotomy

Author, (Reference)	Number of Patients Treated	Main Etiologies	Treatment Success (No Effusion Recurrence)	Follow-up (mo)	Complications
Jneid et al[3] 2016	130	Lung cancer 42.3% Breast cancer 16.2% Nonmalignant 15.4%	85%	5.0 ± 5.8	13% (fever) 15% (larger pleural effusion in preexisting pleural effusions) 9% (large pleural effusion without preexisting pleural effusion)
Di Segni et al,[121] 1995	8	Malignant 87.5% Uremic 12.5%	100%	1–11	12.5% (bleeding)
Galli et al,[123] 1995	10	All malignant	100%	10	None
Chow et al[125] 1996	11	Various etiologies	91%	4.2	Pain or discomfort
Bhardwaj et al,[126] 2015	36	Lung cancer 50% Breast cancer 13.2% Gastrointestinal cancer in 15.7% Nonmalignant 8.3%	94.4%	24	2.8% (fever) 8.3% (large pleural effusion)
Ristić et al,[128] 2000	20	Malignant 100%	90%	4 ± 3.9	10% (large pleural effusion)
Thanopoulos et al,[109] 1997	10	Nonmalignant 100%	90%	14.6	10% (rupture of the balloon and entrapment of its distal part in the pericardium)
Jalisi et al,[130] 2004	17	All with cardiac tamponade and high risk for recurrences	82%	12	None
Ruiz-García et al,[131] 2013, Javier-Irazusta et al,[132] 2017	35	Malignant 97.1%	77.1%	1.9	5.7% (1 large pleural effusion and 1 pseudoaneurysm of the right ventricle)

for either a pericardio–peritoneal or a pericardio–pleural shunt. In most of the studies large, pulmonary valvuloplasty round balloons, 18 to 25 mm in diameter, 30 to 60 mm long (Mansfield, Inoue, Tyshak II, Maxi LD, or Z-MED IIT) have been used.[106–126] Double balloon pericardiotomy has been applied in patients with significant pericardial stiffness,[120,127] although Seferović and Ristić[2,128] used a triple balloon catheter (Schneider Trefoil-Meier, 3×5 or 3×7 mm). Sochman and colleagues[129] successfully applied a cutting pericardiotome for the similar procedure. With this device, great care has to be taken to avoid epicardial trauma.

The fragmentation of the fibroelastic connective tissue of the parietal pericardium was confirmed after percutaneous balloon pericardiotomy.[112] In the first days after the procedure, pericardial fluid is drained to the left pleural or to the peritoneal space. However, there was no difference in the success rate of the procedures in patients in whom pericardio–pleural or pericardio–peritoneal shunts were or were not created.[111,113] The long-term effect could result from the inflammatory fusion of the pericardial layers, which decreases or brings the effusion production to a standstill.[114]

Treatment success and complication rates observed in the US registry on percutaneous balloon pericardiotomy[3] and other series are listed in **Table 3**. There are no randomized studies comparing percutaneous balloon pericardiotomy with pericardiocentesis, prolonged drainage of pericardial effusion, the intrapericardial instillation of cytostatics, radioactive or sclerosing drugs, the surgical creation of a pleuro–pericardial or pleuro–peritoneal window, and systemic chemotherapy and/or radiotherapy.

Virk and colleagues[133] analyzed recurrences of malignant pericardial effusion in 31 studies reporting outcomes of pericardiocentesis (n = 305), pericardiocentesis followed by extended catheter drainage (n = 486), pericardial instillation of sclerosing agents (n = 392), or percutaneous balloon pericardiotomy (n = 157). Isolated pericardiocentesis demonstrated a pooled recurrence rate of 38.3%, extended catheter drainage of 12.1%, pericardial sclerosis of 10.8%, and percutaneous balloon pericardiotomy of 10.3%. Procedure-related mortality ranged from 0.5% to 1.0% across the interventions. The surgical subxiphoid pericardiotomy is more invasive, increases the patient's discomfort and the risk of secondary infections, and has a reported mortality of 1.2%.[134]

PERCUTANEOUS INTRAPERICARDIAL LEFT ATRIAL APPENDAGE LIGATION

Percutaneous left atrial appendage ligation is a novel intrapericardial interventional procedure designed to prevent thromboembolic complications in patients with atrial fibrillation. It is performed after fluoroscopy-guided pericardiocentesis of the normal pericardium using a LARIAT Suture Delivery Device (Sentre HEART, Redwood City, CA).[3,135] A magnet-tipped, 0.025-inch guidewire is advanced into the anterior aspect of the left atrial appendage via femoral vein trans-septally and another magnet-tipped, 0.035-inch wire into the pericardium through a 13.5-F pericardial sheath to form a connection with the magnet-tipped wire, over which the Lariat snare is advanced and closed at the mouth of the appendage. The most recent report from the US multicenter registry included 712 consecutive patients undergoing this procedure at 18 US hospitals.[136] LARIAT was successfully deployed in 95.5% of the patients. A complete closure was achieved in 98%, and 1.8% had a trace leak (<2 mm). There was 1 death related to the procedure (0.14%). Ten patients (1.4%) had cardiac perforation necessitating open heart surgery, and another 14 patients with cardiac perforations (2%) did not need surgery. The risk of cardiac perforation decreased significantly after the introduction of a micropuncture needle for pericardial access. Delayed complications (pericarditis requiring >2 weeks of treatment with nonsteroidal antiinflammatory drugs or colchicine and pericardial and pleural effusion) occurred in 34 patients (4.8%), and the risk decreased significantly with the periprocedural use of colchicine.

INTERVENTIONAL TREATMENT OF PERICARDIAL CYSTS

Pericardial cysts are rare and mostly congenital. Many of them are asymptomatic mediastinal abnormalities. "Spring water cysts," if symptomatic, can be treated with aspiration and alcohol ablation.[4,137] Before ablation with 100% alcohol is performed, a malignancy should be excluded. Absence of communication with the pericardial sac has to be proven by injection of a small amount of contrast medium.

SUMMARY

Percutaneous interventions in pericardial diseases have improved significantly in the last 2 decades, especially with wide use of imaging for guidance, but also with the improvement of technology and our understanding of the technical tips and tricks to improve feasibility and safety. Pericardiocentesis remains the most important procedure; it is life saving in cardiac tamponade and provides essential information in suspected malignant, purulent and tuberculous pericarditis. Pericardiocentesis alone provides immediate symptomatic relief, but subsequent catheter drainage or intrapericardial therapy may be required to minimize recurrences. After establishing the etiology of the pericardial disease, specific intrapericardial treatment can be initiated, which should be associated with systemic therapy in neoplastic or autoreactive pericardial effusions. Percutaneous balloon pericardiotomy may be a potential alternative in managing recurrent effusions. The choice of the most appropriate intervention has to be a part of the individual management strategy based on the clinical status, underlying etiology and the available expertise.

REFERENCES

1. Ristić AD, Imazio M, Adler Y, et al. Triage strategy for urgent management of cardiac tamponade: a position statement of the European Society of Cardiology working group on myocardial and pericardial diseases. Eur Heart J 2014; 35(34):2279–84.

2. Maisch B, Ristić AD, Seferović M, et al. Interventional pericardiology: pericardiocentesis, pericardioscopy, pericardial biopsy, balloon pericardiotomy, and intrapericardial therapy. Heidelberg (Germany): Springer; 2011.

3. Jneid H, Ziskind AA, Palacios IF. Pericardial interventions. In: Topol EJ, Teirstein PS, editors. Textbook of interventional cardiology. 7th Edition. Philadelphia: Elsevier; 2016. p. 861–72.

4. Adler Y, Charron P, Imazio M, et al, European Society of Cardiology (ESC). 2015 ESC Guidelines for the diagnosis and management of pericardial diseases: the Task Force for the diagnosis and management of pericardial diseases of the European Society of Cardiology (ESC) Endorsed by: the European association for Cardio-thoracic surgery (EACTS). Eur Heart J 2015;36(42):2921–64.

5. Sagrista-Sauleda J, Angel J, Permanyer-Miralda G, et al. Long-term follow-up of idiopathic chronic pericardial effusion. N Engl J Med 1999;341:2054–9.

6. Little WC, Freeman GL. Pericardial disease. Circulation 2006;113:1622–32.

7. Halpern DG, Argulian E, Briasoulis A, et al. A novel pericardial effusion scoring index to guide decision for drainage. Crit Pathw Cardiol 2012;11:85–8.

8. El Haddad D, Iliescu C, Yusuf SW, et al. Outcomes of cancer patients undergoing percutaneous pericardiocentesis for pericardial effusion. J Am Coll Cardiol 2015;66(10):1119–28.

9. Iliescu C, Khair T, Marmagkiolis K, et al. Echocardiography and fluoroscopy-guided pericardiocentesis for cancer patients with cardiac tamponade and thrombocytopenia. J Am Coll Cardiol 2016; 68(7):771–3.

10. Tsang T, Enriquez-Sarano M, Freeman W, et al. Consecutive 1127 therapeutic echocardiographically guided pericardiocenteses: clinical profile, practice patterns, and outcomes spanning 21 years. Mayo Clin Proc 2002;77:429–36.

11. Kepez A, Sari I, Cincin A, et al. Pericardiocentesis in patients with thrombocytopenia and high international normalized ratio: case report and review of the literature. Platelets 2014;25(2):140–1.

12. Krikorian JG, Hancock EW. Pericardiocentesis. Am J Med 1978;65(5):808–14.

13. Hayashi T, Tsukube T, Yamashita T, et al. Impact of controlled pericardial drainage on critical cardiac tamponade with acute type A aortic dissection. Circulation 2012;126(11 Suppl 1):S97–101.

14. Cruz I, Stuart B, Caldeira D, et al. Controlled pericardiocentesis in patients with cardiac tamponade complicating aortic dissection: experience of a centre without cardiothoracic surgery. Eur Heart J Acute Cardiovasc Care 2015;4(2):124–8.

15. Maggiolini S, Gentile G, Farina A, et al. Safety, efficacy, and complications of pericardiocentesis by real-time echo-monitored procedure. Am J Cardiol 2016;117(8):1369–74.

16. Ainsworth CD, Salehian O. Echo-guided pericardiocentesis: let the bubbles show the way. Circulation 2011;123(4):e210–1.

17. Battistoni I, Marini M, Angelini L, et al. Safety and efficacy of non-continuous echocardiographic guided pericardiocentesis: a single-center study of 478 patients. Minerva Cardioangiol 2016. [Epub ahead of print].

18. Akyuz S, Zengin A, Arugaslan E, et al. Echo-guided pericardiocentesis in patients with clinically significant pericardial effusion. Outcomes over a 10-year period. Herz 2015;40(Suppl 2):153–9.

19. Kolek M, Brat R. Echocardiography-guided pericardiocentesis as the method of choice for treatment of significant pericardial effusion following cardiac surgery: a 12-year single-centre experience. Minerva Cardioangiol 2017; 65(4):336–47.

20. Jaussaud N, Boignard A, Durand M, et al. Percutaneous drainage of postoperative pericardial effusion in cardiac surgery. J Interv Cardiol 2012; 25(1):95–101.

21. Lindenberg M, Kjellberg M, Karlsson E, et al. Pericardiocentesis guided by 2-D echocardiography: the method of choice for treatment of pericardial effusion. J Intern Med 2003;253:411–7.

22. Vayre F, Lardoux H, Pezzano M, et al. Subxiphoid pericardiocentesis guided by contrast two-dimensional echocardiography in cardiac tamponade: experience of 110 consecutive patients. Eur J Echocardiogr 2000;1:66–71.

23. Duvernoy O, Borowiec J, Helmius G, et al. Complications of percutaneous pericardiocentesis under

fluoroscopic guidance. Acta Radiol 1992;33(4): 309–13.

24. Maisch B, Rupp H, Ristic A, et al. Pericardioscopy and epi- and pericardial biopsy - a new window to the heart improving etiological diagnoses and permitting targeted intrapericardial therapy. Heart Fail Rev 2013;18(3):317–28.

25. Tsang T, El-Najdawi E, Freeman W, et al. Percutaneous echocardiographically guided pericardiocentesis in pediatric patients: evaluation of safety and efficacy. J Am Soc Echocardiogr 1998;11:1072–7.

26. Tsang TS, Freeman WK, Barnes ME, et al. Rescue echocardiographically guided pericardiocentesis for cardiac perforation complicating catheter-based procedures. The Mayo Clinic experience. J Am Coll Cardiol 1998;32(5):1345–50.

27. Tsang T, Barnes M, Hayes S, et al. Clinical and echocardiographic characteristics of significant pericardial effusions following cardiothoracic surgery and outcomes of echo-guided pericardiocentesis for management - Mayo clinic experience, 1979-1998. Chest 1999;116:322–31.

28. Tsang T, Seward J, Barnes M, et al. Outcomes of primary and secondary treatment of pericardial effusion in patients with malignancy. Mayo Clin Proc 2000;75:248–53.

29. Cauduro S, Moder K, Tsang T, et al. Clinical and echocardiographic characteristics of hemodynamically significant pericardial effusions in patients with systemic lupus erythematosus. Am J Cardiol 2003;92:1370–2.

30. Eichler K, Zangos S, Thalhammer A, et al. CT-guided pericardiocenteses: clinical profile, practice patterns and clinical outcome. Eur J Radiol 2010;75(1):28–31.

31. Neves D, Silva G, Morais G, et al. Computed tomography-guided pericardiocentesis - a single-center experience. Rev Port Cardiol 2016;35(5): 285–90.

32. Alraies MC, AlJaroudi W, Yarmohammadi H, et al. Usefulness of cardiac magnetic resonance-guided management in patients with recurrent pericarditis. Am J Cardiol 2015;115(4):542–7.

33. Marmignon C, Chavanon O, Troccaz J. CASPER, a Computer ASsisted PERicardial puncture system: first clinical results. Comput Aided Surg 2005; 10(1):15–21.

34. Ristić AD, Wagner HJ, Maksimović R, et al. Epicardial halo phenomenon: a guide for pericardiocentesis? Heart Fail Rev 2013;18(3):307–16.

35. Petrov I, Dimitrov C. Closing of a right ventricle perforation with a vascular closure device. Catheter Cardiovasc Interv 2009;74(2):247–50.

36. Lauri G, Rossi C, Rubino M, et al. B-type natriuretic peptide levels in patients with pericardial effusion undergoing pericardiocentesis. Int J Cardiol 2016;212:318–23.

37. Imazio M, Belli R, Beqaraj F, et al, DROP Investigators. DRainage or Pericardiocentesis alone for recurrent nonmalignant, nonbacterial pericardial effusions requiring intervention: rationale and design of the DROP trial, a randomized, open-label, multicenter study. J Cardiovasc Med (Hagerstown) 2014;15(6):510–4.

38. Melfi FM, Menconi GF, Chella A, et al. The management of malignant pericardial effusions using permanently implanted devices. Eur J Cardio-thorac Surg 2002;21(2):345–7.

39. Seferovic PM, Ristic AD, Maksimovic R, et al. Diagnostic value of pericardial biopsy: improvement with extensive sampling enabled by pericardioscopy. Circulation 2003;107:978–83.

40. Bishiniotis TS, Antoniadou S, Katseas G, et al. Malignant cardiac tamponade in women with breast cancer treated by pericardiocentesis and intrapericardial administration of triethylenethiophosphoramide (thiotepa). Am J Cardiol 2000; 86(3):362–4.

41. Colleoni M, Martinelli G, Beretta F, et al. Intracavitary chemotherapy with thiotepa in malignant pericardial effusion: an active and well tolerated regimen. J Clin Oncol 1998;16:2371–6.

42. Girardi LN, Ginsberg RJ, Burt ME. Pericardiocentesis and intrapericardial sclerosis: effective therapy for malignant pericardial effusion. Ann Thorac Surg 1997;64:1422–8.

43. Lestuzzi C, Bearz A, Lafaras C, et al. Neoplastic pericardial disease in lung cancer: impact on outcomes of different treatment strategies. A multi-center study. Lung Cancer 2011;72:340–7.

44. Dempke W, Firusian N. Treatment of malignant pericardial effusion with 32 P-colloid. Br J Cancer 1999;80(12):1955–7.

45. Maruyama R, Yokoyama H, Seto T, et al. Catheter drainage followed by the instillation of bleomycin to manage malignant pericardial effusion in non-small cell lung cancer: a multi-institutional phase II trial. J Thorac Oncol 2007;2(1):65–8.

46. Kunitoh H, Tamura T, Shibata T, et al, JCOG Lung Cancer Study Group, Tokyo, Japan. A randomised trial of intrapericardial bleomycin for malignant pericardial effusion with lung cancer (JCOG9811). Br J Cancer 2009;100(3):464–9.

47. Maisch B, Ristic AD, Pankuweit S, et al. Neoplastic pericardial effusion: efficacy and safety of intrapericardial treatment with cisplatin. Eur Heart J 2002; 23:1625–31.

48. Maisch B, Pankuweit S, Brilla C, et al. Intrapericardial treatment of inflammatory and neoplastic pericarditis guided by pericardioscopy and epicardial biopsy—results from a pilot study. Clin Cardiol 1999;22(suppl 1):17–22.

49. Tomkowski W, Szturmowicz M, Fijalkowska A, et al. New approaches to the management and

treatment of malignant pericardial effusion. Support Care Cancer 1997;5(1):64–6.

50. Tondini M, Rocco G, Bianchi C, et al. Intracavitary cisplatin (CDDO) in the treatment of metastatic pericardial involvement from breast and lung cancer. Monaldi Arch Chest Dis 1995;50(2):86–8.

51. Martioni A, Cipolla CM, Cardinale D, et al. Long-term results of intrapericardial chemotherapeutic treatment of malignant pericardial effusions with thiotepa. Chest 2004;126(5):1412–6.

52. Chen D, Zhang Y, Shi F, et al. Intrapericardial bevacizumab safely and effectively treats malignant pericardial effusion in advanced cancer patients. Oncotarget 2016;7(32):52436–41.

53. Numico G, Cristofano A, Occelli M, et al. Prolonged drainage and intrapericardial bleomycin administration for cardiac tamponade secondary to cancer-related pericardial effusion. Medicine (Baltimore) 2016;95(15):e3273.

54. Aitini E, Cavazzini G, Pasquini E, et al. Treatment of primary or metastatic pleural effusion with intracavitary cytosine arabinoside and cisplatin. A phase II study. Acta Oncol 1994;33(2):191–4.

55. Bindi M, Trusso M, Tucci E. Intracavitary cisplatin in malignant cardiac tamponade. Tumori 1987;73(2): 163–5.

56. Pavon-Jimenez R, Garcia-Rubira JC, Garcia-Martinez JT, et al. Intrapericardial cisplatin for malignant tamponade. Rev Esp Cardiol 2000;53(4):587–9.

57. Tomkowski W, Szturmowicz M, Fijalkowska A, et al. Intrapericardial cisplatin for the management of patients with large malignant pericardial effusion. J Cancer Res Clin Oncol 1994;120(7):434–6.

58. Tomkowski WZ, Filipecki S. Intrapericardial cisplatin for the management of patients with large malignant pericardial effusion in the course of the lung cancer. Lung Cancer 1997;16(2–3):215–22.

59. Tomkowski WZ, Filipecki S. Intrapericardial administration of cisplatin in treatment of metastatic pericardial involvement in adenocarcinoma of the lung. Arch Chest Dis 1997;52:221–4.

60. Fiorentino MV, Daniele O, Morandi P, et al. Intrapericardial instillation of platin in malignant pericardial effusion. Cancer 1988;62(9):1904–6.

61. Bischiniotis TS, Lafaras CT, Platogiannis DN, et al. Intrapericardial cisplatin administration after pericardiocentesis in patients with lung adenocarcinoma and malignant cardiac tamponade. Hellenic J Cardiol 2005;46(5):324–9.

62. Thai V, Oneschuk D. Malignant pericardial effusion treated with intrapericardial bleomycin. J Palliat Med 2007;10(2):281–2.

63. Liu G, Crump M, Goss PE, et al. Prospective comparison of the sclerosing agents doxycycline and bleomycin for the primary management of malignant pericardial effusion and cardiac tamponade. J Clin Oncol 1996;14(12):3141–7.

64. van der Gaast A, Kok TC, van der Linden NH, et al. Intrapericardial instillation of bleomycin in the management of malignant pericardial effusion. Eur J Cancer Clin Oncol 1989;25(10):1505–6.

65. Yano T, Yokoyama H, Inoue T, et al. A simple technique to manage malignant pericardial effusion with a local instillation of bleomycin in non-small cell carcinoma of the lung. Oncology 1994;51(6): 507–9.

66. Cormican MC, Nyman CR. Intrapericardial bleomycin for the management of cardiac tamponade secondary to malignant pericardial effusion. Br Heart J 1990;63:61–2.

67. Fukuoka M, Takada M, Tamai S, et al. Local application of anti-cancer drugs for the treatment of malignant pleural and pericardial effusion. Gan To Kagaku Ryoho 1984;11(8):1543–9.

68. Kaira K, Mori M. Intrapericardial instillation of mitomycin C in recurrent cardiac tamponade due to malignant pericardial effusion. Clin Oncol (R Coll Radiol) 2006;18(6):506.

69. Kohnoe S, Maehara Y, Takahashi I, et al. Intrapericardial mitomycin C for the management of malignant pericardial effusion secondary to gastric cancer: case report and review. Chemotherapy 1994;40:57–60.

70. Lee LN, Yang PC, Chang DB, et al. Ultrasound guided pericardial drainage and intrapericardial instillation of mitomycin C for malignant pericardial effusion. Thorax 1994;49(6):594–5.

71. Grau JJ, Estape J, Palombo H, et al. Intracavitary oxytetracycline in malignant peri-cardial tamponade. Oncology 1992;49:489–91.

72. Davis S, Rambotti P, Grignani F. Intrapericardial tetracycline sclerosis in the treatment of malignant pericardial effusion: an analysis of thirty-three cases. J Clin Oncol 1984;2(6):631–6.

73. Maher EA, Shepherd FA, Todd TJ. Pericardial sclerosis as the primary management of malignant pericardial effusion and cardiac tamponade. J Thorac Cardiovasc Surg 1996;112(3): 637–43.

74. Salamon P, Berliner S, Shachner A, et al. Tetracycline treatment for malignant pericardial effusion. Med Interne 1989;27(1):73–4.

75. Shepherd FA, Ginsberg JS, Evans WK, et al. Tetracycline sclerosis in the management of malignant pericardial effusion. J Clin Oncol 1985;3(12): 1678–82.

76. Shepherd FA, Morgan C, Evans WK, et al. Medical management of malignant pericardial effusion by tetracycline sclerosis. Am J Cardiol 1987;60: 1161–6.

77. Musch E, Gremmler B, Nitsch J, et al. Intrapericardial instillation of mitoxantrone in palliative therapy of malignant pericardial effusion. Onkologie 2003; 26:135–9.

78. Norum J, Lunde P, Aasebo U, et al. Mitoxantrone in malignant pericardial effusion. J Chemother 1998; 10(5):399–404.

79. Ammon A, Eiffert H, Reil S, et al. Tumor-associated antigens in effusions of malignant and benign origin. Clin Investig 1993;71(6):437–44.

80. Kuhn K, Purea H, Selbach J, et al. Treatment with locally applied mitoxantrone. Acta Med Austriaca 1989;16(3–4):87–90.

81. Martini N, Freiman AH, Watson RC, et al. Intrapericardial installation of radioactive chromic phosphate in malignant effusion. AJR Am J Roentgenol 1977;128(4):639–41.

82. Firusian N, Dempke W. An early phase II study of intratumoral P-32 chromic phosphate injection therapy for patients with refractory solid tumors and solitary metastases. Cancer 1999;85(4):980–7.

83. Toh U, Fujii T, Seki N, et al. Characterization of IL-2-activated TILs and their use in intrapericardial immunotherapy in malignant pericardial effusion. Cancer Immunol Immunother 2006;55(10):1219–27.

84. Imamura T, Tamura K, Takenaga M, et al. Intrapericardial OK-432 instillation for the management of malignant pericardial effusion. Cancer 1991;68:259–63.

85. Nanjo T. Intracavitary injection of OK-432 for malignant pericardial effusion, a case report. Radiat Med 1990;8(4):155–8.

86. Imamura T, Tamura K, Taguchi T, et al. Intrapericardial instillation of OK-432 for the management of malignant pericardial effusion: report of three cases. Jpn J Med 1989;28(1):62–6.

87. Wakiyama S, Shirabe K, Nagaie T. A case of carcinomatous cardiac tamponade due to breast cancer treated with OK-432 and mitomycin C. Gan To Kagaku Ryoho 2007;34(3):439–41.

88. Furukawa A, Itoh A, Nakamura T, et al. Efficacy of percutaneous balloon pericardiotomy and intrapericardial instillation for the management of refractory pericardial effusion: a case report. J Cardiol 2007; 50(6):389–95.

89. Maisch B, Ristić AD, Pankuweit S. Intrapericardial treatment of autoreactive pericardial effusion with triamcinolone; the way to avoid side effects of systemic corticosteroid therapy. Eur Heart J 2002; 23(19):1503–8.

90. Fuller TJ, Knochel JP, Brennan JP, et al. Reversal of intractable uremic pericarditis by triamcinolone hexacetonide. Arch Intern Med 1976;136(9):979–82.

91. Buselmeier TJ, Davin TD, Simmons RL, et al. Treatment of intractable uremic pericardial effusion. Avoidance of pericardiectomy with local steroid instillation. JAMA 1978;240(13):1358–9.

92. Quigg RJ Jr, Idelson BA, Yoburn DC, et al. Local steroids in dialysis-associated pericardial effusion. A single intrapericardial administration of triamcinolone. Arch Intern Med 1985;145(12):2249–50.

93. Defouilloy C, Meyer G, Starna M, et al. Intrapericardial fibrinolysis: a useful treatment in the management of purulent pericarditis. Intensive Care Med 1997;23(1):5–10.

94. Ustunsoy H, Celkan MA, Sivrikoz MC, et al. Intrapericardial fibrinolytic therapy in purulent pericarditis. Eur J Cardiothorac Surg 2002;22(3):373–6.

95. Schafer M, Lepoir M, Delabays A, et al. Intrapericardial urokinase irrigation and systemic corticosteroids: an alternative to pericardectomy for persistent fibrino-purulent pericarditis. Cardiovasc Surg 2002;10(5):508–11.

96. Ekim H, Demirbag R. Intrapericardial streptokinase for purulent pericarditis. Surg Today 2004; 34:569–72.

97. Tomkowski WZ, Gralec R, Kuca P, et al. Effectiveness of intrapericardial administration of streptokinase in purulent pericarditis. Herz 2004;29(8): 802–5.

98. Cui HB, Chen XY, Cui CC, et al. Prevention of pericardial constriction by transcatheter intrapericardial fibrinolysis with urokinase. Chin Med Sci 2005;20(1):5–10.

99. Kakia A, Wiysonge CS, Ochodo EA, et al. The efficacy and safety of complete pericardial drainage by means of intrapericardial fibrinolysis for the prevention of complications of pericardial effusion: a systematic review protocol. BMJ Open 2016;6(1): e007842.

100. Macris PM, Igo SR. Minimally invasive access of the normal pericardium: initial clinical experience with a novel device. Clin Cardiol 1999;22(suppl 1):I36–9.

101. Rieger PJ, Beaurline CM, Grabek JR. Intrapericardial therapeutics and diagnostics. In: Seferovic PM, Spodick DH, Maisch B, et al, editors. Pericardiology: contemporary answers to continuing challenges. Belgrade (Serbia): Science; 2000. p. 393–406.

102. Maisch B, Ristić AD, Rupp H, et al. Pericardial access using the PerDUCER® and flexible percutaneous pericardioscopy. Am J Cardiol 2001; 88(11):1323–6.

103. Seferovic PM, Ristic AD, Maksimovic R, et al. Initial clinical experience with Per-DUCER®: promising new tool in the diagnosis and treatment of pericardial disease. Clin Cardiol 1999;22(suppl I):I30–5.

104. Rupp H, Rupp TP, Alter P, et al. Intrapericardial procedures for cardiac regeneration by stem cells: need for minimal invasive access (AttachLifter) to the normal pericardial cavity. Herz 2010;35(7): 458–65.

105. Liu X, Feng Y, Xu G, et al. A new strategy for pericardiocentesis with a visual puncture system: the feasibility and efficiency study in a pericardial effusion model. Int J Cardiol 2014;177(3):e128–30.

106. Killu AM, Naksuk N, Desimone CV, et al. Beating heart validation of safety and efficacy of a

percutaneous pericardiotomy tool. J Cardiovasc Electrophysiol 2016;28(3):357–61.

107. Laham RJ, Cohen DJ, Kuntz RE, et al. Pericardial effusion in patients with cancer: outcome with contemporary management strategies. Heart 1996;75(1):67–71.

108. Ovunc K, Aytemir K, Ozer N, et al. Percutaneous balloon pericardiotomy for patients with malignant pericardial effusion including three malignant pleural mesotheliomas. Angiology 2001;52(5): 323–9.

109. Thanopoulos BD, Georgakopoulos D, Tsaousis GS, et al. Percutaneous balloon pericardiotomy for the treatment of large, nonmalignant pericardial effusions in children: immediate and medium-term results. Cathet Cardiovasc Diagn 1997;40:97–100.

110. Aqel R, Mehta D, Zoghbi GJ. Percutaneous balloon pericardiotomy for the treatment of infected pericardial effusion with tamponade. J Invasive Cardiol 2006;18(7):E194–7.

111. Ziskind AA, Pearce AC, Lemmon CC, et al. Percutaneous balloon pericardiotomy for the treatment of cardiac tamponade and large pericardial effusions: description of technique and report of the first 50 cases. J Am Coll Cardiol 1993;21:1–5.

112. Chow LT, Chow WH. Mechanism of pericardial window creation by balloon pericardiotomy. Am J Cardiol 1993;72:1321–2.

113. Bertrand O, Legrand V, Kulbertus H. Percutaneous balloon pericardiotomy: a case report and analysis of mechanism of action. Cathet Cardiovasc Diagn 1996;38:180–2.

114. Sugimoto JT, Little AG, Ferguson MK, et al. Pericardial window: mechanisms of efficacy. Ann Thorac Surg 1990;50:442–5.

115. Palacios IF, Tuzcu EM, Ziskind AA, et al. Percutaneous balloon pericardial window for patients with malignant pericardial effusion and tamponade. Cathet Cardiovasc Diagn 1991;22:244–9.

116. Hajduczok ZD, Ferguson DW. Percutaneous balloon pericardiostomy for non surgical management of recurrent pericardial tamponade: a case report. Intensive Care Med 1991;17:299–301.

117. Jackson G, Keane D, Mishra B. Percutaneous balloon pericardiotomy in the management of recurrent malignant pericardial effusions. Br Heart J 1992;68:613–5.

118. Deb B, Crean P, Graham I. Percutaneous balloon pericardiotomy in the treatment of malignant pericardial effusion. Ir J Med Sci 1993;162:456–7.

119. Jackson G. Cardiology update. Balloon pericardiotomy. Nurs Stand 1994;8:52–3.

120. Iaffaldano RA, Jones P, Lewis BE, et al. Percutaneous balloon pericardiotomy: a double balloon technique. Cathet Cardiovasc Diagn 1995;36: 79–81.

121. Di Segni E, Lavee J, Kaplinsky E, et al. Percutaneous balloon pericardiostomy for treatment of cardiac tamponade. Eur Heart J 1995;16:184–7.

122. Fakiolas CN, Beldekos DI, Foussas SG, et al. Percutaneous balloon pericardiotomy as a therapeutic alternative for cardiac tamponade and recurrent pericardial effusion. Acta Cardiol 1995; 50:65–70.

123. Galli M, Politi A, Pedretti F, et al. Percutaneous balloon pericardiotomy for malignant pericardial tamponade. Chest 1995;108:1499–501.

124. Devlin GP, Smyth D, Charleson HA, et al. Balloon pericardiostomy: a new therapeutic option for malignant pericardial effusion. Aust N Z J Med 1996; 26:556–8.

125. Chow WH, Chow TC, Yip AS, et al. Inoue balloon pericardiotomy for patients with recurrent pericardial effusion. Angiology 1996;47:57–60.

126. Bhardwaj R, Gharib W, Gharib W, et al. Evaluation of safety and feasibility of percutaneous balloon pericardiotomy in hemodynamically significant pericardial effusion (review of 10-years experience in single center). J Interv Cardiol 2015;28(5):409–14.

127. Hsu KL, Tsai CH, Chiang FT, et al. Percutaneous balloon pericardiotomy for patients with recurrent pericardial effusion: using a novel double-balloon technique with one long and one short balloon. Am J Cardiol 1997;80:1635–7.

128. Ristić AD, Seferović PM, Maksimović R, et al. Percutaneous balloon pericardiotomy in neoplastic pericardial effusion. In: Seferović PM, Spodick DH, Maisch B, editors. Pericardiology: contemporary answers to continuing challenges. Beograd (Serbia): Science; 2000. p. 427–38. Maksimović R, Ristić AD (assoc. eds).

129. Sochman J, Peregrin J, Pavcnik D. The cutting pericardiotome: another option for pericardiopleural draining in recurrent pericardial effusion. Initial experience. Int J Cardiol 2001;77(1):69–74.

130. Jalisi FM, Morise AP, Haque R, et al. Primary percutaneous balloon pericardiotomy. W V Med J 2004; 100(3):102–5.

131. Ruiz-García J, Jiménez-Valero S, Moreno R, et al. Percutaneous balloon pericardiotomy as the initial and definitive treatment for malignant pericardial effusion. Rev Esp Cardiol 2013;66(5):357–63.

132. Javier Irazusta F, Jiménez-Valero S, Gemma D, et al. Percutaneous balloon pericardiotomy: treatment of choice in patients with advanced oncological disease and severe pericardial effusion. JACC Cardiovasc Interv 2017;10(Suppl S):CRT-800.48.

133. Virk SA, Chandrakumar D, Villanueva C, et al. Systematic review of percutaneous interventions for malignant pericardial effusion. Heart 2015; 101(20):1619–26.

134. Vaitkus PT, Herrmann HC, LeWinter MM. Treatment of malignant pericardial effusion. JAMA 1994; 272(1):59–64.

135. Bartus K, Han FT, Bednarek J, et al. Percutaneous left atrial appendage suture ligation using the LARIAT device in patients with atrial fibrillation: initial clinical experience. J Am Coll Cardiol 2013; 62(2):108–18.

136. Lakkireddy D, Afzal MR, Lee RJ, et al. Short and long-term outcomes of percutaneous left atrial appendage suture ligation: results from a US multicenter evaluation. Heart Rhythm 2016;13(5): 1030–6.

137. Maisch B. Alcohol ablation of pericardial cysts under pericardioscopical control. Heart Fail Rev 2013;18:361–5.

Neoplastic Pericardial Disease

Joseph J. Maleszewski, MD[a,b,c],*, Nandan S. Anavekar, MB, BCh[b,d]

KEYWORDS

- Tumors • Masses • Cardiac • Epicardium • Thoracic

KEY POINTS

- Pericardial neoplasms are rare and may be primary or secondary, the latter much more common.
- Finding a pericardial mass should always prompt a careful history and may warrant further imaging and/or sampling.
- Imaging plays a critical role in characterizing pericardial masses and can help to narrow the differential diagnosis.

Pericardial tumors include a range of both neoplastic and non-neoplastic entities. Neoplasms of the pericardium can be broadly dichotomized into those that arise within the pericardium (primary pericardial neoplasms) and those that metastasize to involve the pericardium (secondary pericardial neoplasms). Although secondary pericardial neoplasms are, by definition, malignant processes, primary pericardial neoplasms may be either benign or malignant.

In general, involvement of the heart or pericardium by metastatic disease is substantially more common than involvement by a primary neoplastic process. It is estimated that metastatic lesions are greater than 100 times more common, and the pericardium is the most common site of said involvement.[1] In high-stage cancer patients, cardiac involvement has been demonstrated in as many as 14% of cases.[2] Primary pericardial processes, on the other hand, have been estimated to account for between 6% and 10% of primary cardiac tumors but are typically benign.[3]

Involvement of the pericardium by malignant processes can affect cardiac function several important ways, such as pericardial effusion (with or without tamponade physiology), direct myocardial invasion, pericardial constriction, or pericarditis.[4] In general, the most common of these is effusion. Even benign tumors can be large enough to incite hemodynamic compromise by virtue of their size, location, or number.[5–8]

Pericardial tumors may present with a wide range of clinical presentations, ranging from asymptomatic, incidental diagnosis to sudden death. Patients with significant tumor burden in the pericardium may present with dyspnea, orthopnea, pain, edema, or even hemoptysis.[9] Clinical examination can reveal cyanosis, venous distention, hepatomegaly, pleural or pericardial effusion (distant heart sounds or rub), murmur, or electrocardiographic changes.

This review provides an overview of the spectrum of neoplastic pericardial disease and discusses the defining pathologic characteristics as well as the expected findings at imaging. Only brief mention of non-neoplastic entities are made, primarily to round out discussion of the differential diagnosis of pericardial mass-lesions.

Disclosure Statement: The authors have no relevant relationships or financial disclosures to report.
[a] Department of Laboratory Medicine and Pathology, Mayo Clinic, 200 First Street Southwest, Rochester, MN 55905, USA; [b] Department of Cardiovascular Diseases, Mayo Clinic, 200 First Street Southwest, Rochester, MN 55905, USA; [c] Department of Clinical Genomics, Mayo Clinic, 200 First Street Southwest, Rochester, MN 55905, USA; [d] Division of Cardiac Radiology, Department of Radiology, Mayo Clinic, 200 First Street Southwest, Rochester, MN 55905, USA
* Corresponding author. 200 First Street Southwest, Rochester, MN 55905.
E-mail address: maleszewski.joseph@mayo.edu

Cardiol Clin 35 (2017) 589–600
http://dx.doi.org/10.1016/j.ccl.2017.07.011
0733-8651/17/© 2017 Elsevier Inc. All rights reserved.

IMAGING

Pericardial neoplasms may be found incidentally at imaging, surgery, or autopsy or they may be discovered during work-up for symptoms that are considered to have a cardiac etiology. Once discovered, imaging is often integral to the diagnostic work-up. Although plain film radiography and echocardiography are considered the cornerstone of cardiovascular imaging, CT and MRI should be considered frontline in the assessment of pericardial anatomy. Echocardiography may disclose the presence of increased pericardial thickness, nodularity, or discrete mass as well as secondary hemodynamic effects of the lesion, including presence of cardiac tamponade. Beyond these features, the role of echocardiography in the diagnostic evaluation of pericardial tumors remains limited.

CT and MRI have the clear advantage of in their ability to delineate the exact location of the neoplasm, its effects on neighboring cardiac and noncardiac structures; particularly in the setting of CT imaging, the ability to stage disease that can assist in therapeutic planning and surveillance. Despite the advances in cardiovascular imaging, it is important to recognize that in most cases, the evaluation of a primary pericardial tumor requires tissue sampling and remains a pathologic diagnosis.

PERICARDIAL METASTASES

Pericardial metastases are, as discussed previously, the most common cause of pericardial mass-lesions and any findings of a pericardial mass should, therefore, prompt a careful evaluation for underlying malignancy. They may involve the visceral and/or parietal layers. In a series of 60

cases of pericardial metastasis, approximately half of cases had significant cardiovascular compromise as a result.[9] Mechanistically, this is often the result of effusion, but myocardial invasion and tumor encasement were also involved (**Fig. 1**).[10]

The most common malignancies diagnosed, either at biopsy or cytologic sampling, are carcinomas arising from the lung and breast (the most common primary site of origin in women).[11] Involvement of the pericardium is also not uncommon in cases of leukemia/lymphoma. Metastasis from gastrointestinal, genitourinary, and gynecologic malignancies may also occur as well as from extracardiac sarcomas.

Metastatic involvement of the pericardium has nonspecific imaging findings and is often suggested by the diagnosis of the primary noncardiac neoplasm. Imaging findings include presence of effusion, irregular thickening of the pericardium or nodularity, and distinct pericardial masses (see **Fig. 1**).[12] On MRI, most secondary neoplasms to the pericardium have low signal intensity on T1-weighted imaging with the exception of metastatic melanoma, which may have high signal intensity secondary to paramagnetic metals bound by melanin.[13,14] Postcontrast delayed imaging typically discloses pericardial enhancement in the regions of metastases.[12]

Pericardial metastases are often diagnosed in cytologic specimens, rather than biopsy (tissue) specimens.[15] The primary differential, both cytologically and histologically, is between reactive mesothelial hyperplasia and carcinoma — which can have some morphologic overlap. Therefore, it is common to use immunohistochemical studies to help characterize the antigenicity and nature of the cells. If proved a carcinoma, immunohistochemistry

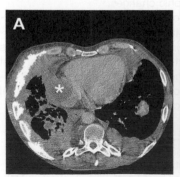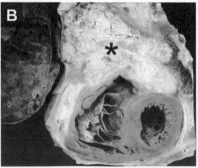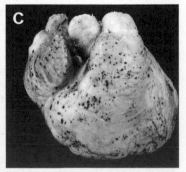

Fig. 1. Pericardial metastases. (*A*) CT scan performed with intravenous iodinated contrast (poor contrast opacification), demonstrating a large pericardial mass (*white asterisk*) with compression of the right atrium with pleural and pulmonary metastases and osteoblastic metastases involving multiple right-sided ribs. The primary tumor was rectal carcinoma. (*B*) Autopsy-derived specimen of a pulmonary adenocarcinoma (*black asterisk*) with direct extension to involve the anterior pericardium (visceral and parietal layers) and the subjacent myocardium. (*C*) Autopsy-derived specimen showing numerous visceral pericardial (epicardial) metastases by metastatic malignant melanoma.

in concert with imaging and clinical findings can usually reveal the site of the primary process.

The presence of a malignant pericardial effusion is an ominous sign, with most patients succumbing to disease in less than a year from diagnosis.[10] Median survival is approximately 5 months to 8 months, depending on the cancer type and therapeutic efficacy.[16,17] In addition to treating the underlying primary tumor, with chemotherapy and/or radiation, pericardiectomy, pericardial window, and sclerotherapy can be used to target the pericardial metastases and their complications.[16,18,19]

PRIMARY PERICARDIAL NEOPLASMS — BENIGN
Lipoma

Pericardial lipomas, like those arising elsewhere in the body, are benign neoplasms composed of mature adipose (fat) tissue. They are rare and are usually incidental findings at the time of imaging, surgery, or autopsy. There are, however, scattered reports of symptomatic epicardial lipomas causing ventricular dysfunction.[20–22]

Cross-sectional imaging is usually diagnostic in the setting of a pericardial lipoma. On CT, these lesions are low (fat) attenuation without contrast enhancement. On MRI, these lesions are nonenhancing and have reduced signal with the use of fat saturation sequences, which indicates the fatty nature of the tumor (**Fig. 2**A).

Grossly, most cardiac lipomas are located on the epicardial surface (see **Fig. 2**B), although myocardial-based and endocardial-based lesions can occur. They can occur in any cardiac chamber. They usually occur singly but have been reported to occur in multiples, particularly in the setting of tuberous sclerosis, where they have

been termed, *fatty foci*, and may be the residuum of involuted rhabdomyomas.[23] Histologically, the lesions are composed of mature adipocytes, typically surrounded by capsule.

These lesions can usually be treated conservatively, but surgical excision may be considered if the patient has obstructive or arrhythmia-induced symptoms.

Pericardial Cyst

Although pericardial cysts are somewhat uncommon in general, they account for approximately a third of all mediastinal cysts.[24] Because they have been reported prenatally, at least a subset of these lesions are congenital in origin.[25,26] Others may form via iatrogenic or idiopathic mechanisms.

Clinically, these lesions are usually asymptomatic. Nevertheless, reports of pericardial cyst that present with pain, dyspnea, obstruction, and hemopericardium/tamponade have all been reported.[6,27,28]

Pericardial cysts are usually found incidentally on chest radiograph (**Fig. 3**A) or echocardiography, and pericardial cysts typically require no further diagnostic work-up, unless considered causing clinical symptoms and surgical resection or percutaneous drainage is considered. CT and MRI can further characterize a lesion as a well-defined, smooth-walled, fluid-filled structure (see **Fig. 3**B, C). On MRI, pericardial cysts typically have signal characteristics typical of fluid, including low signal on T1-weighted imaging; high signal on T2-weighted imaging and no enhancement on postcontrast imaging.

Grossly, these lesions may be uniloculated or multiloculated. They typically contain clear or straw-colored serous fluid but may also contain hemorrhagic fluid (**Fig. 4**). The cyst lining is smooth

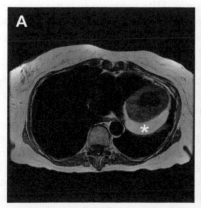
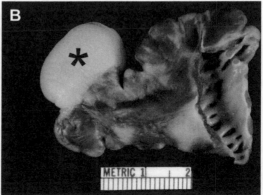

Fig. 2. Pericardial lipoma. (*A*) Cardiac MRI demonstrating a large, well-circumscribed lipoma (*white asterisk*) on the lateral aspect of the left ventricle. The attenuation is notably consistent with adipose tissue. (*B*) Surgically resected left atrial appendage with a well-circumscribed, encapsulated, epicardial lipoma (*black asterisk*).

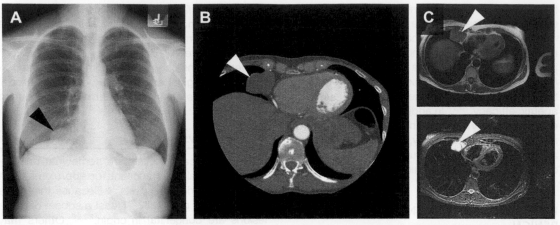

Fig. 3. Pericardial cyst imaging. (*A*) Plain film chest radiograph with a simple cyst (*black arrowhead*) in the right cardiophrenic angle. (*B*) CT imaging in a different patient demonstrates a fluid-filled pericardial cyst (*white arrowhead*) in the right cardiophrenic angle. (*C*) MRI demonstrates fluid characteristics with low intensity signal on T1-weighted image (*top*) and high signal intensity on T2-weighted image (*bottom*) of the same cyst shown in panel B (*white arrowheads*).

and histologically is composed of a single layer of mesothelial cells with a variable quantity of underlying collagen and elastin.

Paraganglioma

Paragangliomas are rare cardiac neoplasms comprised of paraganglion cells. These lesions are thought to arise from the cardiac paraganglia, which reside in the atria along the atrioventricular groove, near the root of the great vessels. Approximately 5% of these tumors will be based in the pericardium itself.[29,30]

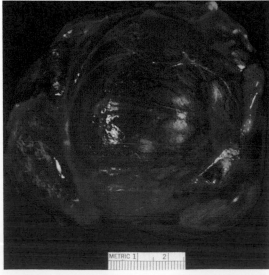

Fig. 4. Pericardial cyst pathology. Intact, surgically resected, multiloculated, pericardial cyst filled with straw-colored fluid.

Patients may be asymptomatic or present with clinical evidence of catecholamine secretion, in which case they are sometimes referred to as cardiac pheochromocytomas. These latter tumors may arise in the context of multiple endocrine neoplasia syndromes (types 2a and 2b, in particular). Those tumors that produce catecholamines have predictable clinical symptoms of headache, palpitations, chest pain, angina, and shortness of breath.

CT and MRI are useful in characterization of the mass and surgical planning. These neoplasms are seen to be enhancing with contrast secondary to its hypervascularity. On occasion, a central area of low attenuation may be observed secondary to necrosis. Functional imaging with indium 111 pentreotide, iodine 131 metaiodobenzylguanidine, or iodine 123 metaiodobenzylguanidine may also be used. [111]In pentreotide is the nuclear medicine agent of choice, with a sensitivity of 94%.[3] Sometimes a feeder vessel may be noted angiographically and can be a clue to the diagnosis.

On gross examination, these tumors usually occur in the atria and tend to be poorly circumscribed. On cut section, they are uniformly tan-yellow and somewhat homogenous. Histologically, they are identical to those that arise outside of the heart, consisting of nests of bland epithelioid cells arranged in anastomosing cords and trabeculae. The organoid character, along with the prominent vasculature and characteristic sustentacular antigenicity with antibodies directed against S100 protein, help make the diagnosis.

Although these lesions are considered benign, malignant degeneration can occur. Surgical resection is, therefore, indicated irrespective of the presence of symptoms (provided the patient is a surgical candidate).

Hemangioma

Hemangiomas are benign tumors of blood vessels that usually resemble capillaries (so-called capillary hemangiomas) but may also consist of larger caliber vessel (cavernous hemangiomas). Those that are located within the pericardium are exceptionally rare with fewer than 200 cases in the reported literature.

These appear as mixed attenuation lesions on noncontrast CT images and rapidly enhance with contrast administration. They may be associated with foci of calcification. With MRI, these lesions are seen to have heterogeneous perfusion characteristics with enhancement observed on delayed postcontrast imaging. Hemangiomas are distinguished from angiosarcomas on imaging based on the presence of reassuring findings, including the presence of well-circumscribed tissue planes without invasion of adjacent structures.[3,31]

Grossly, they are usually red-brown, owing to the abundant blood contained therein (**Fig. 5**). Histologically, variably sized blood vessels are seen throughout the lesion, like hemangiomas found outside of the heart. Cavernous hemangiomas

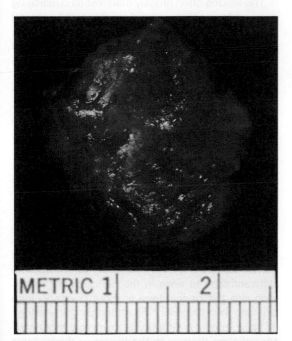

Fig. 5. Pericardial hemangioma. Surgically resected pericardial hemangioma, characterized by a red globular mass that was identified attached to the antero-superior parietal pericardium.

are usually composed of thin-walled or thick-walled vascular structures, whereas capillary hemangiomas are composed of endothelial cells growing in a lobulated fashion. Fat and collagen may be seen scattered throughout.

Because of the possibility of hemorrhage, surgical resection is often attempted and has a high rate of success. Some hemangiomas may be associated with syndromes, such as Kasabach-Merritt, or with extracardiac hemangiomas in general.

PRIMARY PERICARDIAL NEOPLASMS — MALIGNANT
Malignant Mesothelioma

Pericardial malignant mesothelioma is a malignant, neoplastic proliferation of mesothelial cells that arises primarily in the pericardium. The latter qualification necessitates that a careful examination be done for pleural origin to prove that there was not contiguous spread of what is a much more common process. Pericardial mesotheliomas account for less than 2% of cases of mesothelioma.[32] Malignant mesothelioma is the most common primary malignancy of the pericardium but accounts for less than 5% of primary pericardial neoplasms, a testament to the commonality of benign neoplasms. Unlike their pleural counterparts, pericardial mesotheliomas do not share the tight association with asbestos exposure, with only 14% of cases reporting a history of such exposure.[32,33]

Clinical symptoms usually are a consequence of constriction or effusion with tamponade. Unfortunately, from a diagnostic standpoint, examination of the effusion fluid is often insufficient to make the diagnosis cytologically, because tissue invasion must be demonstrated to discriminate between reactive and neoplastic mesothelial cells.

CT and MRI demonstrate increased pericardial thickness with a heterogeneously enhancing pericardial mass and furthermore delineates the extent of cardiac invasion by the tumor (**Fig. 6**). Pericardial mesothelioma can encase the cardiac structures and may demonstrate findings of constrictive physiology on echocardiography and MRI.

Malignant mesotheliomas of the pericardium often diffusely involve the pericardium with complete encasement of the heart (**Fig. 7**). These insidious neoplasms tend to grow along the pericardium and then the pleura and cause a range of secondary complications. Rarely, malignant mesothelioma may be a focal finding or may manifest as a well-differentiated papillary-type, that carries a better prognosis.[34]

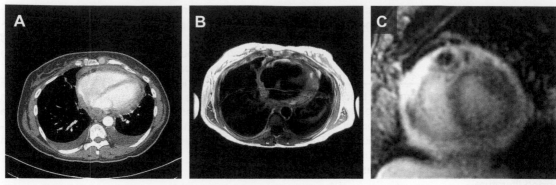

Fig. 6. Pericardial malignant mesothelioma imaging. (*A*) Chest CT with intravenous contrast demonstrates diffusely increased irregular pericardial thickening. (*B*) Cardiac MRI was performed in the same patient (axial imaging plane) similarly demonstrates diffuse and irregular thickening of the pericardium with loss of natural tissue planes. (*C*) Postcontrast delayed imaging (short-axis imaging plane) demonstrates diffuse enhancement of the malignant mesothelioma.

Surgical resection can be attempted but is rarely curative. Newer-generation chemotherapeutics offer some hope for longer survival in mesothelioma patients, generally, but the applicability to pericardial mesothelioma has not been studied owing to the rarity of these lesions.

Lymphoma

Primary pericardial lymphoma is an extranodal lymphoma, with all (or a significant majority) of the tumor located in the pericardium. Lymphomas of the heart affect men twice as commonly as women and usually occur in older individuals.[35] Although uncommon, their incidence is on the rise owing to an association with immunocompromise.

The clinical symptoms of these lesions, like most other pericardial tumors, are highly variable.

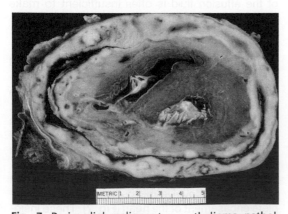

Fig. 7. Pericardial malignant mesothelioma pathology. Autopsy-derived specimen exhibiting diffuse involvement of both the visceral and parietnal pericardial layers by an epithelioid malignant mesothelioma. The diffuse encasement of the heart can lead to constrictive hemodynamics, as it did in this instance.

Arrhythmia, heart failure (obstruction), and B symptoms have all been reported.[35]

On CT imaging, these tumors are usually large and can fill the pericardial space. They can be low attenuation with heterogeneous enhancement after contrast administration. Given their increased metabolism, complementary imaging includes PET-CT, which demonstrates fludeoxyglucose F 18 (FDG) avidity (**Fig. 8**A). Like CT, cardiac MRI may demonstrate pericardial thickening, effusion, and a heterogeneous postcontrast delayed enhancement pattern (see **Fig. 8**B).

The lesions often grossly manifest as coalescing gray-white masses extending along the visceral pericardium, where most of the cardiac lymphatics reside. Histologically, the lesions vary by type of lymphoma, but diffuse large B-cell lymphoma is by far the most common, accounting for greater than 75% of published reports.[35] Systemic lymphoma, however, such as small lymphocytic lymphoma/chronic lymphocytic leukemia, may also be seen and cause primary pericardial disease (see **Fig. 8**C), particularly in older patients.[36]

The prognosis is generally poor, but anthracycline-based chemotherapy has induced remission in some patients.

Angiosarcoma

Pericardial angiosarcomas, along with synovial sarcomas, are the most common sarcomas with differentiation to arise in the pericardium. Extension into the pericardium is more common than primary involvement.[37–39] Although the etiology of these tumors is largely unknown, rare reports after radiation therapy to the breast or thorax have been described.[40,41]

Clinically, these tumors often present with symptoms of heart failure. Pericardial effusion is

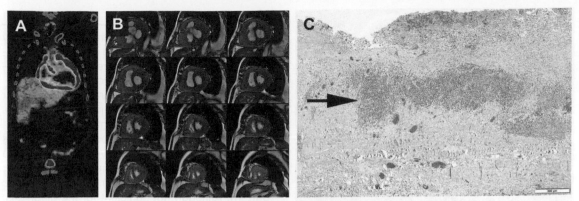

Fig. 8. Pericardial lymphoma. (*A*) PET-CT performed in a patient with pericardial lymphoma, that was later confirmed to be diffuse B-cell lymphoma. On the PET-CT there is hypermetabolism throughout the pericardial mass. (*B*) Cardiac MRI in the same patient (steady state free precession images, in a short-axis imaging plane, from base to apex) demonstrated a large infiltrative mass circumferentially involving the pericardium and blending imperceptibly with the subjacent myocardium. Free-breathing sequences (not shown) demonstrated enhanced ventricular interdependence consistent with constrictive hemodynamics. (*C*) Pericardial thickening secondary to leukemic infiltrate my small lymphocytic lymphoma/chronic lymphocytic leukemia (*black arrow*) (hematoxylin-eosin, original magnification ×100).

common and may be large. Tamponade may also occur, owing to the vascular nature of the tumor.

On CT imaging, these are highly vascular structures with a nodular contour and, therefore, demonstrate avid postcontrast enhancement. CT can also delineate extent of cardiac invasion. Most commonly, cardiac angiosarcoma arises in the region of the right atrioventricular groove. Like other pericardial neoplastic disease, this lesion may be associated with a pericardial effusion; moreover, given the vascular nature of these lesions, hemopericardium may be a manifestation of the disease. On MRI, these are highly vascular structures; on T1-weighted imaging the signal intensity is dependent on the extent of hemorrhage and necrosis in the tumor and is, therefore, heterogeneous (**Fig. 9**). On T2-weighted imaging and steady state free precession images, there is increased signal intensity. On

postcontrast imaging, there is avid tumor enhancement.[42] With diffuse pericardial involvement, there may be secondary hemodynamic effects manifesting as constrictive physiology that may be observed on both MRI and echocardiography.

Grossly, these lesions are usually red brown and hemorrhagic (**Fig. 10**). They are not well circumscribed and may exhibit invasion into the subjacent myocardium or the adjacent lung parenchyma or chest wall. Histologically, they may be epithelioid or spindle cell morphology and immunohistochemistry may, in some cases, be necessary to prove endothelial differentiation.

The prognosis of pericardial angiosarcoma is uniformly poor, with most patients succumbing to disease within months of the diagnosis. Surgical resection can be attempted and is usually

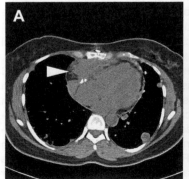
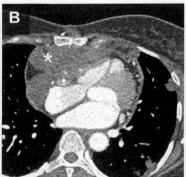
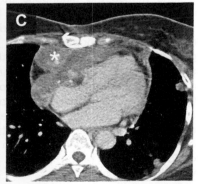

Fig. 9. Pericardial angiosarcoma imaging. (*A*) A noncontrast CT demonstrating a right atrioventricular groove mass (*white arrowhead*). (*B*) This image is taken immediately after contrast administration demonstrating initial contrast enhancement of the mass (*white asterisk*). (*C*) This image is delayed post–contrast imaging demonstrating heterogenous, yet avid, uptake of contrast by the mass (*white asterisk*).

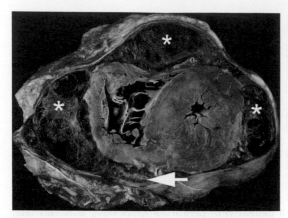

Fig. 10. Pericardial angiosarcoma pathology. Autopsy-derived specimen showing a pericardial angiosarcoma growing in the region of the posterior right atrioventricular groove and extending downward toward the midventricular level (*white arrow*). Tumoral hemorrhage is extensive and causing hemopericardium (*white asterisks*) and clinical tamponade in this instance.

performed primarily for diagnostic and palliative measures.[43]

Synovial Sarcoma

Pericardial synovial sarcoma is a malignant neoplasm associated with a characteristic chromosomal translocation t(X;18). It is an uncommon cardiac neoplasm, but the pericardium is the most common site of origin. Signs and symptoms are typically associated with heart failure, including dyspnea, cough, and sometimes chest pain.

Synovial sarcomas are usually depicted as a solitary mass that is vascular and invasive on cross-sectional imaging with characteristics similar to mesothelioma. The rare nature of these lesions makes the diagnostic utility of imaging limited.

Grossly, like most other pericardial malignancies, they appear smooth surfaced and gray-white to tan. The tumors themselves are usually typed by virtue of their histology as monophasic (single-cell population) or biphasic (containing both spindle-cells and epithelioid cells). Calcification and prominent vasculature also help to characterize this tumor. As discussed previously, demonstration of the translocation or gene fusion product (*SS18-SSX*) is virtually diagnostic.

This malignancy is a high-grade neoplasm that is associated with a poor prognosis. Median survival is slightly longer compared with other pericardial malignancies but still rather poor.

Liposarcoma

Primary pericardial liposarcomas are incredibly rare with only a handful of case reports in the literature. Most that have been reported have presented with constrictive symptoms.

These are rare tumors characterized by their fatty attenuation and invasive nature on imaging. They are usually large at the time of diagnosis.

Grossly, these lesions are bulky, fatty, tumors that exhibit a frankly invasive growth pattern without respect to tissue planes. Histologically, these lesions are typed by cytomorphologic pattern. Although not sufficient for the diagnosis, demonstration of lipoblasts is usually necessary. Careful discrimination must be made from benign conditions, such as excess epicardial fat and lipomatous hypertrophy of the atrial septum, with the latter limited to the limbus of the fossa ovalis in the atrial septum.

Like most other pericardial malignances, prognosis is grim.

Germ Cell Tumor

The anterior mediastinum is the most common site for extragonadal germ cell tumors.[44] Although they usually do not arise in the pericardium proper, intrapericardial location has been described in a rare subset. Nevertheless, even those mediastinal germ cell tumors that arise outside of the pericardium usually involve it by virtue of their proximity.

Germ cell tumors are subclassified into a variety of neoplasms, including teratomas, seminomas, embryonal carcinomas, yolk sac tumors, and choriocarcinomas. Alternatively, multiple histopathologic patterns may be identified, in which cases they are referred to as mixed germ cell tumors. Those tumors arising within the pericardium are usually teratomas or yolk sac tumors, with the former more common in men and the latter more common in young girls.

On cross-sectional imaging in the adult, germ cell tumors are usually well-defined, heterogenous, multilocular masses with areas of calcification and fat[45] and are usually found in an anterior location (**Fig. 11**A). Those that arise within the pericardium are typically located in the region of the great vessels, at the base of the heart. The various components of the tumor dictate the findings on imaging be it CT or MRI. Clinically, these tumors can be found incidentally or present with cardiovascular and respiratory collapse; imaging may reveal an underlying pericardial effusion of hemodynamic significance. These dramatic presentations have usually been described in newborns.[46,47] The advances in

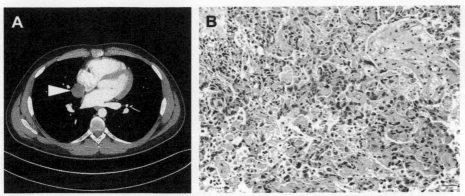

Fig. 11. Pericardial germ cell tumor. (*A*) Chest CT, with intravenous iodinated contrast, demonstrates a right sided, nonenhancing, pericardial mass (*white arrowhead*), with mild distortion of the right atrium. This mass was resected and at pathology was found to be a yolk sac tumor. (*B*) Photomicrograph demonstrating a malignant proliferation of pleomorphic epithelioid cells, morphologically consistent with a yolk sac tumor (hematoxylin-eosin, original magnification ×200).

fetal ultrasonography imaging has also allowed diagnosis of such lesions in utero.[3]

Teratomas are often cystic, owing to the heterologous nature of the tumors (containing tissues from multiple germ cell layers), whereas yolk sac tumors may be solid and hemorrhagic. As is the case with most pericardial lesions, the diagnosis is made on histologic assessment. Histopathologic patterns of pericardial or mediastinal germ cell tumors are identical to their gonadal counterparts (see **Fig. 11**B).

MISCELLANEOUS PERICARDIAL TUMORS
Erdheim-Chester Disease

Erdheim-Chester disease is a form of non-Langerhan cell histiocytosis that presents in middle-aged or older adults. Although the etiology of the disease is unknown, autoimmune and neoplastic etiologies have been posited. The association of the disease with V600 E mutations in the *BRAF* gene certainly adds further support to the notion that the condition is neoplastic. Diagnosis is usually contingent on radiologic and histopathologic findings.

There is a slight male predilection that has been reported.[48] This multisystem disease has myriad clinical manifestations including exophthalmos, xanthelasma, interstitial lung disease, and retroperitoneal fibrosis with renal outflow obstruction secondary to ureteral encasement as well as cardiovascular involvement. Typically the noncardiac symptoms facilitate the diagnostic evaluation and discovery of cardiac involvement. Cardiac involvement is common, approaching 50% in the reported literature,[49,50] and can involve pericardium, myocardium, or endocardium. Of the cardiac

manifestations of the disease, pericardial infiltration has been reported as the most common (44% of patients with cardiac involvement) and in those with pericardial involvement, 15% present with clinical findings of tamponade.[50] Myocardial infiltration, valvular infiltration with predominantly regurgitation (aortic and mitral), myocardial infarction, and heart failure have been reported as secondary effects of tumor involvement.[50] Unfortunately, close to a third of patients succumb to cardiovascular involvement,[50] indicating the poor prognosis of the disease once cardiovascular symptoms manifest.

On cross-sectional imaging, pericardial involvement is represented by a mass-lesion that infiltrates the pericardial space and can encase the coronary vasculature and aorta. They are frequently seen to involve the right atrium and atrioventricular groove.[49] Given the variable cardiac imaging findings, the radiologic diagnosis is best ascertained by a combination of multisystem findings, in particular bone, cerebral, orbital, and renal findings (**Fig. 12**).

Histologically, the disease is characterized by infiltration of the tissue by foamy histiocytes, sometimes with a granulomatous or fibrotic background. These histiocytes are characteristically nonreactive with antibodies directed against CD1a. Due to the rarity of the disease, there are few data on treatment options and their efficacy. Historically, interferon alfa has been used in treatment regimens and most recently moderate clinical efficacy with the use of cladribine in cases without BRAF V600 E mutation has been demonstrated.[51] Due to absence of large clinical trials, however, the efficacy of any treatment strategy for this disease remains unclear.

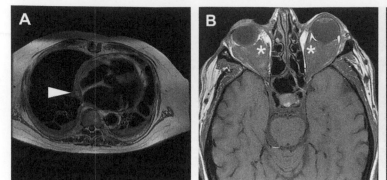
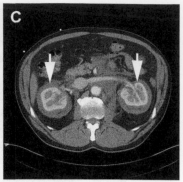

Fig. 12. Pericardial Erdheim-Chester imaging. (*A*) Cardiac MRI disclosed increased pericardial thickening and a mass-like structure along the anterior wall of the upper right atrium (*white arrowhead*). (*B*) Head MRI demonstrates orbital involvement with intraconal soft tissue that fills the intraconal contents and surrounds the optic nerves bilaterally (*white asterisks*). (*C*) Abdominal CT demonstrates a mildly enhancing infiltrative soft tissue process in the upper abdomen and retroperitoneum involving the visualized abdominal aorta and the bilateral kidneys (*white arrows*).

IgG4-Related Disease

IgG4-related disease is an increasingly recognized form of systemic inflammatory disease and has been reported to cause pericardial thickening in a subset of patients with pericarditis.[52] The disease is characterized by increased serum IgG4 levels and tissue infiltration by IgG4-reactive plasma cells, associated with fibrosis and inflammation (**Fig. 13**). Classical manifestations include pancreatitis, sialadenitis, and (in some cases) aortitis. Reporting of cardiovascular manifestations are limited in number but have included inflammatory aortic abdominal aneurysm, coronary arteritis, pericarditis, and pulmonary hypertension.[53]

The assessment of cardiovascular involvement by imaging requires a multimodality approach and remains heterogeneous. Echocardiography has been a mainstay because it allows for assessment of cardiac structure and function. In terms of pericardial involvement, it provides an evaluation of pericardial effusion, underlying constrictive physiology, if present, and may identify cardiac pseudotumors.[53] As discussed previously, however, limitations of echocardiography in the assessment of pericardial structures has led to the use of CT and MRI for further evaluation of this disease. CT can assess periaortitis/periarteritis, which manifests as smooth tissue thickening encircling these vascular structures with intraluminal irregularities as well as pericardial involvement, which may manifest as increased thickness, areas of calcification, and postcontrast enhancement.[54] FDG-PET/CT imaging may be useful in staging IgG4-related disease and may offer an assessment of treatment response at

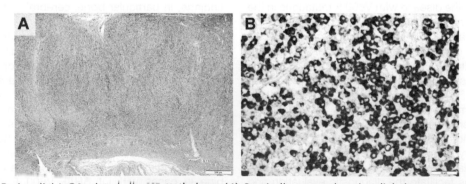

Fig. 13. Pericardial IgG4-related disease pathology. (*A*) Surgically resected pericardial tissue, removed in the setting of pericardial constriction demonstrates diffuse involvement of the parietal pericardium by a proliferation of plasma cells (hematoxylin-eosin, original magnification ×100). (*B*) Many of these plasma cells were reactive with antibodies directed against IgG4 and the serum IgG4 level was also elevated, in keeping with involvement by IgG4-related disease (original magnification ×400).

follow-up.[55] MRI can also be used to assess cardiac involvement, specifically evaluating pericardial and myocardial involvement. The imaging characteristics are nonspecific, and it is the constellation of findings, including pericardial and multisystem vascular involvement, that suggests the diagnosis.[53]

Although too few cases exist to draw firm conclusions regarding presentation or prognosis, at least a subset of these lesions present with constrictive hemodynamics.[56]

REFERENCES

1. Butany J, Leong SW, Carmichael K, et al. A 30-year analysis of cardiac neoplasms at autopsy. Can J Cardiol 2005;21(8):675–80.
2. Bussani R, De-Giorgio F, Abbate A, et al. Cardiac metastases. J Clin Pathol 2007;60(1):27–34.
3. Restrepo CS, Vargas D, Ocazionez D, et al. Primary pericardial tumors. Radiographics 2013; 33(6):1613–30.
4. Thurber DL, Edwards JE, Achor RW. Secondary malignant tumors of the pericardium. Circulation 1962; 26:228–41.
5. Satur CM, Hsin MK, Dussek JE. Giant pericardial cysts. Ann Thorac Surg 1996;61(1):208–10.
6. Sokouti M, Halimi M, Golzari SE. Pericardial cyst presented as chronic cough: a rare case report. Tanaffos 2012;11(4):60–2.
7. Feigin DS, Fenoglio JJ, McAllister HA, et al. Pericardial cysts. A radiologic-pathologic correlation and review. Radiology 1977;125(1):15–20.
8. Sankar NM, Thiruchelvam T, Thirunavukkaarasu K, et al. Symptomatic lipoma in the right atrial free wall. A case report. Tex Heart Inst J 1998;25(2): 152–4.
9. Adenle AD, Edwards JE. Clinical and pathologic features of metastatic neoplasms of the pericardium. Chest 1982;81(2):166–9.
10. Garcia-Riego A, Cuinas C, Vilanova JJ. Malignant pericardial effusion. Acta Cytol 2001;45(4):561–6.
11. Gupta RK, Kenwright DN, Fauck R, et al. The usefulness of a panel of immunostains in the diagnosis and differentiation of metastatic malignancies in pericardial effusions. Cytopathology 2000;11(5): 312–21.
12. Wang ZJ, Reddy GP, Gotway MB, et al. CT and MR imaging of pericardial disease. Radiographics 2003; 23:S167–80.
13. Enochs WS, Petherick P, Bogdanova A, et al. Paramagnetic metal scavenging by melanin: MR imaging. Radiology 1997;204(2):417–23.
14. Mousseaux E, Meunier P, Azancott S, et al. Cardiac metastatic melanoma investigated by magnetic resonance imaging. Magn Reson Imaging 1998; 16(1):91–5.
15. Wilkes JD, Fidias P, Vaickus L, et al. Malignancy-related pericardial effusion. 127 cases from the Roswell Park Cancer Institute. Cancer 1995;76(8): 1377–87.
16. Quraishi MA, Costanzi JJ, Hokanson J. The natural history of lung cancer with pericardial metastases. Cancer 1983;51(4):740–2.
17. Swanepoel E, Apffelstaedt JP. Malignant pericardial effusion in breast cancer: terminal event or treatable complication? J Surg Oncol 1997;64(4):308–11.
18. Olson JE, Ryan MB, Blumenstock DA. Eleven years' experience with pericardial-peritoneal window in the management of malignant and benign pericardial effusions. Ann Surg Oncol 1995;2(2): 165–9.
19. Fiocco M, Krasna MJ. The management of malignant pleural and pericardial effusions. Hematol Oncol Clin North Am 1997;11(2):253–65.
20. Wu S, Teng P, Zhou Y, et al. A rare case report of giant epicardial lipoma compressing the right atrium with septal enhancement. J Cardiothorac Surg 2015; 10:150.
21. King SJ, Smallhorn JF, Burrows PE. Epicardial lipoma: imaging findings. AJR Am J Roentgenol 1993;160(2):261–2.
22. Vyas SJ, Pramesh CS, Sharma S, et al. Giant pericardial lipoma: unusual cause of intrathoracic mass. Ann Acad Med Singapore 2003;32(6):832–4.
23. Adriaensen ME, Schaefer-Prokop CM, Duyndam DA, et al. Fatty foci in the myocardium in patients with tuberous sclerosis complex: common finding at CT. Radiology 2009;253(2):359–63.
24. Davis RD Jr, Oldham HN Jr, Sabiston DC Jr. Primary cysts and neoplasms of the mediastinum: recent changes in clinical presentation, methods of diagnosis, management, and results. Ann Thorac Surg 1987;44(3):229–37.
25. Lewis KM, Sherer DM, Goncalves LF, et al. Mid-trimester prenatal sonographic diagnosis of a pericardial cyst. Prenat Diagn 1996;16(6):549–53.
26. Bernasconi A, Yoo SJ, Golding F, et al. Etiology and outcome of prenatally detected paracardial cystic lesions: a case series and review of the literature. Ultrasound Obstet Gynecol 2007;29(4):388–94.
27. Borges AC, Gellert K, Dietel M, et al. Acute right-sided heart failure due to hemorrhage into a pericardial cyst. Ann Thorac Surg 1997;63(3):845–7.
28. Hekmat M, Ghaderi H, Tatari H, et al. Giant pericardial cyst: a case report and review of literature. Iran J Radiol 2016;13(1):e21921.
29. Grebenc ML, Rosado de Christenson ML, Burke AP, et al. Primary cardiac and pericardial neoplasms: radiologic-pathologic correlation. Radiographics 2000;20(4):1073–103 [quiz: 1110–1, 1112].
30. Pacheco Gomez N, Marcos Gomez G, Garciperez de Vargas FJ, et al. Intrapericardial paraganglioma. Rev Esp Cardiol 2010;63(1):116–7.

31. Ediae J, Lim PS, Addonizio VP, et al. Pericardial hemangioma taking origin from the posterior wall of the left atrium. Ann Thorac Surg 2009;87(6):e54–6.

32. Thomason R, Schlegel W, Lucca M, et al. Primary malignant mesothelioma of the pericardium. Case report and literature review. Tex Heart Inst J 1994; 21(2):170–4.

33. Roggli VL. Pericardial mesothelioma after exposure to asbestos. N Engl J Med 1981;304(17):1045.

34. Sane AC, Roggli VL. Curative resection of a well-differentiated papillary mesothelioma of the pericardium. Arch Pathol Lab Med 1995;119(3):266–7.

35. Petrich A, Cho SI, Billett H. Primary cardiac lymphoma: an analysis of presentation, treatment, and outcome patterns. Cancer 2011;117(3):581–9.

36. Habboush HW, Dhundee J, Okati DA, et al. Constrictive pericarditis in B cell chronic lymphatic leukaemia. Clin Lab Haematol 1996;18(2):117–9.

37. Kupsky DF, Newman DB, Kumar G, et al. Echocardiographic features of cardiac angiosarcomas: the Mayo Clinic experience (1976-2013). Echocardiography 2016;33(2):186–92.

38. Leduc C, Jenkins SM, Sukov WR, et al. Cardiac angiosarcoma: histopathologic, immunohistochemical, and cytogenetic analysis of 10 cases. Hum Pathol 2017;60:199–207.

39. Fatima J, Duncan AA, Maleszewski JJ, et al. Primary angiosarcoma of the aorta, great vessels, and the heart. J Vasc Surg 2013;57(3):756–64.

40. Sharma A, DeValeria PA, Scherber RM, et al. Angiosarcoma causing cardiac constriction late after radiation therapy for breast carcinoma. Tex Heart Inst J 2016;43(1):81–3.

41. Killion MJ, Brodovsky HS, Schwarting R. Pericardial angiosarcoma after mediastinal irradiation for seminoma. A case report and a review of the literature. Cancer 1996;78(4):912–7.

42. Yahata S, Endo T, Honma H, et al. Sunray appearance on enhanced magnetic resonance image of cardiac angiosarcoma with pericardial obliteration. Am Heart J 1994;127(2):468–71.

43. Ma GT, Liu JZ, Miao Q, et al. Angiosarcoma of the pericardium: a case report. Int J Clin Exp Pathol 2015;8(10):13568–70.

44. Nichols CR. Mediastinal germ cell tumors. Clinical features and biologic correlates. Chest 1991;99(2): 472–9.

45. Lamba G, Frishman WH. Cardiac and pericardial tumors. Cardiol Rev 2012;20(5):237–52.

46. MacKenzie S, Loken S, Kalia N, et al. Intrapericardial teratoma in the perinatal period. Case report and review of the literature. J Pediatr Surg 2005; 40(12):e13–8.

47. Sbragia L, Paek BW, Feldstein VA, et al. Outcome of prenatally diagnosed solid fetal tumors. J Pediatr Surg 2001;36(8):1244–7.

48. Drier A, Haroche J, Savatovsky J, et al. Cerebral, facial, and orbital involvement in Erdheim-Chester disease: CT and MR imaging findings. Radiology 2010;255(2):586–94.

49. Haroche J, Amoura Z, Dion E, et al. Cardiovascular involvement, an overlooked feature of Erdheim-Chester disease: report of 6 new cases and a literature review. Medicine (Baltimore) 2004;83(6):371–92.

50. Haroche J, Cluzel P, Toledano D, et al. Images in cardiovascular medicine. Cardiac involvement in Erdheim-Chester disease: magnetic resonance and computed tomographic scan imaging in a monocentric series of 37 patients. Circulation 2009;119(25):e597–8.

51. Goyal G, Shah MV, Call TG, et al. Clinical and radiologic responses to cladribine for the treatment of Erdheim-Chester Disease. JAMA Oncol 2017. [Epub ahead of print].

52. Mori K, Yamada K, Konno T, et al. Pericardial involvement in IgG4-related disease. Intern Med 2015;54(10):1231–5.

53. Mavrogeni S, Markousis-Mavrogenis G, Kolovou G. IgG4-related cardiovascular disease. The emerging role of cardiovascular imaging. Eur J Radiol 2017; 86:169–75.

54. Inoue D, Zen Y, Abo H, et al. Immunoglobulin G4-related periaortitis and periarteritis: CT findings in 17 patients. Radiology 2011;261(2):625–33.

55. Ebbo M, Grados A, Guedj E, et al. Usefulness of 2-[18F]-fluoro-2-deoxy-D-glucose-positron emission tomography/computed tomography for staging and evaluation of treatment response in IgG4-related disease: a retrospective multicenter study. Arthritis Care Res (Hoboken) 2014;66(1):86–96.

56. Sugimoto T, Morita Y, Isshiki K, et al. Constrictive pericarditis as an emerging manifestation of hyper-IgG4 disease. Int J Cardiol 2008;130(3):e100–1.

Congenital Abnormalities of the Pericardium

Yuvrajsinh J. Parmar, MD[a], Ankit B. Shah, MD, MPH[b], Michael Poon, MD[a], Itzhak Kronzon, MD, FESC[a],*

KEYWORDS

- Congenital abnormalities of the pericardium • Congenital absence of the pericardium
- Pericardial cysts and diverticula • Congenital defects

KEY POINTS

- Congenital abnormalities of the pericardium are a rare group of disorders that include congenital absence of the pericardium, pericardial cysts, and diverticula.
- These congenital defects result from alterations in the embryologic formation and structure of the pericardium.
- Most cases go undetected or are found incidentally, but occasionally present as symptomatic, life threatening disease.

INTRODUCTION

Congenital abnormalities of the pericardium are a rare group of disorders that include congenital absence of the pericardium, pericardial cysts, and diverticula. These congenital defects result from alterations in the embryologic formation and structure of the pericardium. Although many cases go undetected or are incidentally found, they can occasionally present as symptomatic, life-threatening disease. Owing to their rarity, many cases are inappropriately diagnosed as other, more common conditions. Alterations in the embryologic formation and structure of the pericardium may result in the formation of these congenital abnormalities of the pericardium. We review the presentation, diagnosis, and management of congenital absence of the pericardium, pericardial cysts and diverticula. A summary of their multimodality imaging features is also provided (**Tables 1** and **2**).

Embryology of the Normal Pericardium

The intraembryonic coelom gives rise to 3 body cavities during the fourth week of embryogenesis: the pericardial cavity, peritoneal cavity, and 2 pleuropericardial canals. Each cavity contains a parietal and visceral layer that are lined with mesothelium derived from the mesoderm. The pericardial and peritoneal cavities are separated by the growth of the septum transversum, the primordium of the central tendon of the diaphragm. As the bronchial bud grows, the pleuropericardial canals separate the pleural cavities from the pericardial cavity via the growth and fusion of the right and left pleuropericardial membranes, which contain the common cardinal veins (ducts of Cuvier) and phrenic nerves. The pleuropericardial membrane later becomes the fibrous pericardium.[1–4] Congenital lesions of the pericardium arise from defects in the fusion of the pericardial cavity. The anatomy and functions of the pericardium are detailed in Brian D. Hoit's article, "Anatomy and Physiology of the Pericardium," in this issue.

CONGENITAL ABSENCE OF THE PERICARDIUM

Congenital absence of the pericardium results from a failure of pleuropericardial membranes to fuse completely on one or both sides. The

The authors have no conflicts of interest.
[a] Department of Cardiovascular Medicine, Lenox Hill Hospital, Northwell Health, 100 East 77th Street, New York, NY 10075, USA; [b] Division of Cardiology, Massachusetts General Hospital, 55 Fruit Street, Boston, MA 02114, USA
* Corresponding author. Lenox Hill Hospital, 100 East 77th Street, 2nd Floor Noninvasive Cardiology, New York, NY 10075.
E-mail address: kronzon@aol.com

Table 1
Summary of imaging findings of congenital absence of the pericardium

Image Modality	Findings
Chest radiograph	• Posteroanterior view with levorotation of the heart • Lateral view with a posterior shift of the heart • Elongation of the left ventricular contour (Snoopy's sign) • Prominent pulmonary artery • Radiolucency (lung tissue) between the base of the heart and the diaphragm or between the aortic knob and main pulmonary artery • An obscured right heart border • Radiopaque bulge from herniated cardiac tissue
Echocardiography	• Unusual imaging windows • Cardiac hypermobility • Right ventricular dilatation • Sharp angulation of the atrioventricular groove • Elongated atria with widened ventricles (teardrop shape) on apical 4-chamber view • Tricuspid insufficiency seen on Doppler echocardiography • Paradoxic septal motion seen on M-mode imaging • Increased angle of the longitudinal axis of the left ventricular posterior wall in the PLAX view in the left lateral decubitus position that disappears in the right lateral decubitus position • Increased distance between the starting point of the ultrasound beam to the most distal portion of the left ventricular posterior wall in the PSAX view in the left lateral decubitus position that disappears in the right lateral decubitus position
CCT and CMR	• Direct visualization of absent pericardium • Leftward and posterior displacement of the heart • Greater degree of clockwise rotation (>60°) • Whole heart volume change of >13%
Angiography	• Normal caliber vessels with an abrupt focal kink or angulation that results from external compression by the rim of the partial pericardial defect

Abbreviations: CCT, cardiac computed tomography; CMR, cardiac magnetic resonance; PLAX, parasternal long axis; PSAX, parasternal short axis.

Adapted from Klein AL, Abbara S, Agler DA, et al. American Society of Echocardiography clinical recommendations for multimodality cardiovascular imaging of patients with pericardial disease: endorsed by the Society for Cardiovascular Magnetic Resonance and Society of Cardiovascular Computed Tomography. J Am Soc Echocardiogr 2013;26:1004; with permission.

resultant pericardial defects can be described as a complete absence of the entire pericardium, complete absence of the left- or right-sided pericardium, partial foramen-type absence of the left- or right-sided pericardium, or diaphragmatic absence of the pericardium.[5] This distinction is important, because patients with partial defects are more likely to present with symptoms and complications than those with complete absence of the pericardium. Left-sided defects are the most commonly encountered defects (70%). Less common are diaphragmatic defects (17%), bilateral or complete defects (9%), and right-sided defects (4%).[6]

Congenital absence of the pericardium was first observed by Columbus in 1559 and first described by Baillie in 1793.[7] Congenital defects of the pericardium are exceedingly rare, with an incidence between 0.007% and 0.044% as reported by autopsies and surgical case series.[8] The first of 2 large autopsy series conducted in 1909 identified 2 cases in 13,000 autopsies. The second series conducted in 1938 identified only 1 case in 14,000 autopsies.[9–11] More contemporary data suggest that the early autopsy series may have underestimated its true incidence: a surgical series discovered 15 cases in 34,000 cardiothoracic surgeries performed between 1952 and 1991 at the Mayo Clinic.[8,10] Thus, the true prevalence of this abnormality is likely underestimated because the majority of patients are asymptomatic and go undetected or are incidentally found. Historical data report a 3:1 male predominance; however, data from the Mayo Clinic suggests no clear gender predominance.[7] Familial occurrence of this defect is rare.[12]

Table 2
Summary of imaging findings of pericardial cysts[a]

Image Modality	Findings
Chest radiograph	• Ovid, well-circumscribed, radiopaque mass bordering the heart
Echocardiography	• Round, echolucent cavities • Apical and subcostal views may differentiate cystic margins • Lack of vascular flow on Doppler imaging
CCT	• Homogenous cystic fluid contents near water density (0–20 Hounsfield units) • Lack of enhancement with intravenous contrast
CMR	• Homogenous low to intermediate intensity on T1-weighted images • Homogenous high intensity on T2-weighted images • Lack of enhancement with administration of gadolinium

Abbreviations: CCT, cardiac computed tomography; CMR, cardiac magnetic resonance.

[a] Pericardial diverticula have the same characteristics, except that a communication with the pericardial space can be seen and the size of the diverticula can change with different body positions and phases of respiratory cycle.

Associations

Of patients with congenital absence of the pericardium, 30% to 50% have associated cardiac or noncardiac birth defects.[13] Bilateral and right-sided defects are more often seen with associated congenital anomalies. Cardiac anomalies that have been reported include atrial septal defects, patent ductus arteriosus, tetralogy of Fallot, and sinus venous defects with partial anomalous pulmonary venous drainage.[10,13] Aortic connective tissue disorders, such as Marfan syndrome, and bicuspid aortic valve have also been linked to this defect. Several type A aortic dissections have been reported as well. In such cases, cardiac tamponade or pericardial effusion may not be present, and patients instead present with hypovolemic shock owing to large left hemothoraces that result from the absence of the pericardium that would normally restrict fluid drainage into the thorax.[14–16] Noncardiac anomalies include bronchogenic cysts, pulmonary sequestration, aberrant lobes of the lung, and pectus excavatum.[11,17] Diaphragmatic defects may be associated with partial diaphragmatic aplasia with abdominal organs herniating into the pericardial sac.[6] Other reported associations are with VATER syndrome (vertebral defects, anal atresia, tracheoesophageal fistula, radial and renal dysplasia), and Pallister-Killian syndrome (mental retardation, hypopigmentation or hyperpigmentation, and facial anomalies).[18,19]

Clinical Presentation

The majority of patients with congenital absence of the pericardium are asymptomatic and cases are typically found incidentally on imaging, during a surgical procedure, or postmortem. Clinical findings and symptoms result from the lack of constraint on the heart and loss of isolation from surrounding structures that the normal pericardium provides. Patients may present with a wide range of nonspecific symptoms, of which the most common is atypical, sharp, or stabbing chest pain, which is usually left sided and nonexertional in nature. Pain may also be positional because, in the absence of pericardial tissue, the heart is subject to increased mobility and its relationship to surrounding structures can be changed. Although not well-understood, this chest pain may result from torsion of the great vessels at the base of the heart, lack of pericardial cushioning, or tension from pleuropericardial adhesions. In partial defects, chest pain can be due to ischemia from cardiac herniation or pressure from the rim of remaining pericardial tissue.[6,11,13] Dyspnea and trepopnea (dyspnea while in the lateral decubitus position on 1 side but not the other) have also been reported and may result from compression of the lower left pulmonary vein between the left atrium and the descending aorta.[6,20] Other presenting symptoms may include palpitations, dizziness, and syncope. The most feared presentation, sudden cardiac death, can result from strangulation of cardiac tissue and compression of coronary vessels through left-sided partial foramen-type defects. The most common site of herniation is the left atrial appendage; however, herniation of the entire left atrium and both ventricles has been reported.[11]

Physical Examination and Electrocardiogram

A wide differential diagnosis exists for the symptomatic patient with congenital absence of the pericardium owing to the nonspecific nature of the complaints reported. Symptoms can mimic a plethora of other conditions, such as acute coronary syndromes, pericarditis, myocarditis, cardiac aneurysms, tumors of the lung or heart, mitral valve disease, atrial septal defects, pulmonic stenosis, idiopathic dilation of pulmonary artery, and hilar lymphadenopathy.[8,13] The physical examination and electrocardiogram in patients with congenital absence of the pericardium are nonspecific. Examination can reveal a lateral displacement of the apical impulse and a systolic ejection murmur at the second left intercostal space or the left sternal boarder. The electrocardiogram can show right axis deviation, incomplete right bundle branch block, poor R-wave progression in the precordial leads, and bradycardia from vagal stimulation.[21,22] In partial defects, ST segment elevation can be seen when there is external compression of coronary arteries in a herniated segment of myocardium by the pericardial rim (**Fig. 1**A).[13]

Chest Radiograph

In 1959, Ellis and colleagues[5,8] reported the first case of congenital absence of the pericardium diagnosed on chest radiography. Suspicious of the diagnosis, the authors produced an iatrogenic pneumothorax by injecting air into the pleural space to confirm the condition by showing a subsequent pneumopericardium. This invasive confirmatory technique has fallen out of favor given the associated risks and with the development of more sensitive and less invasive diagnostic modalities.[11] There are characteristic findings of complete bilateral or left-sided pericardial absence on chest radiography. The cardiac silhouette may demonstrate levoposition of the heart in the posteroanterior view, posterior shift of the cardiac silhouette in the lateral view, elongation of the left ventricular contour (referred to as Snoopy's sign), prominent pulmonary artery, radiolucency (lung tissue) between the base of the heart and the diaphragm or between the aortic knob and main pulmonary artery (previously referred to as a "tongue" of tissue), or an obscured right heart border owing to a superimposed spine (**Fig. 2**A). Importantly, despite all of the cardiac rotation seen, this condition does not cause tracheal deviation and thus all of these findings are noted with a midline trachea. In partial or foramen-type defects, herniation of the left atrial appendage can be seen as a radiopaque bulge of the left upper heart border (see **Fig. 2**B).[11,21]

Even with the additional support of radiographic findings, the diagnosis often remains elusive. The most likely reason for this underdiagnosis is a low suspicion for this exceedingly rare disease. In addition, much of the findings mentioned are nonspecific and may fit a variety of other disease states. For this reason, use of advanced imaging techniques is necessary to make the diagnosis while excluding other diagnoses in the symptomatic patient with congenital absence of the pericardium.

Additional noninvasive imaging techniques such as echocardiography, cardiac computed tomography (CCT) and cardiac magnetic resonance (CMR) imaging have improved the ability to recognize and characterize this defect. Echocardiography may be nondiagnostic because the pericardium is difficult to visualize, but can provide certain clues to the diagnosis. CMR and CCT are the diagnostic modalities of choice given their enhanced tomographic visualization of the pericardium along with a functional assessment and tissue characterization ability.[8]

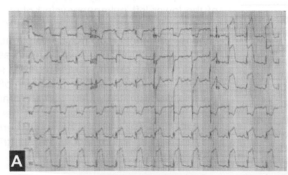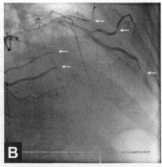

Fig. 1. (*A*) Electrocardiogram showing ST elevations in a patient admitted with chest pain found to have a partial foramen-type defect. (*B*) Coronary angiography of the same patient showing significant stenosis (*arrows*) and abrupt angulation of the left anterior descending artery, diagonal arteries, and obtuse marginal arteries owing to external compression from a partial foramen-type defect. Otherwise, the coronary arteries are of normal caliber and appearance.

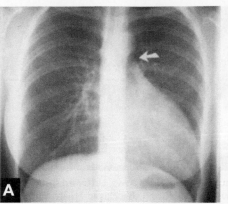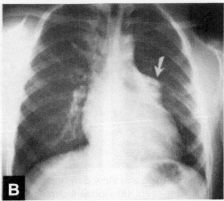

Fig. 2. (*A*) Posteroanterior radiograph of a patient with complete congenital absence of left pericardium. There is a "tongue" of lung tissue interposing between the main pulmonary artery and aorta (*arrow*). Also, there is marked levoposition of the cardiac silhouette, loss of right heart border, and prominent main pulmonary artery. (*B*) Posteroanterior radiograph from a patient with a partial foramen-type defect. A herniated left atrial appendage can be seen on the left heart border (*arrow*). (*Reprinted from* Gatzoulis MA, Munk MD, Merchant N, et al. Isolated congenital absence of the pericardium: clinical presentation, diagnosis, and management. Ann Thorac Surg 2000;69:1210–12; with permission from Elsevier.)

Coronary Angiography

Coronary angiography may occasionally be pursued if the workup shows evidence of electrocardiographic ischemic changes, inducible ischemia on stress perfusion imaging, or positive biomarkers that result from coronary artery compression. Coronary evaluation can show normal caliber vessels with an abrupt focal kink or angulation that result from external compression by the rim of the partial pericardial defect (see **Fig. 1**B). Catheter-induced coronary vasospasm and cardiopulmonary support during angioplasty have also been reported to have similar appearances. Focal narrowing from external compression will not respond to administration of intracoronary nitroglycerin, excluding vasospasm from the differential diagnosis.[13]

Echocardiography

Echocardiography demonstrates features of an unrestrained heart and the altered geometry that results from complete absence of the left pericardium. Nontraditional cardiac windows may be needed to appropriately assess the cardiac structure owing to the levoposition and cardiac hypermobility (cardiopstosis). As seen on chest radiography, leftward and posterior displacement produces an off-axis view of the right ventricle. In the traditional parasternal long axis view, the leftward shift allows more of the right ventricle to be seen, thus giving the appearance of right ventricular dilatation (**Fig. 3**A).[11] However, the absence of other causes for right ventricular dilatation, such as an atrial septal defect, tricuspid insufficiency,

anomalous pulmonary venous drainage, or pulmonic insufficiency, can help the clinician to narrow the differential diagnosis. In the apical windows, there is marked lateral displacement of the heart and the appearance of compressed atria. The typical findings in complete absence of the pericardium in the apical 4-chamber view are a "teardrop" shape of the heart, bulbous left ventricle, elongated atria, and a sharp angulation of the atrioventricular groove (see **Fig. 3**B).[23–26] Varying degrees of tricuspid insufficiency can be seen from the altered anatomy of an unrestrained heart. The leftward and posterior displacement stretches the anterior right ventricular wall distorting the geometry of the tricuspid annulus and potentially causing chordal rupture.[8,27,28] Paradoxic motion of the interventricular septum can be seen owing to the exaggerated posterior left ventricular wall motion causing an anterior displacement of the interventricular septum. The characteristic M-mode findings demonstrate paradoxic septal motion and right ventricular enlargement (see **Fig. 3**C).[23,26] Instances of cardiac herniation may demonstrate bulging of tissue through a partial defect. If coronary blood flow is compromised, regional wall motion abnormalities or edema from coronary venous obstruction may be appreciated.[13] Evaluation of speckle tracking showed a decrease in ventricular torsion, but strain and strain rates showed no difference in the absence of ischemia when compared with controls. This finding suggests that absence of the pericardium does not alter left ventricular function.[11,29] Given the nonspecific nature of these echocardiographic findings, Kim and colleagues[30] compared positional changes of normal patients,

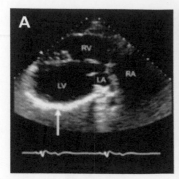
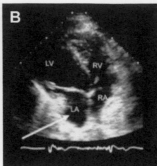
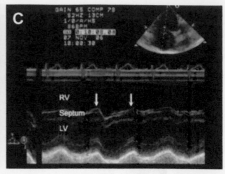

Fig. 3. (*A*) Parasternal long axis view demonstrating unusual cardiac windows. Leftward shift of the heart allows more of the RV to be seen. (*B*) Apical 4-chamber view demonstrating the classic "teardrop" appearance with elongated atria and widened ventricles. Sharp angulation can be seen between the LA and LV (*arrow*) (*C*) M-Mode of the parasternal long axis view showing abnormal septal motion (*arrows*). The septum paradoxically moves anteriorly during systole. LA, left atrium; LV, left ventricle; RA, right atrium; RV, right ventricle. (*Reproduced from [A, B]* Abbas AE, Appleton CP, Liu PT, et al. Congenital absence of the pericardium: case presentation and review of literature. Int J Cardiol 2005;98(1):23; with permission from Elsevier; and [C] Kronzon I, Srichai MB. Rare pericardial disorders. In: Lang RM, Goldstein SA, Kronzon I, et al, editors. Dynamic echocardiography. 1st edition. St Louis (MO): Elsevier; 2011. p. 263; with permission from Elsevier.)

patients with an atrial septal defect, and patients with total or left congenital absence of the pericardium to aid in making the diagnosis. In this study, right ventricular enlargement was observed in patients with an atrial septal defect and congenital absence of the pericardium. The angle of the longitudinal axis of the left ventricular posterior wall in the parasternal long axis view and distance between the starting point of the ultrasound beam to the most distal portion of the left ventricular posterior wall in the parasternal short axis view were measured in the left lateral decubitus position and right lateral decubitus position. The authors demonstrated a significant difference in both the angle of the longitudinal axis of the left ventricular posterior wall and the distance from the starting point of the ultrasound beam to the left ventricular posterior wall when compared with normal patients and patients with an atrial septal defect. This significant difference was eliminated when these parameters were measured in the right lateral decubitus position. The posterior displacement of the heart seen in congenital absence of the pericardium in the left lateral decubitus position resolved once the patient shifted to the right lateral decubitus position and the heart moved more anteriorly. These measurements and maneuvers may help to diagnose congenital absence of the pericardium when standard echocardiographic findings are nonspecific and clinical suspicion remains high.

Cardiac Computed Tomography and Cardiac Magnetic Resonance

Because echocardiography remains limited in the evaluation of the pericardium, CMR and

CCT have emerged as the diagnostic modalities of choice owing to increased resolution of the pericardium and unlimited viewing angle. Compared with CCT, CMR is more accurate for soft tissue characterization with better contrast resolution, greater temporal resolution for functional evaluation, and avoiding exposure to ionizing radiation.[31] CMR is therefore considered the gold standard for the evaluation of pericardial diseases. The pericardium can be visualized directly on T1-weighted and T2-weighted spin-echo images as a dark, curvilinear line between the medium-intensity myocardium and high-intensity pericardial fat.[11,32,33] Visualization becomes increasingly difficult with less pericardial fat, particularly in younger individuals. In addition, a paucity of surrounding fat along the lateral left cardiac wall makes visualization of the pericardium difficult in this area, which is the most frequent location of pericardial defects.[31] An inability to visualize the pericardium may lead to an erroneous diagnosis in 10% of patients and it is therefore important to rely on other morphologic and functional signs that can aid in the diagnosis.[8] Common morphologic findings include leftward and posterior displacement of the heart (**Fig. 4**A) and interposition of lung tissue in areas of absent pericardium, most commonly between the aorta and pulmonary artery or between the base of the heart and the diaphragm (see **Fig. 4**B, C). Partial foramen type defects can show a cardiac indentation that results from external pressure exerted by the rim (see **Fig. 4**D) or direct herniation of cardiac tissue.[31] In such cases, edema seen as increased wall thickness may result from coronary venous

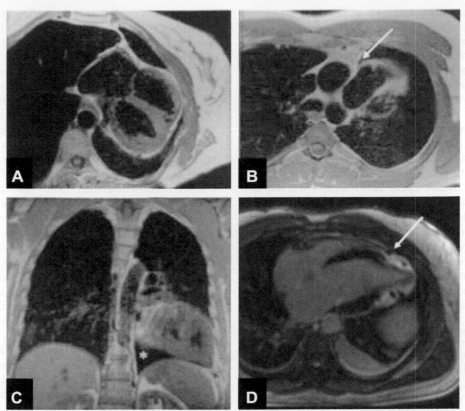

Fig. 4. Cardiac magnetic resonance findings in congenital absence of the pericardium. (*A*) Axial T1-weighted spin-echo image of complete absence of the left pericardium demonstrating marked leftward and posterior displacement. (*B*) Axial T1-weighted spin-echo image demonstrating interposition of lung tissue in between the aorta and pulmonary artery (*arrow*). (*C*) Coronal T1-weighted spin-echo image demonstrating interposition of lung tissue in between the diaphragm and the heart (*asterisk*). (*D*) Delayed postcontrast sequences showing microvascular damage at the apex. An indentation can be seen at the sight of the partial foramen-type defect (*arrow*). (*Reprinted from [A–C]* Gatzoulis MA, Munk MD, Merchant N, et al. Isolated congenital absence of the pericardium: clinical presentation, diagnosis, and management. Ann Thorac Surg 2000;69:1210–1; with permission from Elsevier.)

congestion as a consequence of external compression.[13]

Cine sequences provide a functional cardiac assessment in which cardiac hypermobility is frequently the initial finding. Macaione and colleagues[31] analyzed 9 patients with congenital absence of the left pericardium that underwent CMR and proposed 2 quantitative parameters to increase diagnostic sensitivity. Levorotation of the heart is a typical finding in patients with complete left-sided defects. In diastole, the heart is located deeper within the thorax when compared with normal individuals. In systole, the cardiac apex swings anteriorly with the base serving as a fulcrum. Levorotation itself is not pathognomonic for congenital absence of the pericardium and may be seen in disease states that cause right ventricular overload. A greater degree of clockwise rotation, with a proposed cut off of 60°, may

distinguish complete absence of the left pericardium from right ventricular overload. Another proposed quantitative parameter is whole heart volume change, measured as the changed in volume at the end of systole and end of diastole. It has been shown that complete absence of the left pericardium has a larger whole heart volume change, with a proposed cutoff of 13%, when compared with other disease states such as right ventricular overload, hypertrophic cardiomyopathy, and dilated cardiomyopathy. The increased volume change seen in this condition may be explained by the lack of pericardial constraint allowing for increased compliance and dilation of the ventricles during diastole and atria during systole.[31]

Diagnostic accuracy of CCT when compared with CMR is probably similar. The pericardium, best visualized in systole, can be seen on both noncontrast and contrast-enhanced images. Its visibility is enhanced against the low attenuation of surrounding adipose tissue, and therefore subject to limitations similar to CMR. CCT can also demonstrate the morphologic and functional findings seen on CMR, including the quantitative parameters proposed by Macaione and colleagues.[31] The advantages of CCT are the speed of the examination and better spatial resolution, but these come at the expense of increased radiation exposure, especially with retrospective scanning to visualize the pericardium throughout the entire cardiac cycle. With the advent of modern computed tomography scanners and a prospective electrocardiogram-triggered protocol, this exposure can be limited. In the workup of atypical chest pain and nonspecific symptoms, nongated chest computed tomography is often obtained and can incidentally diagnose pericardial defects without the need for further workup based on the image quality.[8]

Management and Treatment

The rarity of this disease precludes any large controlled study to help guide management. Therefore, recommendations are based on case reports and observations. This condition remains clinically silent in the majority of patients and does not require treatment. In complete bilateral or unilateral defects, cardiac function and life expectancy were suggested to be similar when compared with controls; therefore, conservative management is recommended.[7,11,29] Surgery is generally reserved for partial foramen-type defects when patients are symptomatic or have high-risk features, such as cardiac herniation or coronary artery ischemia. Surgical options include pericardioplasty (dilation of the pericardial defect to prevent strangulation), pericardectomy, or patch closure of the defect. In cases of left atrial appendage herniation, the left atrial appendage can be excised and the defect can be closed with a patch.[10,11] Of these options, pericardioplasty is the most commonly cited procedure with low morbidity.[20]

CONGENITAL PERICARDIAL CYSTS AND DIVERTICULA

Pericardial cysts and diverticula were first described during postmortem examinations in the 19th century. The first reported pericardial diverticulum and cyst were described in 1837 and 1891, respectively. Initially thought to be separate conditions, it was not until 1903 that Rohn, from the Charles University of Prague, realized the association between cysts and diverticula. He concluded that pericardial cysts and diverticula represent different stages of the same developmental process.[34] Congenital lesions may result from incomplete fusion of one or several lacunae that create the pericardial cavity that causes weakness in the defective region. Herniation or protrusion of the weak region in the pericardium ultimately led to the formation of a diverticulum or cyst.[35] Although cysts and diverticula arise from similar processes, they can be distinguished from each other based on their relationship with the pericardial sac. Pericardial diverticula are outpouchings from the pericardium that maintain communication with the pericardial space through a wide or narrow neck. Thin-walled cysts are formed when the communication between the pericardial space and diverticulum is obliterated.[35] Therefore, cysts do not communicate with the pericardial space. Cysts can be distinguished from diverticula in that their size remains constant, whereas the size of diverticula can change with position and respirations.[36] Cysts are reported to be 3 times more common than diverticula, and although the majority of cysts range from 1 to 15 cm, giant cysts as large as 37 cm have been reported.[36–38] Because cysts and diverticula result from a common embryologic process, symptoms and complications are similar, and the distinction between the two in the literature are vague, they are discussed together.

Because the majority of cases are clinically silent, advances in radiographic imaging have increased the characterization and diagnostic yield for these conditions. In 1958, during a mass chest radiograph campaign, 3 of 300,000 individuals were identified to have a pericardial cyst, making the reported incidence of this rare disorder 1 in 100,000 with a 3:2 male predominance.[39] These lesions comprise 6% of all mediastinal masses and 33% of all mediastinal cysts. The other common mediastinal cysts include bronchogenic, enteric, and thymic cysts.[40] The right cardiophrenic angle (70%) is most commonly involved, followed by the left cardiophrenic angle (22%) and other parts of the mediastinum (8%).[36,41,42] Cysts are generally benign, unilocular intrathoracic lesions that contain serous fluid, although multilocular lesions can be seen.[39] Cysts and diverticula have been discovered in patients of all ages, from early adolescence to advanced ages with the majority of cases being reported in the fourth decade of life.[36,39] The majority of pericardial cysts and diverticula are congenital, but they can also be acquired secondary to pericarditis, or increased intrapericardial pressure from an effusion resulting in herniation, surgery, and trauma. Parasitic infections with Echinococcus granulosus can cause cystic lesions that are typically seen in the lung and liver; however, cardiac involvement can be seen in 0.2% to 2.0% of cases.[37]

Clinical Presentation and Complications

Up to 75% of pericardial cysts and diverticula remain clinically silent and are found serendipitously.[39] The remaining 25% of these patients may develop symptoms as the lesion enlarges and exerts pressure on adjacent structures, such as lung, trachea, thoracic wall, diaphragm, esophagus, and heart. Symptoms are often vague and can encompass a wide differential diagnosis. The most common symptoms reported are retrosternal chest pressure or tightness, dyspnea, and chronic cough.[39,41] These symptoms generally result from the interaction with surrounding organs; however, rare cases of torsion at the neck of the diverticula or cyst causing chest pain have been reported.[43–45] Pleuritic chest pain can be present in cases of ruptured pericardial cysts that cause pleuropericarditis and pneumonitis.[46] The compression of pulmonary hilar structures can cause repeated respiratory infections, cough, dyspnea, and cyanosis.[47] In situations where the esophagus is involved, dysphagia, indigestion, and epigastric pain may be present.[39] Palpitations from atrial arrhythmias, most commonly fibrillation, have been reported from the compression of the atria, pulmonary vein, or sinoatrial node.[48,49] Other reported findings include hemoptysis, atelectasis, and pneumothorax.[39,41,50] More serious complications are rare and also arise from mass effect by the cyst itself or from cystic contents. Cystic growth may alter the cardiac geometry by encroaching on cardiac chambers. In addition to congestive heart failure from right atrial and ventricular compression, valvular diseases have been observed as a result of this altered geometry. Distortion of the mitral valve annulus can subsequently cause mitral valve prolapse and mitral regurgitation,[51] whereas compression of the right ventricular outflow tract can result in subpulmonic stenosis.[52] Other rare complications include cyst infection, compression of the superior vena cava, compression of the left atrium, hemorrhage or rupture into the pericardial space causing cardiac tamponade, right mainstem bronchus obstruction, erosion into adjacent structures such as the superior vena cava and right ventricular wall, and sudden death.[52–59]

Physical Examination and Electrocardiography

Physical examination and electrocardiography are generally unrevealing in the diagnosis of this condition. However, in certain complicated cysts, specific physical examination findings may be appreciated. For example, when compression of the superior vena cava or cardiac chambers occur, signs of superior vena cava syndrome or right heart failure may be present. Given the vague presentation, imaging is essential to make the diagnosis.[35,60]

Chest Radiograph

Chest radiographs classically demonstrate an ovoid, well-circumscribed, radiopaque mass bordering the cardiac silhouette, most often at the right cardiophrenic angle abutting the diaphragm (Fig. 5). Other locations such as the left

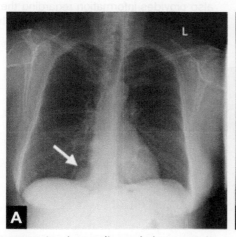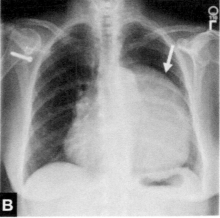

Fig. 5. Posteroanterior chest radiograph demonstrating a right cardiophrenic (*A*) and giant left-sided (*B*) pericardial cyst (*arrows*). (*Reproduced from* [*A*] Kronzon I, Srichai MB. Rare pericardial disorders. In: Lang RM, Goldstein SA, Kronzon I, et al, editors. Dynamic Echocardiography. St Louis (MO): Elsevier; 2011. p. 263; with permission from Elsevier; and [*B*] Jain S, Gorscan J III, Mankad SV. Chapter 145. Pericardial cysts and congenital absence of the pericardium. In: Lang MR, Goldstein SA, Kronzon I, et al, editors. ASE's Comprehensive Echocardiography. Second Edition. Philadelphia: Elsevier; 2016. p. 615; with permission from Elsevier.)

cardiophrenic angle, hila, superior, or posterior mediastinum can also be seen. Because position and respiration can alter the size and shape of diverticula, differences may be noted between radiographs.[39,41] Ruptured pericardial cysts can result in complete disappearance of the mass with possible pleural effusions seen on chest radiographs.[35,46] Findings on chest radiography are not specific to pericardial cysts or diverticula and differentiation from other diseases is necessary. Multiple solid tumors, angiomas, lipomas, neurogenic tumors, sarcomas, granulomatous lesions, and abscesses can mimic pericardial cysts and are a key limitation to the use of radiographs to diagnose pericardial cysts and diverticula. Other mediastinal cysts that must be considered are bronchogenic cysts, enteric cysts, thymic cysts, and lypmhangiomas.[41] In addition, diaphragmatic hernia, ventricular aneurysm, aortic aneurysm, prominent fat pad, prominent left atrial appendage, and enlarged diaphragmatic lymph nodes may have a similar appearance.[36] Given this broad differential diagnosis, supplemental imaging is necessary.

Echocardiography

On echocardiography, pericardial cysts are round, echolucent cavities typically seen at the right heart border. Apical and subcostal windows allow for the differentiation of cystic margins from the cardiac boarder (**Fig. 6**).[53] Depending on the location, cysts may mimic other diseases. For instance, cysts located in the right cardiophrenic angle may be confused with diaphragmatic hernias, whereas cysts in the left cardiophrenic angle may be confused with ventricular aneurysms.[36] The differential diagnosis can also include pericardial sinuses, malignant lesions, pseudoaneurysms, aortic aneurysms, prominent fat pad, prominent

left atrial appendage, and a loculated pericardial effusion.[53] Cystic lesions do not contain vascular flow; thus, the use of color Doppler, pulse wave Doppler, and contrast can aid in narrowing the differential diagnosis.[36,61] Large cysts may encroach on surrounding structures and distort their appearance, such as compression of right-sided heart chambers. Pericardial diverticula share similar properties to pericardial cysts, but their distinction may be possible when the pericardial lining can be seen.[61] Lesions in atypical locations may go unnoticed on transthoracic echocardiography; thus, transesophageal echocardiography can be useful when transthoracic echocardiography is suboptimal.[60] Although echocardiography can aid in the diagnosis, its narrow window of visualization limits its sensitivity. CCT and CMR provide greater resolution when visualizing the pericardium and surrounding structures and are, therefore, considered the imaging modalities of choice.[36]

Cardiac Computed Tomography and Cardiac Magnetic Resonance

On CCT, pericardial cysts are spherical, thin-walled structures that are well-circumscribed. Cystic contents are generally homogenous with their attenuation near that of water (0–20 Hounsfield units) and fail to enhance with intravenous contrast administration (**Fig. 7**).[62,63] Limitations arise when their attenuation exceeds that of water (20–40 Houndsfield units) as a result of higher proteinaceous material. Higher attenuations make it increasingly difficult to differentiate cysts between soft tissue masses and hematomas.[36,62–66] CCT also provides information regarding the anatomic location of the lesion and its relationship to surrounding structures.

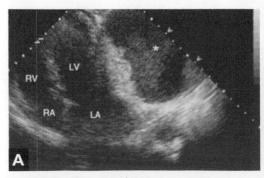 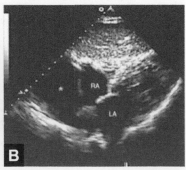

Fig. 6. (*A*) Apical 4 chamber view showing an ovoid, echolucent space (*asterisk*) adjacent to the left sided heart chambers consistent with a pericardial cyst. (*B*) Subcostal view showing a pericardial cyst (*asterisk*) adjacent to the RA. LA, left atrium; LV, left ventricle; RA, right atrium; RV, right ventricle. (*Reproduced from* Jain S, Gorscan J III, Mankad SV. Chapter 145. Pericardial cysts and congenital absence of the pericardium. In: Lang MR, Goldstein SA, Kronzon I, et al, editors. ASE's Comprehensive Echocardiography. Second Edition. Philadelphia: Elsevier; 2016. p. 614; with permission from Elsevier.)

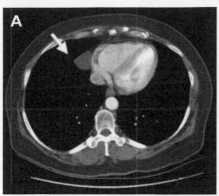
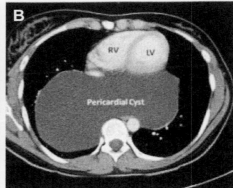

Fig. 7. (*A*) Computed tomography (CT) scan of the chest showing a pericardial cyst with low-density fluid (*arrow*) at the right cardiophrenic angle. (*B*) CT scan showing a giant pericardial cyst with low-density fluid. LV, left ventricle; RV, right ventricle. (*Reproduced from* [A] Kronzon I, Srichai MB. Rare pericardial disorders. In: Lang RM, Goldstein SA, Kronzon I, et al, editors. Dynamic Echocardiography. St Louis (MO): Elsevier; 2011. p. 263; with permission from Elsevier; and [B] Thanneer L, Saric M, Perk G, et al. A giant pericardial cyst. J Am Coll Cardiol 2011;57(17):1784; with permission.)

CMR is also effective at the diagnosis of pericardial cysts with similar characteristics and limitations as CCT. Cystic fluid typically has a low to intermediate signal intensity on T1-weighted images and homogenous high intensity on T2-weighted images (**Fig. 8**). Cysts generally do not enhance with administration of gadolinium-based contrast. As in CCT, atypical contents of the cystic fluid alter the appearance on CMR imaging. Cysts with hemorrhagic components or highly proteinaceous fluid decrease T2-weighted signals and increase T1-weighted signals. In such cases,

differentiation of cysts from hematomas or soft tissue masses may prove to be difficult and diffusion weighted MRI can be helpful.[36,65–68] The distinction between pericardial diverticula and cysts can be made on CCT or CMR when a complete wall around the circumference mass cannot be identified.[61]

Treatment

The approach to management depends on presenting symptoms, cyst or diverticulum size, and

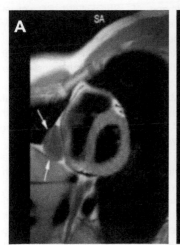
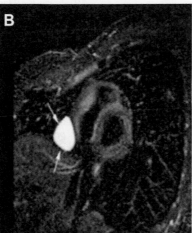
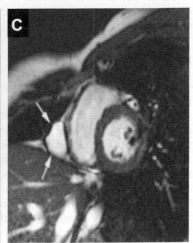

Fig. 8. Cardiac magnetic resonance (CMR) images of pericardial cysts. The cystic contents are homogenous and have signal characteristics of water. (*A*) A short axis T1-weighted spin-echo image shows a pericardial cyst (*arrows*) with low signal intensity. (*B*) A short axis T2-weighted spin-echo image shows a pericardial cyst (*arrows*) with high signal intensity. (*C*) Cine CMR image of a pericardial cyst (*arrows*). (*Reproduced from* Bogaert J, Francone M. Cardiovascular magnetic resonance in pericardial diseases. J Cardiovasc Magn Reson 2009;11(1):14, published under license to BioMed Central Ltd under the Creative Commons Attribution License.)

impact on surrounding structures. In general, asymptomatic patients with cysts that do not impact surrounding structures can be safely monitored with serial imaging with CCT or CMR every 1 to 2 years. CMR is preferred if there are concerns about radiation.[61] Spontaneous resolution of lesions has been reported, likely as a result of rupture.[60,69,70] Symptomatic lesions, an unclear diagnosis, large lesions, or lesions that compress surrounding structures require more definitive treatment by either percutaneous aspiration or surgical resection. Image-guided percutaneous aspiration with ethanol sclerosis of lesions has been reported with excellent results.[53,65,71–74] Therefore, the European Society of Cardiology recommends a percutaneous approach as the initial treatment of congenital pericardial cysts. Surgical resections with thoracotomy or video-assisted thoracotomy are also effective and may be necessary for recurrent cysts or if the diagnosis is not completely established.[53,65,75–77] Video-assisted thoracotomy compared with standard surgical resection is associated with less trauma and earlier postoperative recovery.[53,60,65] Similarly, pericardial diverticula in asymptomatic patients can be monitored safely with serial CCT or CMR. Surgical resection is recommended for symptomatic patients, lesions with an unclear diagnosis, and complicated lesions.[61] Recommendations of this rare disease are based on observational data and long-term follow-up of these recommendations are inadequate, requiring a tailored management approach to each case. Treatment options should be individualized and based on symptoms, the size of the lesion, evidence of compression of surrounding structures, and prevention of life-threatening complications.

SUMMARY

Congenital pericardial abnormalities in the form of absence of the pericardium, cysts, and diverticula are rare disorders and generally of little clinical significance, but can be important sources of morbidity and even mortality. In each condition, patients are generally asymptomatic and many cases go undetected as symptoms, clinical examination, and electrocardiography are nondiagnostic. Life-threatening complications can occur rarely, and timely diagnosis is therefore paramount. When complications or symptoms do occur, advanced imaging with CMR or CCT remains the gold standard for diagnosis. Treatment is generally reserved for symptomatic patients or those with impending complications. Management strategies should be tailored to each patient's presentation, risk, and condition.

REFERENCES

1. Moore KL, Persaud TV. The developing human: clinically oriented embryology. 7th edition. Philadelphia: Saunders Company; 2003. p. 188–200.
2. Kronzon I. 2nd edition. Introduction to pericardial diseases, ASE's Comprehensive Echocardiography, vol. 139. Philadelphia: Elsevier Health Sciences; 2016. p. 593–5.
3. Giovannone S, Donnino R, Saric M. 2nd edition. Normal pericardial anatomy, ASE's Comprehensive Echocardiography, vol. 140. Philadelphia: Elsevier Health Sciences; 2016. p. 595–9.
4. Bogaert J, Francone M. Pericardial disease: value of CT and MR imaging. Radiology 2013;267:340–56.
5. Ellis K, Leeds NE, Himmelstein A. Congenital deficiencies in the parietal pericardium: a review with 2 new cases including successful diagnosis by plain roentgenography. Am J Roentgenol 1959;82:125–32.
6. Garnier F, Eicher JC, Phillip JL, et al. Congenital complete absence of the left pericardium: a rare cause of chest pain or pseudo-right heart overload. Clin Cardiol 2010;33:E52–7.
7. Nasser WK. Congenital diseases of the pericardium. Cardiovasc Clin 1976;7:271–86.
8. Lopez D, Asher CR. Congenital absence of the pericardium. Prog Cardiovasc Dis 2016;136(4):270–8.
9. Southworth H, Stevenson CS. Congenital defects of the pericardium. Arch Intern Med 1938;61:223–40.
10. Van Son JA, Danielson GK, Schaff HV, et al. Congenital partial and complete absence of the pericardium. Mayo Clin Proc 1993;68(8):743–7.
11. Shah AB, Kronzon I. Congenital defects of the pericardium: a review. Eur Heart J Cardiovasc Imaging 2015;16(8):821–7.
12. Taysi K, Hartmann AF, Shackelford GD, et al. Congenital absence of left pericardium in a family. Am J Med Genet 1985;21(1):77–85.
13. Wilson SR, Kronzon I, Machnicki SC, et al. A constrained heart: a case of sudden onset unrelenting chest pain. Circulation 2014;130:1625–31.
14. Matsuda N, Marumoto A, Nakashima H, et al. Congenital pericardial defect associated with ruptured type A aortic dissection. Ann Thorac Surg 2004;77:1069–70.
15. Furui M, Ohashi T, Hirai Y, et al. Congenital pericardial defect with ruptured acute type A aortic dissection. Interact Cardiovasc Thorac Surg 2012;15:912–4.
16. Nakajima M, Tsuchiya K, Naito Y, et al. Partial pericardial defect associated with ruptured aortic dissection of the ascending aorta: a rare feature presenting severe left hemothorax without cardiac tamponade. Ann Thorac Surg 2004;77:1066–8.
17. Hipona FA, Crummy AB. Congenital pericardial defect associated with tetralogy of Fallot: herniation of normal lung into the pericardial cavity. Circulation 1964;29:132–5.

18. Lu C, Ridker PM. Echocardiographic diagnosis of congenital absence of the pericardium in a patient with VATER association defects. Clin Cardiol 1994; 17:503–4.

19. Zakowski MF, Wright Y, Ricci AJ. Pericardial agenesis and focal aplasia cutis intetrasomy 12p (Pallister-Killian syndrome). Am J Med Genet 1992;42:323–5.

20. Gatzoulis MA, Munk MD, Merchant N, et al. Isolated congenital absence of the pericardium: clinical presentation, diagnosis and management. Ann Thorac Surg 2000;69:1209–15.

21. Nasser WK, Helmen C, Tavel ME, et al. Congenital absence of the left pericardium. Clinical, electrocardiographic, radiographic, hemodynamic, and angiographic findings in six cases. Circulation 1970;41: 469–78.

22. Ahn C, Hosier DM, Vasko JS. Congenital pericardial defect with herniation of the left atrial appendage. Ann Thorac Surg 1969;7:369–84.

23. Candan I, Erol Q, Sonel A. Cross sectional echocardiographic appearance in presumed congenital absence of the left pericardium. Br Heart J 1986;55:405–7.

24. Abbas AE, Appleton CP, Liu PT, et al. Congenital absence of the pericardium: case presentation and review of literature. Int J Cardiol 2005;98:21–5.

25. Feigenbaum H. Pericardial disease. In: Feigenbaum H, editor. Echocardiography. 4th edition. Philadelphia: Lea and Febiger; 1986. p. 575.

26. Jain S, Gorscan JIII, Mankad SV. Chapter 145. Pericardial cysts and congenital absence of the pericardium. In: Lang MR, Goldstein SA, Kronzon I, et al, editors. ASE's Comprehensive Echocardiography. Second Edition. Philadelphia: Elsevier; 2016. p. 614–6.

27. Goetz WA, Liebold A, Vogt F, et al. Tricuspid valve repair in a case with congenital absence of left thoracic pericardium. Eur J Cardiothorac Surg 2004;26(4):848–9.

28. Scheuermann-Freestone M, Orchard E, Francis J, et al. Partial congenital absence of the pericardium. Circulation 2007;116(6):e126–9.

29. Tanaka H, Oishi Y, Mizuguchi Y, et al. Contribution of the pericardium to left ventricular torsion and regional myocardial function in patients with total absence of the left pericardium. J Am Soc Echocardiogr 2008;21:268–74.

30. Kim MJ, Kim HK, Jung JH, et al. Echocardiographic diagnosis of total or left congenital pericardial absence with positional change. Heart 2017; 103(15):1203–9.

31. Macaione F, Barison A, Pescetelli I, et al. Quantitative criteria for the diagnosis of congenital absence of pericardium by cardiac magnetic resonance. Eur J Radiol 2016;85:83–92.

32. Sechtem U, Tscholakoff D, Higgins CB. MRI of the normal pericardium. Am J Roentgenol 1986;147: 239–44.

33. Bremerich J, Reddy GP, Higgins CB. Magnetic resonance image of cardiac structure. In: Pohost GM, O'Rourke RA, Berman D, et al, editors. Imaging in cardiovascular disease. Philadelphia: Lippincott Williams & Wilkins; 2000. p. 409, 756.

34. Schweigert M, Dubecz A, Beron M, et al. The tale of spring water cysts: a historical outline of surgery for congenital pericardial diverticula and cysts. Tex Heart Inst J 2012;39:330–4.

35. King JF, Crosby I, Pugh D, et al. Rupture of pericardial cyst. Chest 1971;60:611–2.

36. Tower-Rader A, Kwon D. Pericardial masses, cysts and diverticula: a comprehensive review using multimodality imaging. Prog Cardiovasc Dis 2017;59(4): 389–97.

37. Kronzon I, Srichai MB. Rare pericardial disorders. In: Lang RM, Goldstein SA, Kronzon I, et al, editors. Dynamic echocardiography. 1st edition. St Louis (MO): Elsevier; 2011. p. 262–5.

38. Satur CM, Hsin MK, Dussek JE. Giant pericardial cysts. Ann Thorac Surg 1996;61(1):208–10.

39. Le Roux BT. Pericardial coelomic cysts. Thorax 1959;14:27–35.

40. Maisch B, Seferovic PM, Ristic AD, et al. Guidelines on the diagnosis and management of pericardial diseases executive summary; the Task Force on the Diagnosis and Management of Pericardial Diseases of the European Society of Cardiology. Eur Heart J 2004;25:587–610.

41. Feign DS, Fenoglio JJ, McAllister HA, et al. Pericardial cysts. A radiologic-pathologic correlation and review. Radiology 1977;125:15–20.

42. Unverferth DV, Wooley CF. The differential diagnosis of paracardiac lesions: pericardial cysts. Cathet Cardiovasc Diagn 1979;5:31–40.

43. Borges AC, Gellert K, Dietel M, et al. Acute right-sided heart failure due to hemorrhage into a pericardial cyst. Ann Thorac Surg 1997;63(3):845–7.

44. Liaquat HB, Ali L, Ara J. Pericardial cyst: a rare congenital anomaly. Pak J Med Sci 2009;25:1018–20.

45. Maier HC. Diverticulum of the pericardium. Circulation 1957;16(6):1040–5.

46. Frisoli T, Grosu H, Paul S, et al. Recurrent rupture of a pericardial cyst presenting as Syncope, pleuropericarditis, and pneumonitis. Chest 2011;140(4_MeetingAbstracts):90A.

47. Pader E, Kirschner PA. Pericardial diverticulum. Dis chest 1969;55(4):344–6.

48. Vlay SC, Hartman AR. Mechanical treatment of atrial fibrillation: removal of pericardial cyst by thoracoscopy. Am Heart J 1995;129(3):616–8.

49. Generali T, Garatti A, Gagliardotto P, et al. Right mesothelial pericardial cyst determining intractable atrial arrhythmias. Interact Cardiovasc Thorac Surg 2011;12(5):837–9.

50. De Roover P, Maisin J, Lacquet A. Congenital pleuro-pericardial cysts. Thorax 1963;18(2):146–50.

51. Gibson JY. A large intrapericardial cyst presenting as a cardiac abnormality 1. Radiology 1976;119(1):49–50.

52. Ng AF, Olak J. Pericardial cyst causing right ventricular outflow tract obstruction. Ann Thorac Surg 1997;63(4):1147–8.

53. Najib MQ, Chaliki HP, Raizada A, et al. Symptomatic pericardial cyst: a case series. Eur J Echocardiogr 2011;12:E43.

54. Chopra PS, Duke DJ, Pellett JR, et al. Pericardial cyst with partial erosion of the right ventricular wall. Ann Thorac Surg 1991;51(5):840–1.

55. Mastroroberto P, Chello M, Bevacqua E, et al. Pericardial cyst with partial erosion of the superior vena cava. An unusual case. J Cardiovasc Surg 1996;37(3):323–4.

56. Davis WC, German JD, Johnson NJ. Pericardial diverticulum causing pulmonary obstruction. Arch Surg 1961;82(2):285–9.

57. Shiraishi I, Yamagishi M, Kawakita A, et al. Acute cardiac tamponade caused by massive hemorrhage from pericardial cyst. Circulation 2000;101(19):e196–7.

58. Fredman CS, Parsons SR, Aquino TI, et al. Sudden death after a stress test in a patient with a large pericardial cyst. Am Heart J 1994;127(4):946–50.

59. Seo GW, Seol SH, Jeong HJ, et al. A large pericardial cyst compressing the left atrium presenting as a pericardiopleural effusion. Heart Lung Circ 2014;23(12):e273–5.

60. Patel J, Park C, Michaels J, et al. Pericardial cyst: case reports and a literature review. Echocardiography 2004;21:269–72.

61. Klein AL, Abbara S, Agler DA, et al. American Society of Echocardiography clinical recommendations for multimodality cardiovascular imaging of patients with pericardial disease: endorsed by the Society for Cardiovascular Magnetic Resonance and Society of Cardiovascular Computed Tomography. J Am Soc Echocardiogr 2013;26:965–1012.e15.

62. Kutlay H, Yavuzer I, Han S, et al. Atypically located pericardial cysts. Ann Thorac Surg 2001;72(6):2137–9.

63. Stoller JK, Shaw C, Matthay RA. Enlarging, atypically located pericardial cyst: recent experience and literature review. Chest 1986;89(3):402–6.

64. Pugatch RD, Braver JH, Robbins AH, et al. CT diagnosis of pericardial cysts. Am J Roentgenol 1978;131(3):515–6.

65. Kar SK, Ganguly T, Dasgupta S, et al. Pericardial cyst: a review of historical perspective and current concept of diagnosis and management. Interv Cardiol J 2015.

66. Wang ZJ, Reddy GP, Gotway MB, et al. CT and MR imaging of pericardial disease. Radiographics 2003;23:S167–80.

67. Bogaert J, Francone M. Cardiovascular magnetic resonance in pericardial diseases. J Cardiovasc Magn Reson 2009;11(1):14.

68. Jeung MY, Gasser B, Gangi A, et al. Imaging of cystic masses of the mediastinum. Radiographics 2002;22 Spec No:S79–93.

69. Kruger SR, Michaud J, Cannom DS. Spontaneous resolution of a pericardial cyst. Am Heart J 1985;109(6):1390–1.

70. Ambalavanan SK, Mehta JB, Taylor RA, et al. Spontaneous resolution of a large pericardial cyst. Tenn Med J Tenn Med Assoc 1997;90(3):97–8.

71. Kinoshita Y, Shimada T, Murakami Y, et al. Ethanol sclerosis can be a safe and useful treatment for pericardial cyst. Clin Cardiol 1996;19(10):833–5.

72. Maisch B. Alcohol ablation of pericardial cysts under pericardioscopical control. Heart Fail Rev 2013;18(3):361–5.

73. Butz T, Faber L, Langer C, et al. Echocardiography-guided percutaneous aspiration of a large pericardial cyst. Circulation 2007;116(18):e505–7.

74. Sharma R, Harden S, Peebles C, et al. Percutaneous aspiration of a pericardial cyst: an acceptable treatment for a rare disorder. Heart 2007;93(1):22.

75. Klatte EC, Yune HY. Diagnosis and treatment of pericardial cysts. Radiology 1972;104:541–4.

76. Horita K, Sakao Y, Itoh T. Excision of a recurrent pericardial cyst using video-assisted thoracic surgery. Chest 1998;114(4):1203–4.

77. Thanneer L, Saric M, Perk G, et al. A giant pericardial cyst. J Am Coll Cardiol 2011;57(17):1784.

Tuberculous and Infectious Pericarditis

Sung-A Chang, MD, PhD

KEYWORDS

- Infectious pericarditis • Viral pericarditis • Bacterial pericarditis • Fungal pericarditis
- Tuberculosis pericarditis

KEY POINTS

- The clinical presentation dictates whether comprehensive assessment for infective pericarditis is necessary. Viral pericarditis presents as acute pericarditis with chest pain but rarely progresses to constrictive pericarditis. The most common clinical manifestations of tuberculous pericarditis are dyspnea and pericardial effusion. Purulent pericarditis is rare but should be suspected if fever or sepsis is present.
- Viral pericarditis is the most common infectious pericarditis and is often classified as idiopathic pericarditis. It can be treated with aspirin or nonsteroidal anti-inflammatories. Steroid therapy should be reserved for refractory cases.
- The presentation of tuberculous pericarditis is variable. It is typically fatal in immunocompromised hosts, if untreated. However, in immunocompetent patients, tuberculous pericarditis often improves spontaneously and progresses to chronic constrictive pericarditis. Steroid therapy along with antituberculosis treatment can rescue these patients.
- Bacterial and fungal pericarditis are fatal if untreated and are rare in the current era. Microbiologic diagnosis and appropriate antibacterial/antifungal treatment should be followed by drainage of the purulent pericardial effusion.

INTRODUCTION

The diagnosis and treatment of pericarditis has been largely empirical because of lack of clinical trials and to the fact that infectious pericarditis may present in a way that is similar to noninfectious pericarditis. However, pericarditis caused by certain infectious pathogens should be managed differently because it can be fatal or result in severe complications if treatment is delayed.

All infectious forms of pericarditis can present as acute pericarditis, pericardial effusion, tamponade, or constrictive pericarditis. Initial management should be based on the severity of the

presentation and the clinical scenario (eg, if bacterial pericarditis is suspected). Environmental factors and host factors, including other underlying diseases, should be considered when assessing potential etiologies of infectious pericarditis.

TUBERCULOUS PERICARDITIS
Epidemiology

Tuberculous pericarditis is caused by *Mycobacterium tuberculosis* and is found in 1% to 2% of people who have pulmonary tuberculosis in endemic areas.[1] Tuberculous pericarditis is more prevalent in Africa and East Asia. Although tuberculous pericarditis is rare in Europe and North America (less

Disclosure Statement: None.
Division of Cardiology, Department of Medicine, Samsung Medical Center, Sungkyunkwan University School of Medicine, Heart Vascular and Stroke Institute Imaging Center, 81 Irwon-ro, Gangnam-gu, Seoul 06351, Republic of Korea
E-mail address: elisabet.chang@gmail.com

Cardiol Clin 35 (2017) 615–622
http://dx.doi.org/10.1016/j.ccl.2017.07.013

than 5% of all pericardial disease[2]), it should be suspected in patients who have immigrated from those areas that have a higher prevalence. In Africa, human immunodeficiency virus infection/acquired immune deficiency syndrome (HIV/AIDS) have a relatively high prevalence, which, in turn, leads to a relatively high prevalence of tuberculous pericarditis. In fact, tuberculous pericarditis is the cause for up to 70% of cases referred for diagnostic pericardiocentesis.[2] Mortality and morbidity is high for untreated cases, especially in patients with HIV/AIDS (30%–60%), who have a 3-fold higher mortality rate when compared with patients without HIV/AIDS.[3] In Asian countries, most patients with tuberculous pericarditis do not have HIV/AIDS and are immunocompetent. Therefore, spontaneous regression with subsequent fibrosis is not unusual.

Clinical Features

Clinical presentations of tuberculous pericarditis include pericardial effusion, effusive-constrictive pericarditis, or constrictive pericarditis. Symptomatic pericardial effusion is more common among HIV/AIDS patients and its prevalence is reported to be as high as 80% in patients referred for pericardiocentesis.[4] The classic presentation of acute pericarditis with sudden-onset chest pain and typical electrocardiographic changes is rare in tuberculous pericarditis. Instead, systemic symptoms and signs are common, such as cough (94%), dyspnea (88%), chest pain (76%), fever (70%), night sweats (56%), orthopnea (53%), and weight loss (48%).[1,5] Constrictive pericarditis develops after acute infection has resolved and can linger for many years, eventually resulting in heart failure; surgical pericardiectomy should be reserved for these patients. Progression to constrictive pericarditis, even with optimal antituberculosis therapy (without corticosteroid therapy), is reported in up to 30% of cases.

Pathogenesis

Tuberculous pericarditis has various clinical presentations that are associated with 4 pathologic stages[6]: (1) fibrinous exudation with initial polymorphonuclear leukocytosis, relatively abundant mycobacteria, and early granuloma formation with loose organization of macrophages and T cells; (2) serosanguineous effusion with a predominantly lymphocytic exudate with monocytes and foam cells; (3) effusion absorption with organization of granulomatous caseation and pericardial thickening caused by fibrin, collagenosis, and ultimately, fibrosis; and (4) constrictive scarring, which involves fibrosis of the visceral and parietal pericardium. The scarred (and sometimes calcified) pericardium encases the heart in a fibrocalcific skin that impedes diastolic filling and causes the classic constrictive pericarditis syndrome.

In HIV/AIDS patients, fewer granulomas were observed than in non-HIV patients because of severely depleted CD4+ lymphocytes.[7] This finding correlates with clinical findings of fewer effusive-constrictive pericarditis cases in HIV/AIDS patients than in non-HIV patients.

Diagnosis

Diagnosing tuberculous pericarditis is not simple in most cases. In countries in which tuberculosis is not endemic, treatment should be reserved for patients with proven diagnosis or high likelihood of having tuberculous pericarditis. The tuberculin skin test can be a diagnostic clue in countries with low tuberculosis prevalence. However, in areas in which tuberculosis is prevalent, this is of little value, given the high prevalence of primary tuberculosis, mass Bacillus Calmette–Guérin immunization, and the likelihood of cross-sensitization from the environment.[8] Among patients who are at risk for tuberculosis, a presumptive diagnosis of tuberculous pericarditis is enough for initiation of therapy, given the high risk of not treating when tuberculosis is the etiology. The European Society of Cardiology 2015 guidelines suggested that, if pericardial fluid is not accessible in cases from endemic areas, a diagnostic score of ≥ 6, based on the following criteria, indicates tuberculous pericarditis and warrants presumptive treatment: fever (1), night sweats (1), weight loss (2), globulin level greater than 40 g/L (3), and peripheral leukocyte count less than 10×10^9/L.[3,9]

Clinical features and risk factors should be considered at initial evaluation. Acute chest pain with electrocardiographic abnormalities is rarely found in tuberculous pericarditis patients. Risk factors for patients include HIV/AIDS[10] and long-term use of steroids or immunosuppressive agents.[11] Echocardiography is the initial diagnostic tool for most cases, allowing for assessment of pericardial effusion and constrictive physiology. Electrocardiographic results are abnormal in most cases; however, these results are nondiagnostic because most ST-segment and T-wave abnormalities are nonspecific. PR-segment deviation and ST-segment elevation are found in only 10% of cases.[12,13] Pericardial effusion with fibrinous material of porridgelike appearance on echocardiography is a typical finding for tuberculous pericarditis but is not sufficiently specific to make the diagnosis.

In addition to echocardiography, chest computerized tomography is helpful in the evaluation, typically showing mediastinal lymph node enlargement (>10 mm).[14] Cardiac MRI allows for visualization of the pericardium, assessment of pericardial inflammation, and development of effusive-constrictive pericarditis and pericardial abscess (**Fig. 1**). Fludeoxyglucose F 18 can be helpful to discriminate tuberculous pericarditis from idiopathic pericarditis,[15] but differentiation between physiologic and pathologic cardiac fludeoxyglucose uptake by positron emission tomography/computed tomography remains challenging.[16]

Active pulmonary tuberculosis accompanies 30% of cases, and pleural effusion is present in 40% to 60% of cases[1,2,17]; therefore, sputum culture, gastric aspirate, and urine for *Mycobacterium tuberculosis* should be evaluated for each patient.

Pericardiocentesis for drainage and analysis of pericardial effusion is recommended for all patients when tuberculous pericarditis is suspected. Pericardial effusions are usually a lymphocyte-dominant, protein-rich exudate. Bloody effusion accounts for 80% of tuberculous pericarditis cases; however, bloody effusion is also common in malignant effusion or traumatic effusion, thus rendering it a nonspecific finding.

Definite and direct methods for diagnosing tuberculous pericarditis involve identifying acid-fast bacilli (AFB) in any body site.[2] Positive staining for AFB in sputum, lymph nodes, or pericardial effusion would be sufficient to directly confirm the diagnosis. A problem with this method is that detection rates of tuberculous bacilli in direct smears range from 0% to 42%. AFB culture can increase the diagnostic yield, but the results are not available for weeks, limiting its value in the immediate decision-making process.

Pericardial biopsy may be helpful for diagnosing tuberculosis. Pericardial biopsy can be performed

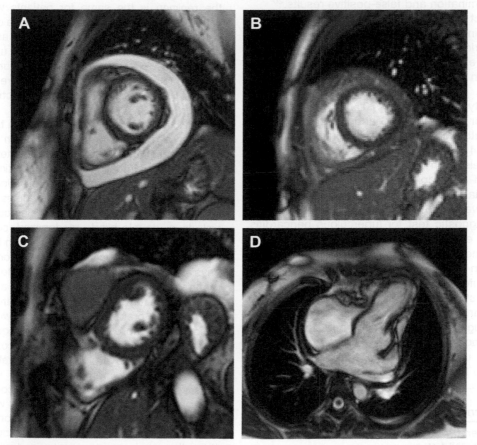

Fig. 1. Cardiac MRI of tuberculous pericarditis with different stages: (*A*) Pericardial effusion without pericardial thickening. (*B*) Development of effusive constrictive pericarditis. (*C*) Pericardial abscess. None of the patients had a history of antituberculous medication. Patient A and B presented with dyspnea. Patient C presented with a pericardial effusion 3 months prior, which was thought to be viral pericarditis. (*D*) Pericardial calcification and distortion of the left ventricular shape in a patient with chronic constrictive pericarditis who had a history of pulmonary tuberculosis. Pericardiectomy was successfully performed for this patient.

easily but is inferior to pericardiotomy or a video-assisted thoracoscopic approach. Typical histology with caseous necrosis and granulomatous inflammation or positive AFB staining can confirm the diagnosis. AFB culture increases the diagnostic yield. Diagnostic efficacy of pericardial biopsy ranges from 10% to 64%,[18,19] which is slightly greater than analysis of the pericardial effusion. However, with late-stage tuberculous pericarditis, typical microscopy findings can disappear, and only fibrotic changes and chronic inflammation are seen. Moreover, surgical procedures for pericardial biopsy can be troublesome in the presence of pericardial adhesions without effusion. Therefore, consideration of pericardial biopsy should be individualized based on the patient's clinical course. Polymerase chain reaction (PCR) has been suggested as a rapid diagnostic test with high sensitivity in tissue (80%) but not in pericardial fluid (15%). However, the specificity of PCR is a concern because of a high possibility of contamination and false-positive results.[20]

Indirect diagnostic methods have also been applied in the diagnosis of tuberculous pericarditis. Pericardial adenosine deaminase (ADA) activity is elevated in tuberculous infections and, based on a range of cutoff values from 30 to 60 IU/L, its sensitivity is approximately 90% and specificity approximately 70%.[19,21] ADA level is useful for both HIV/AIDS and non-HIV/AIDS patients, although advanced HIV patients with severe CD4 lymphocyte depletion can have lower ADA levels. High ADA levels may be a strong predictor of developing constrictive pericarditis in pericardial tuberculosis.[22] Pericardial lysozyme cutoff level of 6.5 μg/dL has also been proposed as a diagnostic test for tuberculous pericarditis, with an estimated sensitivity and specificity of 100% and 91%, respectively.[23] Measurement of interferon-γ levels in pericardial tissue also provides information for rapid early diagnosis. Another study of 30 patients with diverse causes of pericardial effusion showed its diagnostic efficacy, suggesting a sensitivity and specificity of 100% each if a cutoff value of greater than 200 pg/L is used.[21] However, technical capability can be a hurdle for these methods in developing countries.

Treatment

Antituberculosis medications and corticosteroid therapy

Treatment of tuberculous pericarditis requires a multidisciplinary team approach that includes a cardiologist, an infection specialist, and, sometimes, a pulmonologist, because pulmonary tuberculosis frequently coexists. For patients living in endemic areas, even when there is no definite evidence of tuberculous pericarditis, clinical suspicion can justify starting empirical antituberculosis medication if no other obvious cause is found. However, for patients living in nonendemic areas, empiric anti tuberculous treatment is not recommended when systematic investigations fail to yield a tuberculous pericarditis diagnosis.[9]

A treatment regimen for tuberculous pericarditis includes the following 4-drug regimen[6,24]:

- Isoniazid (300 mg orally once daily)
- Rifampicin (600 mg orally once daily; 10 mg/kg/d)
- Ethambutol (15–25 mg/kg orally once daily)
- Pyrazinamide (15–30 mg/kg/d up to 2 g/d given as a single dose)

After the initial 4-drug therapy for 8 weeks, a 2-drug regimen with isoniazid and rifampin should be continued for another 6 months. The length of the regimen is the same for patients with and without HIV/AIDS. For patients who have concomitant extrapulmonary tuberculosis, such as lymphadenitis, treatment can be extended for up to 9 to 12 months. Extension of treatment duration or changes in antibiotics in cases of severe side effects should be discussed with an infectious diseases specialist.

Adjunctive corticosteroid therapy can be beneficial in avoiding severe inflammation from a paradoxical immunologic response after antituberculosis treatment. Adjunctive corticosteroid therapy may also prevent complications from constrictive pericarditis after tuberculous pericarditis treatment. However, this remains controversial. In a double-blind, randomized controlled trial in South Africa,[25] 143 patients with tuberculous pericarditis and clinical signs of constrictive physiology were randomly assigned to receive prednisolone or placebo in addition to antituberculosis drugs for their first 11 weeks of treatment. Although the prednisolone group showed more rapid clinical improvement, a lower requirement for pericardiectomy (relative risk, 0.66; confidence interval, 0.34–1.29) and a lower mortality from pericarditis at 24 months compared with the nonsteroid group (relative risk, 0.31; confidence interval, 0.07–1.43), these differences were not statistically significant. In their study, constriction resolved within 6 months after antituberculosis chemotherapy in most patients, and only 29 of the 114 patients (25%) required pericardiectomy for persistent or worsening constriction follow-up. These benefits were maintained for up to 10 years.[17]

Corticosteroid therapy potentially causes complications, including aggravation of diabetes, hypertension, Cushingoid features, infection risk, osteoporosis, acne, and insomnia. Also, corticosteroid therapy can increase cancer risk for HIV/AIDS patients. A combination of 6-week adjunctive therapy with prednisolone and 3-month intradermal *Mycobacterium indicus pranii* immunotherapy for tuberculous pericarditis did not show a significant effect on the combined all-cause death outcome. However, the use of adjunctive glucocorticoids reduced the incidence of pericardial constriction and hospitalization.[26] Another double-blind, randomized, placebo-controlled trial of adjunctive prednisolone for treatment of effusive tuberculous pericarditis in HIV seropositive patients (n = 58) found that adjunctive prednisolone produced a pronounced reduction in mortality.[27]

The suggested dosage for corticosteroid is 1 mg/kg/d for 4 weeks, 0.5 mg/kg/d for 4 weeks, 0.25 mg/kg/d for 2 weeks, and 0.125 mg/kg/d for 2 weeks, all with prednisolone.[25]

Surgical treatment

Constrictive pericarditis is the most important complication from tuberculous pericarditis. It has been reported to occur in 30% to 60% of patients, even including those who have been treated with corticosteroids.[2] A pericardiectomy is recommended if the patient's condition does not improve or deteriorates after 4 to 8 weeks of antituberculosis therapy.[9] For chronic constrictive pericarditis as a complication of a remote episode of tuberculous pericarditis, extended pericardiectomy is the treatment of choice.

VIRAL PERICARDITIS
Clinical Features

Viral pericarditis is presumed to be the most common type of acute pericarditis. Clinically, it is indistinguishable from idiopathic pericarditis. If recent history of viral illness is present, a presumed diagnosis of viral pericarditis is frequently made. Currently, there are no proven effective therapies for viral causes of pericarditis and, therefore, antiviral agents are not recommended. Viral pericarditis is self-limiting in most cases and rarely leads to cardiac tamponade or constrictive pericarditis. However, progression to tamponade might occur in high-risk patients.[28]

Recurrence rates after an initial episode of viral or idiopathic pericarditis ranges from 15% to 30%,[29,30] and most recurrences are associated with inadequate treatment of the first pericarditis episode. In up to 20% of viral pericarditis recurrences, the viral etiology is detected when additional virologic assays have been conducted on pericardial fluid or tissue.[31]

Pathogenesis

Cardiotropic viruses can cause pericardial and myocardial inflammation. Their mechanism of action includes cytolytic or cytotoxic effects or T- or B-cell–derived immune-mediated mechanisms. If viral nucleic acids persist, they perpetuate the inflammation and produce effusions via an immune process directed against specific cardiac proteins by molecular mimicry.[32] Common viruses that can cause acute pericarditis include enteroviruses (coxsackieviruses, echoviruses), herpesviruses (Epstein-Barr virus, cytomegalovirus, human herpesvirus-6), adenoviruses, and parvovirus B19 (including a possible overlap with myocarditis).

Diagnosis

Most viral pericarditis cases involve limited disease, and their treatment is similar to that for pericarditis of other etiologies; thus, a definite diagnosis of viral pericarditis is not necessary. However, for an immunocompromised patient, identifying specific viral agents, such as cytomegalovirus in HIV/AIDS patients, can be helpful. A definitive diagnosis for viral pericarditis involves a comprehensive workup, including histology, cytology, and immunologic and molecular evaluations of pericardial fluid and tissue.[32] Serologic tests are easier to perform; however, there is no correlation between antiviral antibodies in serum, virus isolated from the throat, or rectal swabs with PCR analysis in pericardial fluid.[33] Because of the complexity, cost, invasiveness, and limited availability, investigations into specific viral etiologies are rarely performed in clinical settings.

Treatment

Most viral pericarditis is self-limiting, and the first treatment of choice is usually aspirin or nonsteroidal anti-inflammatory drugs. Colchicine as adjunctive therapy has been found to reduce recurrence.[29,30]

Some experts suggest antiviral treatments that are similar to those used for myocarditis (intravenous immunoglobulin therapy for acute systemic enterovirus, cytomegalovirus, Epstein-Barr virus, or parvovirus B19 infection; oral valganciclovir for herpesvirus-6 perimyocarditis; interferon-α for enteroviral pericarditis). However, these treatments are still under investigation and are rarely used clinically because of a lack of clinical evidence for their efficacy. Furthermore, until recently, no therapy was available to treat persistent viral proteins and associated inflammation, particularly when induced by herpes viruses or parvovirus B19.[32] Importantly, corticosteroid therapy is not recommended for viral pericarditis.[9]

PURULENT PERICARDITIS
Clinical Features

Purulent pericarditis can occur from bacterial or fungal infections. Both are rare in the current era, however, they occur more frequently in immunocompromised hosts, such as patients undergoing chemotherapy or patients who have been treated with immunosuppressant agents. Other risk factors include chronic alcoholism and history of chest trauma, including thoracic/cardiac surgery. Before the antibiotic era, purulent pericarditis was usually associated with contiguous infection from adjacent organs, particularly pneumonia. Currently, more than 70% of purulent pericarditis cases are secondary to seeding from other sites in the body, and less than 25% of these patients have pneumonia.[34] Fever is the most common clinical manifestation of purulent pericarditis, and chest pain does not always co-occur. Dyspnea associated with effusive-constrictive pericarditis is common, and pericardial effusions are present in most cases.[34] Cardiac tamponade is common, and purulent pericarditis can lead to rapid clinical deterioration via septic shock if left untreated.

Pathogenesis

Gram-positive infections are the most common cause of purulent pericarditis, and other pathogenic origins, including gram-negative and fungal infections are increasing. Bacterial pericarditis can be caused by Coxiella burnetii, Borrelia burgdorferi, and, rarely, by Pneumococcus spp, Meningococcus spp, Gonococcus spp, Streptococcus spp, Staphylococcus spp, Haemophilus spp, Chlamydia spp, Mycoplasma spp, Legionella spp, Leptospira spp, Listeria spp, and Providencia stuartii. Fungal pericarditis is extremely rare but is highly fatal if untreated. Histoplasma spp are the most common organisms found in immunocompetent patients. Fungal pericarditis associated with Aspergillus, Blastomyces, and Candida spp are more likely to be seen in immunocompromised hosts.

Diagnosis

Purulent pericarditis commonly presents with fever, often with sepsis. Concomitant infections, particularly pneumonia, are common. The presence of a complicated pericardial effusion (pericardial effusion with treadlike material, effusion with high echogenicity, and multiple septations in the pericardial space), and the clinical features of sepsis, strongly indicate purulent pericarditis. When purulent pericarditis is suspected, the pericardial fluid should be drained immediately and the fluid cultured for bacterial or fungal presence. Blood and sputum cultures are also recommended. Typically, the pericardial fluid is very thick and purulent, and the pericardial-fluid analysis finds a low pericardial/serum glucose ratio (mean, 0.3) and an elevated white blood cell count with a high proportion of neutrophils (mean cell count, 2800 µg/mL; 92% neutrophils).[35] Chest computed tomography scan can also be helpful to recognize the adjacent infection.

Treatment

Immediate empirical intravenous broad-spectrum antibiotics should be started if the patient is septic, or purulent pericarditis is otherwise suspected. Pericardial fluid would ideally be drained before initiation of antibiotics to increase the potential diagnostic yield. Intrapericardial administration of antibiotics is not necessary; intravenous antibiotics are sufficient to achieve the target antibiotic delivery level. Possible regimens may include[24]: (1) vancomycin plus ceftriaxone, cefotaxime, or gentamicin; (2) a carbapenem (such as imipenem or meropenem); (3) a combination of penicillin plus a β-lactamase inhibitor, such as ticarcillin clavulanate, piperacillin, tazobactam, or ampicillin sulbactam; or (4) cefepime.

In severely immunocompromised hosts, empirical therapy with fluconazole (200–400 mg once daily intravenously) is prudent while awaiting culture results. After identification of the specific underlying pathogens, antibiotics should be adjusted accordingly.

If purulent pericarditis is suspected, pericardiocentesis should be performed for diagnostic and therapeutic purposes. In patients with a rapidly deteriorating condition that is not responsive to medical therapy, particularly in the setting of residual complicated effusion, surgical drainage of the pericardial fluid (subxiphoid pericardiotomy or video-assisted thoracic surgery) is recommended. The risk of progression to constrictive pericarditis is high in bacterial pericarditis cases (20%–30%), especially purulent pericarditis [28,36] When constrictive pericarditis is chronic and persists after completion of antibiotics/fungal treatment, pericardiectomy is the treatment of choice.

REFERENCES

1. Fowler NO. Tuberculous pericarditis. JAMA 1991; 266:99–103.

2. Sagrista-Sauleda J, Permanyer-Miralda G, Soler-Soler J. Tuberculous pericarditis: ten year experience with a prospective protocol for diagnosis and treatment. J Am Coll Cardiol 1988;11:724–8.

3. Mayosi BM, Wiysonge CS, Ntsekhe M, et al. Mortality in patients treated for tuberculous pericarditis in sub-Saharan Africa. S Afr Med J 2008;98:36–40.

4. Mayosi BM, Wiysonge CS, Ntsekhe M, et al. Clinical characteristics and initial management of patients with tuberculous pericarditis in the HIV era: the Investigation of the Management of Pericarditis in Africa (IMPI Africa) registry. BMC Infect Dis 2006;6:2.

5. Gooi H, Smith JM. Tuberculous pericarditis in Birmingham. Thorax 1978;33:94–6.

6. Mayosi BM, Burgess LJ, Doubell AF. Tuberculous pericarditis. Circulation 2005;112:3608–16.

7. Reuter H, Burgess L, Schneider J, et al. The role of histopathology in establishing the aetiology of pericardial effusions in the presence of HIV. J Lab Clin Med 2005;48:295–302.

8. Ng T, Strang J, Wilkins E. Serodiagnosis of pericardial tuberculosis. QJM 1995;88:317–20.

9. Adler Y, Charron P, Imazio M, et al. 2015 ESC guidelines for the diagnosis and management of pericardial diseases: the Task Force for the diagnosis and management of pericardial diseases of the European Society of Cardiology (ESC)Endorsed by: The European Association for Cardio-Thoracic Surgery (EACTS). Eur Heart J 2015;36:2921–64.

10. Sunderam G, McDonald RJ, Maniatis T, et al. Tuberculosis as a manifestation of the acquired immunodeficiency syndrome (AIDS). JAMA 1986; 256:362–6.

11. Katz I, Rosenthal T, Michaeli D. Undiagnosed tuberculosis in hospitalized patients. Chest 1985; 87:770–4.

12. Habashy AG, Mittal A, Ravichandran N, et al. The electrocardiogram in large pericardial effusion: the forgotten "P" wave and the influence of tamponade, size, etiology, and pericardial thickness on QRS voltage. Angiology 2004;55:303–7.

13. Rooney JJ, Crocco JA, Lyons HA. Tuberculous pericarditis. Ann Intern Med 1970;72:73–8.

14. Cherian G. Diagnosis of tuberculous aetiology in pericardial effusions. Postgrad Med J 2004;80: 262–6.

15. Dong A, Dong H, Wang Y, et al. 18F-FDG PET/CT in differentiating acute tuberculous from idiopathic pericarditis: preliminary study. Clin Nucl Med 2013; 38:e160–5.

16. Lobert P, Brown R, Dvorak R, et al. Spectrum of physiological and pathological cardiac and pericardial uptake of FDG in oncology PET-CT. Clin Radiol 2013;68:e59–71.

17. Strang J, Nunn A, Johnson D, et al. Management of tuberculous constrictive pericarditis and tuberculous pericardial effusion in Transkei: results at 10 years follow-up. QJM 2004;97:525–35.

18. Schepers GW. Tuberculous pericarditis. Am J Cardiol 1962;9:248–76.

19. Koh KK, Kim EJ, Cho CH, et al. Adenosine deaminase and carcinoembryonic antigen in pericardial effusion diagnosis, especially in suspected tuberculous pericarditis. Circulation 1994;89:2728–35.

20. Cegielski JP, Devlin BH, Morris AJ, et al. Comparison of PCR, culture, and histopathology for diagnosis of tuberculous pericarditis. J Clin Microbiol 1997;35:3254–7.

21. Burgess LJ, Reuter H, Carstens ME, et al. The use of adenosine deaminase and interferon-γ as diagnostic tools for tuberculous pericarditis. Chest 2002;122:900–5.

22. Komsuoglu B, Göldeli Ö, Kulan K, et al. The diagnostic and prognostic value of adenosine deaminase in tuberculous pericarditis. Eur Heart J 1995; 16:1126–30.

23. Aggeli C, Pitsavos C, Brili S, et al. Relevance of adenosine deaminase and lysozyme measurements in the diagnosis of tuberculous pericarditis. Cardiology 2001;94:81–5.

24. Imazio M, Brucato A, Mayosi BM, et al. Medical therapy of pericardial diseases: part I: idiopathic and infectious pericarditis. J Cardiovasc Med 2010;11: 712–22.

25. Strang J, Gibson D, Nunn A, et al. Controlled trial of prednisolone as adjuvant in treatment of tuberculous constrictive pericarditis in Transkei. Lancet 1987; 330:1418–22.

26. Mayosi BM, Ntsekhe M, Bosch J, et al. Prednisolone and Mycobacterium indicus pranii in tuberculous pericarditis. N Engl J Med 2014;371:1121–30.

27. Hakim J, Ternouth I, Mushangi E, et al. Double blind randomised placebo controlled trial of adjunctive prednisolone in the treatment of effusive tuberculous pericarditis in HIV seropositive patients. Heart 2000; 84:183–8.

28. Imazio M, Brucato A, Adler Y, et al. Prognosis of idiopathic recurrent pericarditis as determined from previously published reports. Am J Cardiol 2007;100: 1026–8.

29. Imazio M, Bobbio M, Cecchi E, et al. Colchicine in addition to conventional therapy for acute pericarditis. Circulation 2005;112:2012–6.

30. Imazio M, Brucato A, Cemin R, et al. A randomized trial of colchicine for acute pericarditis. N Engl J Med 2013;369:1522–8.

31. Pankuweit S, Stein A, Karatolios K, et al. Viral genomes in the pericardial fluid and in peri-and epicardial biopsies from a German cohort of patients with large to moderate pericardial effusions. Heart Fail Rev 2013;18: 329–36.

32. Maisch B, Rupp H, Ristic A, et al. Pericardioscopy and epi-and pericardial biopsy—a new window to the heart improving etiological diagnoses and permitting targeted intrapericardial therapy. Heart Fail Rev 2013;18:317–28.

33. Mahfoud F, Gärtner B, Kindermann M, et al. Virus serology in patients with suspected myocarditis: utility or futility? Eur Heart J 2011;32:897–903.

34. Sagristà-Sauleda J, Barrabés JA, Permanyer-Miralda G, et al. Purulent pericarditis: review of a 20-year experience in a general hospital. J Am Coll Cardiol 1993;22:1661–5.

35. Ben-Horin S, Bank I, Shinfeld A, et al. Diagnostic value of the biochemical composition of pericardial effusions in patients undergoing pericardiocentesis. Am J Cardiol 2007;99: 1294–7.

36. Imazio M, Brucato A, Maestroni S, et al. Risk of constrictive pericarditis after acute pericarditis. Circulation 2011;124(11):1270–5.

UNITED STATES POSTAL SERVICE®

Statement of Ownership, Management, and Circulation
(All Periodicals Publications Except Requester Publications)

1. Publication Title	2. Publication Number	3. Filing Date
CARDIOLOGY CLINICS	000 – 701	9/18/2017

4. Issue Frequency	5. Number of Issues Published Annually	6. Annual Subscription Price
FEB, MAY, AUG, NOV	4	$326.00

7. Complete Mailing Address of Known Office of Publication (Not printer) (Street, city, county, state, and ZIP+4®)

ELSEVIER INC.
230 Park Avenue, Suite 800
New York, NY 10169

Contact Person
STEPHEN R. BUSHING

Telephone (Include area code)
215-239-3688

8. Complete Mailing Address of Headquarters or General Business Office of Publisher (Not printer)

ELSEVIER INC.
230 Park Avenue, Suite 800
New York, NY 10169

9. Full Names and Complete Mailing Addresses of Publisher, Editor, and Managing Editor (Do not leave blank)

Publisher (Name and complete mailing address)
ADRIANNE BRIGIDO, ELSEVIER INC.
1600 JOHN F KENNEDY BLVD. SUITE 1800
PHILADELPHIA, PA 19103-2899

Editor (Name and complete mailing address)
STACY EASTMAN, ELSEVIER INC.
1600 JOHN F KENNEDY BLVD. SUITE 1800
PHILADELPHIA, PA 19103-2899

Managing Editor (Name and complete mailing address)
PATRICK MANLEY, ELSEVIER INC.
1600 JOHN F KENNEDY BLVD. SUITE 1800
PHILADELPHIA, PA 19103-2899

10. Owner (Do not leave blank. If the publication is owned by a corporation, give the name and address of the corporation immediately followed by the names and addresses of all stockholders owning or holding 1 percent or more of the total amount of stock. If not owned by a corporation, give the names and addresses of the individual owners. If owned by a partnership or other unincorporated firm, give its name and address as well as those of each individual owner. If the publication is published by a nonprofit organization, give its name and address.)

Full Name	Complete Mailing Address
WHOLLY OWNED SUBSIDIARY OF REED/ELSEVIER, US HOLDINGS	1600 JOHN F KENNEDY BLVD. SUITE 1800 PHILADELPHIA, PA 19103-2899

11. Known Bondholders, Mortgagees, and Other Security Holders Owning or Holding 1 Percent or More of Total Amount of Bonds, Mortgages, or Other Securities. If none, check box ➤ ☐ None

Full Name	Complete Mailing Address
N/A	

12. Tax Status (For completion by nonprofit organizations authorized to mail at nonprofit rates) (Check one)
The purpose, function, and nonprofit status of this organization and the exempt status for federal income tax purposes:
☒ Has Not Changed During Preceding 12 Months
☐ Has Changed During Preceding 12 Months (Publisher must submit explanation of change with this statement)

13. Publication Title	14. Issue Date for Circulation Data Below
CARDIOLOGY CLINICS	AUGUST 2017

PS Form 3526, July 2014 [Page 1 of 4 (see instructions page 4)] PSN: 7530-01-000-9631   PRIVACY NOTICE: See our privacy policy on www.usps.com

---

15. Extent and Nature of Circulation			Average No. Copies Each Issue During Preceding 12 Months	No. Copies of Single Issue Published Nearest to Filing Date
a. Total Number of Copies (Net press run)			377	411
b. Paid Circulation (By Mail and Outside the Mail)	(1)	Mailed Outside-County Paid Subscriptions Stated on PS Form 3541 (Include paid distribution above nominal rate, advertiser's proof copies, and exchange copies)	175	177
	(2)	Mailed In-County Paid Subscriptions Stated on PS Form 3541 (Include paid distribution above nominal rate, advertiser's proof copies, and exchange copies)	0	0
	(3)	Paid Distribution Outside the Mails Including Sales Through Dealers and Carriers, Street Vendors, Counter Sales, and Other Paid Distribution Outside USPS®	78	94
	(4)	Paid Distribution by Other Classes of Mail Through the USPS (e.g. First-Class Mail®)	0	0
c. Total Paid Distribution (Sum of 15b (1), (2), (3), and (4))			253	271
d. Free or Nominal Rate Distribution (By Mail and Outside the Mail)	(1)	Free or Nominal Rate Outside-County Copies included on PS Form 3541	32	40
	(2)	Free or Nominal Rate In-County Copies included on PS Form 3541	0	0
	(3)	Free or Nominal Rate Copies Mailed at Other Classes Through the USPS (e.g. First-Class Mail)	0	0
	(4)	Free or Nominal Rate Distribution Outside the Mail (Carriers or other means)	32	40
e. Total Free or Nominal Rate Distribution (Sum of 15d (1), (2), (3) and (4))			32	40
f. Total Distribution (Sum of 15c and 15e)			285	311
g. Copies not Distributed (See instructions to Publishers #4 (page 83))			92	100
h. Total (Sum of 15f and g)			377	411
i. Percent Paid (15c divided by 15f times 100)			88.77%	87.14%

* If you are claiming electronic copies, go to line 16 on page 3. If you are not claiming electronic copies, skip to line 17 on page 3.

16. Electronic Copy Circulation		Average No. Copies Each Issue During Preceding 12 Months	No. Copies of Single Issue Published Nearest to Filing Date
a. Paid Electronic Copies	➤	0	0
b. Total Paid Print Copies (Line 15c) + Paid Electronic Copies (Line 16a)	➤	253	271
c. Total Print Distribution (Line 15f) + Paid Electronic Copies (Line 16a)	➤	285	311
d. Percent Paid (Both Print & Electronic Copies) (16b divided by 16c × 100)	➤	88.77%	87.14%

☒ I certify that 50% of all my distributed copies (electronic and print) are paid above a nominal price.

17. Publication of Statement of Ownership
☒ If the publication is a general publication, publication of this statement is required. Will be printed in the NOVEMBER 2017 issue of this publication. ☐ Publication not required.

18. Signature and Title of Editor, Publisher, Business Manager, or Owner

STEPHEN R. BUSHING - INVENTORY DISTRIBUTION CONTROL MANAGER

Date
9/18/2017

I certify that all information furnished on this form is true and complete. I understand that anyone who furnishes false or misleading information on this form or who omits material or information requested on the form may be subject to criminal sanctions (including fines and imprisonment) and/or civil sanctions (including civil penalties).

PS Form 3526, July 2014 (Page 3 of 4)   PRIVACY NOTICE: See our privacy policy on www.usps.com

Moving?

Make sure your subscription moves with you!

To notify us of your new address, find your **Clinics Account Number** (located on your mailing label above your name), and contact customer service at:

Email: journalscustomerservice-usa@elsevier.com

800-654-2452 (subscribers in the U.S. & Canada)
314-447-8871 (subscribers outside of the U.S. & Canada)

Fax number: 314-447-8029

Elsevier Health Sciences Division
Subscription Customer Service
3251 Riverport Lane
Maryland Heights, MO 63043

*To ensure uninterrupted delivery of your subscription, please notify us at least 4 weeks in advance of move.

Printed and bound by CPI Group (UK) Ltd, Croydon, CR0 4YY

03/10/2024

01040302-0015